M000239042

FREE Study Skills Videos/DVD Offer

Dear Customer,

Thank you for your purchase from Mometrix! We consider it an honor and a privilege that you have purchased our product and we want to ensure your satisfaction.

As part of our ongoing effort to meet the needs of test takers, we have developed a set of Study Skills Videos that we would like to give you for <u>FREE</u>. These videos cover our *best practices* for getting ready for your exam, from how to use our study materials to how to best prepare for the day of the test.

All that we ask is that you email us with feedback that would describe your experience so far with our product. Good, bad, or indifferent, we want to know what you think!

To get your FREE Study Skills Videos, you can use the **QR code** below, or send us an **email** at <u>studyvideos@mometrix.com</u> with *FREE VIDEOS* in the subject line and the following information in the body of the email:

- The name of the product you purchased.
- Your product rating on a scale of 1-5, with 5 being the highest rating.
- Your feedback. It can be long, short, or anything in between. We just want to know your impressions and experience so far with our product. (Good feedback might include how our study material met your needs and ways we might be able to make it even better. You could highlight features that you found helpful or features that you think we should add.)

If you have any questions or concerns, please don't hesitate to contact me directly.

Thanks again!

Sincerely,

Jay Willis
Vice President
<u>jay.willis@mometrix.com</u>
1-800-673-8175

National Certified
Medical
Assistant
Exam Secrets
Study Guide

NCCT Test Review for the National Center for Competency Testing Exam

Copyright © 2022 by Mometrix Media LLC

All rights reserved. This product, or parts thereof, may not be reproduced, stored in a retrieval system, or transmitted in any form or by any means—electronic, mechanical, photocopy, recording, scanning, or other—except for brief quotations in critical reviews or articles, without the prior written permission of the publisher.

Written and edited by Mometrix Test Prep

Printed in the United States of America

This paper meets the requirements of ANSI/NISO Z39.48-1992 (Permanence of Paper).

Mometrix offers volume discount pricing to institutions. For more information or a price quote, please contact our sales department at sales@mometrix.com or 888-248-1219.

Mometrix Media LLC is not affiliated with or endorsed by any official testing organization. All organizational and test names are trademarks of their respective owners.

Paperback
ISBN 13: 978-1-61072-227-8
ISBN 10: 1-6107-2227-2

DEAR FUTURE EXAM SUCCESS STORY

First of all, **THANK YOU** for purchasing Mometrix study materials!

Second, congratulations! You are one of the few determined test-takers who are committed to doing whatever it takes to excel on your exam. **You have come to the right place.** We developed these study materials with one goal in mind: to deliver you the information you need in a format that's concise and easy to use.

In addition to optimizing your guide for the content of the test, we've outlined our recommended steps for breaking down the preparation process into small, attainable goals so you can make sure you stay on track.

We've also analyzed the entire test-taking process, identifying the most common pitfalls and showing how you can overcome them and be ready for any curveball the test throws you.

Standardized testing is one of the biggest obstacles on your road to success, which only increases the importance of doing well in the high-pressure, high-stakes environment of test day. Your results on this test could have a significant impact on your future, and this guide provides the information and practical advice to help you achieve your full potential on test day.

Your success is our success

We would love to hear from you! If you would like to share the story of your exam success or if you have any questions or comments in regard to our products, please contact us at **800-673-8175** or **support@mometrix.com**.

Thanks again for your business and we wish you continued success!

Sincerely,
The Mometrix Test Preparation Team

Need more help? Check out our flashcards at:
http://MometrixFlashcards.com/NCCT

Copyright © 2022 by Mometrix Media LLC. All rights reserved.
Written and edited by the Mometrix Exam Secrets Test Prep Team
Printed in the United States of America

TABLE OF CONTENTS

Introduction

Thank you for purchasing this resource! You have made the choice to prepare yourself for a test that could have a huge impact on your future, and this guide is designed to help you be fully ready for test day. Obviously, it's important to have a solid understanding of the test material, but you also need to be prepared for the unique environment and stressors of the test, so that you can perform to the best of your abilities.

For this purpose, the first section that appears in this guide is the **Secret Keys**. We've devoted countless hours to meticulously researching what works and what doesn't, and we've boiled down our findings to the five most impactful steps you can take to improve your performance on the test. We start at the beginning with study planning and move through the preparation process, all the way to the testing strategies that will help you get the most out of what you know when you're finally sitting in front of the test.

We recommend that you start preparing for your test as far in advance as possible. However, if you've bought this guide as a last-minute study resource and only have a few days before your test, we recommend that you skip over the first two Secret Keys since they address a long-term study plan.

If you struggle with **test anxiety**, we strongly encourage you to check out our recommendations for how you can overcome it. Test anxiety is a formidable foe, but it can be beaten, and we want to make sure you have the tools you need to defeat it.

Copyright © Mometrix Media. You have been licensed one copy of this document for personal use only. Any other reproduction or redistribution is strictly prohibited. All rights reserved. This content is provided for test preparation purposes only and does not imply an endorsement by Mometrix of any particular political, scientific, or religious point of view.

Secret Key #1 – Plan Big, Study Small

There's a lot riding on your performance. If you want to ace this test, you're going to need to keep your skills sharp and the material fresh in your mind. You need a plan that lets you review everything you need to know while still fitting in your schedule. We'll break this strategy down into three categories.

Information Organization

Start with the information you already have: the official test outline. From this, you can make a complete list of all the concepts you need to cover before the test. Organize these concepts into groups that can be studied together, and create a list of any related vocabulary you need to learn so you can brush up on any difficult terms. You'll want to keep this vocabulary list handy once you actually start studying since you may need to add to it along the way.

Time Management

Once you have your set of study concepts, decide how to spread them out over the time you have left before the test. Break your study plan into small, clear goals so you have a manageable task for each day and know exactly what you're doing. Then just focus on one small step at a time. When you manage your time this way, you don't need to spend hours at a time studying. Studying a small block of content for a short period each day helps you retain information better and avoid stressing over how much you have left to do. You can relax knowing that you have a plan to cover everything in time. In order for this strategy to be effective though, you have to start studying early and stick to your schedule. Avoid the exhaustion and futility that comes from last-minute cramming!

Study Environment

The environment you study in has a big impact on your learning. Studying in a coffee shop, while probably more enjoyable, is not likely to be as fruitful as studying in a quiet room. It's important to keep distractions to a minimum. You're only planning to study for a short block of time, so make the most of it. Don't pause to check your phone or get up to find a snack. It's also important to **avoid multitasking**. Research has consistently shown that multitasking will make your studying dramatically less effective. Your study area should also be comfortable and well-lit so you don't have the distraction of straining your eyes or sitting on an uncomfortable chair.

 The time of day you study is also important. You want to be rested and alert. Don't wait until just before bedtime. Study when you'll be most likely to comprehend and remember. Even better, if you know what time of day your test will be, set that time aside for study. That way your brain will be used to working on that subject at that specific time and you'll have a better chance of recalling information.

Finally, it can be helpful to team up with others who are studying for the same test. Your actual studying should be done in as isolated an environment as possible, but the work of organizing the information and setting up the study plan can be divided up. In between study sessions, you can discuss with your teammates the concepts that you're all studying and quiz each other on the details. Just be sure that your teammates are as serious about the test as you are. If you find that your study time is being replaced with social time, you might need to find a new team.

Copyright © Mometrix Media. You have been licensed one copy of this document for personal use only. Any other reproduction or redistribution is strictly prohibited. All rights reserved. This content is provided for test preparation purposes only and does not imply an endorsement by Mometrix of any particular political, scientific, or religious point of view.

Secret Key #2 – Make Your Studying Count

You're devoting a lot of time and effort to preparing for this test, so you want to be absolutely certain it will pay off. This means doing more than just reading the content and hoping you can remember it on test day. It's important to make every minute of study count. There are two main areas you can focus on to make your studying count.

Retention

It doesn't matter how much time you study if you can't remember the material. You need to make sure you are retaining the concepts. To check your retention of the information you're learning, try recalling it at later times with minimal prompting. Try carrying around flashcards and glance at one or two from time to time or ask a friend who's also studying for the test to quiz you.

To enhance your retention, look for ways to put the information into practice so that you can apply it rather than simply recalling it. If you're using the information in practical ways, it will be much easier to remember. Similarly, it helps to solidify a concept in your mind if you're not only reading it to yourself but also explaining it to someone else. Ask a friend to let you teach them about a concept you're a little shaky on (or speak aloud to an imaginary audience if necessary). As you try to summarize, define, give examples, and answer your friend's questions, you'll understand the concepts better and they will stay with you longer. Finally, step back for a big picture view and ask yourself how each piece of information fits with the whole subject. When you link the different concepts together and see them working together as a whole, it's easier to remember the individual components.

Finally, practice showing your work on any multi-step problems, even if you're just studying. Writing out each step you take to solve a problem will help solidify the process in your mind, and you'll be more likely to remember it during the test.

Modality

Modality simply refers to the means or method by which you study. Choosing a study modality that fits your own individual learning style is crucial. No two people learn best in exactly the same way, so it's important to know your strengths and use them to your advantage.

For example, if you learn best by visualization, focus on visualizing a concept in your mind and draw an image or a diagram. Try color-coding your notes, illustrating them, or creating symbols that will trigger your mind to recall a learned concept. If you learn best by hearing or discussing information, find a study partner who learns the same way or read aloud to yourself. Think about how to put the information in your own words. Imagine that you are giving a lecture on the topic and record yourself so you can listen to it later.

For any learning style, flashcards can be helpful. Organize the information so you can take advantage of spare moments to review. Underline key words or phrases. Use different colors for different categories. Mnemonic devices (such as creating a short list in which every item starts with the same letter) can also help with retention. Find what works best for you and use it to store the information in your mind most effectively and easily.

3

Copyright © Mometrix Media. You have been licensed one copy of this document for personal use only. Any other reproduction or redistribution is strictly prohibited. All rights reserved.
This content is provided for test preparation purposes only and does not imply an endorsement by Mometrix of any particular political, scientific, or religious point of view.

Secret Key #3 – Practice the Right Way

Your success on test day depends not only on how many hours you put into preparing, but also on whether you prepared the right way. It's good to check along the way to see if your studying is paying off. One of the most effective ways to do this is by taking practice tests to evaluate your progress. Practice tests are useful because they show exactly where you need to improve. Every time you take a practice test, pay special attention to these three groups of questions:

- The questions you got wrong
- The questions you had to guess on, even if you guessed right
- The questions you found difficult or slow to work through

This will show you exactly what your weak areas are, and where you need to devote more study time. Ask yourself why each of these questions gave you trouble. Was it because you didn't understand the material? Was it because you didn't remember the vocabulary? Do you need more repetitions on this type of question to build speed and confidence? Dig into those questions and figure out how you can strengthen your weak areas as you go back to review the material.

 Additionally, many practice tests have a section explaining the answer choices. It can be tempting to read the explanation and think that you now have a good understanding of the concept. However, an explanation likely only covers part of the question's broader context. Even if the explanation makes perfect sense, **go back and investigate** every concept related to the question until you're positive you have a thorough understanding.

As you go along, keep in mind that the practice test is just that: practice. Memorizing these questions and answers will not be very helpful on the actual test because it is unlikely to have any of the same exact questions. If you only know the right answers to the sample questions, you won't be prepared for the real thing. **Study the concepts** until you understand them fully, and then you'll be able to answer any question that shows up on the test.

It's important to wait on the practice tests until you're ready. If you take a test on your first day of study, you may be overwhelmed by the amount of material covered and how much you need to learn. Work up to it gradually.

On test day, you'll need to be prepared for answering questions, managing your time, and using the test-taking strategies you've learned. It's a lot to balance, like a mental marathon that will have a big impact on your future. Like training for a marathon, you'll need to start slowly and work your way up. When test day arrives, you'll be ready.

Start with the strategies you've read in the first two Secret Keys—plan your course and study in the way that works best for you. If you have time, consider using multiple study resources to get different approaches to the same concepts. It can be helpful to see difficult concepts from more than one angle. Then find a good source for practice tests. Many times, the test website will suggest potential study resources or provide sample tests.

Copyright © Mometrix Media. You have been licensed one copy of this document for personal use only. Any other reproduction or redistribution is strictly prohibited. All rights reserved.
This content is provided for test preparation purposes only and does not imply an endorsement by Mometrix of any particular political, scientific, or religious point of view.

Practice Test Strategy

If you're able to find at least three practice tests, we recommend this strategy:

UNTIMED AND OPEN-BOOK PRACTICE

Take the first test with no time constraints and with your notes and study guide handy. Take your time and focus on applying the strategies you've learned.

TIMED AND OPEN-BOOK PRACTICE

Take the second practice test open-book as well, but set a timer and practice pacing yourself to finish in time.

TIMED AND CLOSED-BOOK PRACTICE

Take any other practice tests as if it were test day. Set a timer and put away your study materials. Sit at a table or desk in a quiet room, imagine yourself at the testing center, and answer questions as quickly and accurately as possible.

Keep repeating timed and closed-book tests on a regular basis until you run out of practice tests or it's time for the actual test. Your mind will be ready for the schedule and stress of test day, and you'll be able to focus on recalling the material you've learned.

Copyright © Mometrix Media. You have been licensed one copy of this document for personal use only. Any other reproduction or redistribution is strictly prohibited. All rights reserved.
This content is provided for test preparation purposes only and does not imply an endorsement by Mometrix of any particular political, scientific, or religious point of view.

Secret Key #4 – Pace Yourself

Once you're fully prepared for the material on the test, your biggest challenge on test day will be managing your time. Just knowing that the clock is ticking can make you panic even if you have plenty of time left. Work on pacing yourself so you can build confidence against the time constraints of the exam. Pacing is a difficult skill to master, especially in a high-pressure environment, so **practice is vital**.

Set time expectations for your pace based on how much time is available. For example, if a section has 60 questions and the time limit is 30 minutes, you know you have to average 30 seconds or less per question in order to answer them all. Although 30 seconds is the hard limit, set 25 seconds per question as your goal, so you reserve extra time to spend on harder questions. When you budget extra time for the harder questions, you no longer have any reason to stress when those questions take longer to answer.

Don't let this time expectation distract you from working through the test at a calm, steady pace, but keep it in mind so you don't spend too much time on any one question. Recognize that taking extra time on one question you don't understand may keep you from answering two that you do understand later in the test. If your time limit for a question is up and you're still not sure of the answer, mark it and move on, and come back to it later if the time and the test format allow. If the testing format doesn't allow you to return to earlier questions, just make an educated guess; then put it out of your mind and move on.

On the easier questions, be careful not to rush. It may seem wise to hurry through them so you have more time for the challenging ones, but it's not worth missing one if you know the concept and just didn't take the time to read the question fully. Work efficiently but make sure you understand the question and have looked at all of the answer choices, since more than one may seem right at first.

Even if you're paying attention to the time, you may find yourself a little behind at some point. You should speed up to get back on track, but do so wisely. Don't panic; just take a few seconds less on each question until you're caught up. Don't guess without thinking, but do look through the answer choices and eliminate any you know are wrong. If you can get down to two choices, it is often worthwhile to guess from those. Once you've chosen an answer, move on and don't dwell on any that you skipped or had to hurry through. If a question was taking too long, chances are it was one of the harder ones, so you weren't as likely to get it right anyway.

On the other hand, if you find yourself getting ahead of schedule, it may be beneficial to slow down a little. The more quickly you work, the more likely you are to make a careless mistake that will affect your score. You've budgeted time for each question, so don't be afraid to spend that time. Practice an efficient but careful pace to get the most out of the time you have.

Copyright © Mometrix Media. You have been licensed one copy of this document for personal use only. Any other reproduction or redistribution is strictly prohibited. All rights reserved.
This content is provided for test preparation purposes only and does not imply an endorsement by Mometrix of any particular political, scientific, or religious point of view.

Secret Key #5 – Have a Plan for Guessing

When you're taking the test, you may find yourself stuck on a question. Some of the answer choices seem better than others, but you don't see the one answer choice that is obviously correct. What do you do?

The scenario described above is very common, yet most test takers have not effectively prepared for it. Developing and practicing a plan for guessing may be one of the single most effective uses of your time as you get ready for the exam.

In developing your plan for guessing, there are three questions to address:

- When should you start the guessing process?
- How should you narrow down the choices?
- Which answer should you choose?

When to Start the Guessing Process

Unless your plan for guessing is to select C every time (which, despite its merits, is not what we recommend), you need to leave yourself enough time to apply your answer elimination strategies. Since you have a limited amount of time for each question, that means that if you're going to give yourself the best shot at guessing correctly, you have to decide quickly whether or not you will guess.

Of course, the best-case scenario is that you don't have to guess at all, so first, see if you can answer the question based on your knowledge of the subject and basic reasoning skills. Focus on the key words in the question and try to jog your memory of related topics. Give yourself a chance to bring the knowledge to mind, but once you realize that you don't have (or you can't access) the knowledge you need to answer the question, it's time to start the guessing process.

It's almost always better to start the guessing process too early than too late. It only takes a few seconds to remember something and answer the question from knowledge. Carefully eliminating wrong answer choices takes longer. Plus, going through the process of eliminating answer choices can actually help jog your memory.

Summary: Start the guessing process as soon as you decide that you can't answer the question based on your knowledge.

Copyright © Mometrix Media. You have been licensed one copy of this document for personal use only. Any other reproduction or redistribution is strictly prohibited. All rights reserved. This content is provided for test preparation purposes only and does not imply an endorsement by Mometrix of any particular political, scientific, or religious point of view.

How to Narrow Down the Choices

The next chapter in this book (**Test-Taking Strategies**) includes a wide range of strategies for how to approach questions and how to look for answer choices to eliminate. You will definitely want to read those carefully, practice them, and figure out which ones work best for you. Here though, we're going to address a mindset rather than a particular strategy.

Your odds of guessing an answer correctly depend on how many options you are choosing from.

Number of options left	5	4	3	2	1
Odds of guessing correctly	20%	25%	33%	50%	100%

You can see from this chart just how valuable it is to be able to eliminate incorrect answers and make an educated guess, but there are two things that many test takers do that cause them to miss out on the benefits of guessing:

- Accidentally eliminating the correct answer
- Selecting an answer based on an impression

We'll look at the first one here, and the second one in the next section.

To avoid accidentally eliminating the correct answer, we recommend a thought exercise called **the $5 challenge**. In this challenge, you only eliminate an answer choice from contention if you are willing to bet $5 on it being wrong. Why $5? Five dollars is a small but not insignificant amount of money. It's an amount you could afford to lose but wouldn't want to throw away. And while losing

$5 once might not hurt too much, doing it twenty times will set you back $100. In the same way, each small decision you make—eliminating a choice here, guessing on a question there—won't by itself impact your score very much, but when you put them all together, they can make a big difference. By holding each answer choice elimination decision to a higher standard, you can reduce the risk of accidentally eliminating the correct answer.

The $5 challenge can also be applied in a positive sense: If you are willing to bet $5 that an answer choice *is* correct, go ahead and mark it as correct.

Summary: Only eliminate an answer choice if you are willing to bet $5 that it is wrong.

8

Copyright © Mometrix Media. You have been licensed one copy of this document for personal use only. Any other reproduction or redistribution is strictly prohibited. All rights reserved.
This content is provided for test preparation purposes only and does not imply an endorsement by Mometrix of any particular political, scientific, or religious point of view.

Which Answer to Choose

You're taking the test. You've run into a hard question and decided you'll have to guess. You've eliminated all the answer choices you're willing to bet $5 on. Now you have to pick an answer. Why do we even need to talk about this? Why can't you just pick whichever one you feel like when the time comes?

The answer to these questions is that if you don't come into the test with a plan, you'll rely on your impression to select an answer choice, and if you do that, you risk falling into a trap. The test writers know that everyone who takes their test will be guessing on some of the questions, so they intentionally write wrong answer choices to seem plausible. You still have to pick an answer though, and if the wrong answer choices are designed to look right, how can you ever be sure that you're not falling for their trap? The best solution we've found to this dilemma is to take the decision out of your hands entirely. Here is the process we recommend:

Once you've eliminated any choices that you are confident (willing to bet $5) are wrong, select the first remaining choice as your answer.

Whether you choose to select the first remaining choice, the second, or the last, the important thing is that you use some preselected standard. Using this approach guarantees that you will not be enticed into selecting an answer choice that looks right, because you are not basing your decision on how the answer choices look.

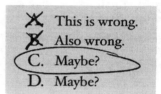

This is not meant to make you question your knowledge. Instead, it is to help you recognize the difference between your knowledge and your impressions. There's a huge difference between thinking an answer is right because of what you know, and thinking an answer is right because it looks or sounds like it should be right.

Summary: To ensure that your selection is appropriately random, make a predetermined selection from among all answer choices you have not eliminated.

9

Copyright © Mometrix Media. You have been licensed one copy of this document for personal use only. Any other reproduction or redistribution is strictly prohibited. All rights reserved.
This content is provided for test preparation purposes only and does not imply an endorsement by Mometrix of any particular political, scientific, or religious point of view.

Test-Taking Strategies

This section contains a list of test-taking strategies that you may find helpful as you work through the test. By taking what you know and applying logical thought, you can maximize your chances of answering any question correctly!

It is very important to realize that every question is different and every person is different: no single strategy will work on every question, and no single strategy will work for every person. That's why we've included all of them here, so you can try them out and determine which ones work best for different types of questions and which ones work best for you.

Question Strategies

☑ READ CAREFULLY

Read the question and the answer choices carefully. Don't miss the question because you misread the terms. You have plenty of time to read each question thoroughly and make sure you understand what is being asked. Yet a happy medium must be attained, so don't waste too much time. You must read carefully and efficiently.

☑ CONTEXTUAL CLUES

Look for contextual clues. If the question includes a word you are not familiar with, look at the immediate context for some indication of what the word might mean. Contextual clues can often give you all the information you need to decipher the meaning of an unfamiliar word. Even if you can't determine the meaning, you may be able to narrow down the possibilities enough to make a solid guess at the answer to the question.

☑ PREFIXES

If you're having trouble with a word in the question or answer choices, try dissecting it. Take advantage of every clue that the word might include. Prefixes can be a huge help. Usually, they allow you to determine a basic meaning. *Pre-* means before, *post-* means after, *pro-* is positive, *de-* is negative. From prefixes, you can get an idea of the general meaning of the word and try to put it into context.

☑ HEDGE WORDS

Watch out for critical hedge words, such as *likely, may, can, sometimes, often, almost, mostly, usually, generally, rarely,* and *sometimes*. Question writers insert these hedge phrases to cover every possibility. Often an answer choice will be wrong simply because it leaves no room for exception. Be on guard for answer choices that have definitive words such as *exactly* and *always*.

☑ SWITCHBACK WORDS

Stay alert for *switchbacks*. These are the words and phrases frequently used to alert you to shifts in thought. The most common switchback words are *but, although,* and *however*. Others include *nevertheless, on the other hand, even though, while, in spite of, despite,* and *regardless of.* Switchback words are important to catch because they can change the direction of the question or an answer choice.

Copyright © Mometrix Media. You have been licensed one copy of this document for personal use only. Any other reproduction or redistribution is strictly prohibited. All rights reserved. This content is provided for test preparation purposes only and does not imply an endorsement by Mometrix of any particular political, scientific, or religious point of view.

☑ FACE VALUE

When in doubt, use common sense. Accept the situation in the problem at face value. Don't read too much into it. These problems will not require you to make wild assumptions. If you have to go beyond creativity and warp time or space in order to have an answer choice fit the question, then you should move on and consider the other answer choices. These are normal problems rooted in reality. The applicable relationship or explanation may not be readily apparent, but it is there for you to figure out. Use your common sense to interpret anything that isn't clear.

Answer Choice Strategies

☑ ANSWER SELECTION

The most thorough way to pick an answer choice is to identify and eliminate wrong answers until only one is left, then confirm it is the correct answer. Sometimes an answer choice may immediately seem right, but be careful. The test writers will usually put more than one reasonable answer choice on each question, so take a second to read all of them and make sure that the other choices are not equally obvious. As long as you have time left, it is better to read every answer choice than to pick the first one that looks right without checking the others.

☑ ANSWER CHOICE FAMILIES

An answer choice family consists of two (in rare cases, three) answer choices that are very similar in construction and cannot all be true at the same time. If you see two answer choices that are direct opposites or parallels, one of them is usually the correct answer. For instance, if one answer choice says that quantity x increases and another either says that quantity x decreases (opposite) or says that quantity y increases (parallel), then those answer choices would fall into the same family. An answer choice that doesn't match the construction of the answer choice family is more likely to be incorrect. Most questions will not have answer choice families, but when they do appear, you should be prepared to recognize them.

☑ ELIMINATE ANSWERS

Eliminate answer choices as soon as you realize they are wrong, but make sure you consider all possibilities. If you are eliminating answer choices and realize that the last one you are left with is also wrong, don't panic. Start over and consider each choice again. There may be something you missed the first time that you will realize on the second pass.

☑ AVOID FACT TRAPS

Don't be distracted by an answer choice that is factually true but doesn't answer the question. You are looking for the choice that answers the question. Stay focused on what the question is asking for so you don't accidentally pick an answer that is true but incorrect. Always go back to the question and make sure the answer choice you've selected actually answers the question and is not merely a true statement.

☑ EXTREME STATEMENTS

In general, you should avoid answers that put forth extreme actions as standard practice or proclaim controversial ideas as established fact. An answer choice that states the "process should be used in certain situations, if..." is much more likely to be correct than one that states the "process should be discontinued completely." The first is a calm rational statement and doesn't even make a definitive, uncompromising stance, using a hedge word *if* to provide wiggle room, whereas the second choice is far more extreme.

11

Copyright © Mometrix Media. You have been licensed one copy of this document for personal use only. Any other reproduction or redistribution is strictly prohibited. All rights reserved.
This content is provided for test preparation purposes only and does not imply an endorsement by Mometrix of any particular political, scientific, or religious point of view.

⊘ BENCHMARK

As you read through the answer choices and you come across one that seems to answer the question well, mentally select that answer choice. This is not your final answer, but it's the one that will help you evaluate the other answer choices. The one that you selected is your benchmark or standard for judging each of the other answer choices. Every other answer choice must be compared to your benchmark. That choice is correct until proven otherwise by another answer choice beating it. If you find a better answer, then that one becomes your new benchmark. Once you've decided that no other choice answers the question as well as your benchmark, you have your final answer.

⊘ PREDICT THE ANSWER

Before you even start looking at the answer choices, it is often best to try to predict the answer. When you come up with the answer on your own, it is easier to avoid distractions and traps because you will know exactly what to look for. The right answer choice is unlikely to be word-for-word what you came up with, but it should be a close match. Even if you are confident that you have the right answer, you should still take the time to read each option before moving on.

General Strategies

⊘ TOUGH QUESTIONS

If you are stumped on a problem or it appears too hard or too difficult, don't waste time. Move on! Remember though, if you can quickly check for obviously incorrect answer choices, your chances of guessing correctly are greatly improved. Before you completely give up, at least try to knock out a couple of possible answers. Eliminate what you can and then guess at the remaining answer choices before moving on.

⊘ CHECK YOUR WORK

Since you will probably not know every term listed and the answer to every question, it is important that you get credit for the ones that you do know. Don't miss any questions through careless mistakes. If at all possible, try to take a second to look back over your answer selection and make sure you've selected the correct answer choice and haven't made a costly careless mistake (such as marking an answer choice that you didn't mean to mark). This quick double check should more than pay for itself in caught mistakes for the time it costs.

⊘ PACE YOURSELF

It's easy to be overwhelmed when you're looking at a page full of questions; your mind is confused and full of random thoughts, and the clock is ticking down faster than you would like. Calm down and maintain the pace that you have set for yourself. Especially as you get down to the last few minutes of the test, don't let the small numbers on the clock make you panic. As long as you are on track by monitoring your pace, you are guaranteed to have time for each question.

⊘ DON'T RUSH

It is very easy to make errors when you are in a hurry. Maintaining a fast pace in answering questions is pointless if it makes you miss questions that you would have gotten right otherwise. Test writers like to include distracting information and wrong answers that seem right. Taking a little extra time to avoid careless mistakes can make all the difference in your test score. Find a pace that allows you to be confident in the answers that you select.

Copyright © Mometrix Media. You have been licensed one copy of this document for personal use only. Any other reproduction or redistribution is strictly prohibited. All rights reserved. This content is provided for test preparation purposes only and does not imply an endorsement by Mometrix of any particular political, scientific, or religious point of view.

⊘ Keep Moving

Panicking will not help you pass the test, so do your best to stay calm and keep moving. Taking deep breaths and going through the answer elimination steps you practiced can help to break through a stress barrier and keep your pace.

Final Notes

The combination of a solid foundation of content knowledge and the confidence that comes from practicing your plan for applying that knowledge is the key to maximizing your performance on test day. As your foundation of content knowledge is built up and strengthened, you'll find that the strategies included in this chapter become more and more effective in helping you quickly sift through the distractions and traps of the test to isolate the correct answer.

Now that you're preparing to move forward into the test content chapters of this book, be sure to keep your goal in mind. As you read, think about how you will be able to apply this information on the test. If you've already seen sample questions for the test and you have an idea of the question format and style, try to come up with questions of your own that you can answer based on what you're reading. This will give you valuable practice applying your knowledge in the same ways you can expect to on test day.

Good luck and good studying!

Copyright © Mometrix Media. You have been licensed one copy of this document for personal use only. Any other reproduction or redistribution is strictly prohibited. All rights reserved.
This content is provided for test preparation purposes only and does not imply an endorsement by Mometrix of any particular political, scientific, or religious point of view.

Copyright © Mometrix Media. You have been licensed one copy of this document for personal use only. Any other reproduction or redistribution is strictly prohibited. All rights reserved.
This content is provided for test preparation purposes only and does not imply an endorsement by Mometrix of any particular political, scientific, or religious point of view.

Pharmacology

Principles of Pharmacology

SIX RIGHTS OF MEDICATION ADMINISTRATION

Six rights of medication administration include the following:

- **Right patient**: The medication should be prescribed specifically for the patient and the medical assistant should check two identifiers before giving medications.
- **Right medication**: The medication should be the correct choice for patient's condition and should match the prescription. Always verify that the medication is correct. Check the medication label when obtaining the medication, when preparing it, and before administering it.
- **Right route**: Administration should be the route that is appropriate for patient's condition and the type of medications (oral, sub-lingual, rectal, injection [IV, IM, or SC], etc.).
- **Right dose**: The dose must be as prescribed and appropriate for age, weight, and condition. If the medication is provided in a different dose from that prescribed, check calculations with a nurse.
- **Right time**: Medication should not be expired (always check date) and must be administered at the time ordered, such as "stat" (immediately) or "every 5 minutes times three."
- **Right documentation**: Documentation should be done immediately after administration and recorded in the correct format.

ACTIONS REQUIRED IF PATIENT BRINGS THEIR OWN MEDICATIONS FOR SELF-ADMINISTRATION

A patient may **bring his or her own medications** into the facility for self-administration, for example, an Epi-pen, asthma inhaler, insulin, pain pump, or nitroglycerin. This means that the patient gets instant treatment, but it also represents a liability to the facility. The drugs could be improperly stored, shared, stolen, or mistakenly administered to another patient. The syringes used to administer the medication may be disposed of incorrectly in the regular garbage, instead of a sharps container, and present a hazard to cleaning staff.

The medical assistant may assist the patient with self-administration to the extent of:

- Checking the label and dosage to ensure it is taken as directed
- Opening the case and placing the medication in the patient's hand
- Ensuring safe disposal of sharps (e.g., broken ampoules, needles)

However, the medical assistant may not actually inject or otherwise administer the medication without the doctor's expressed instructions. The medical assistant's liability is greatest for medications marked "as needed" (prn). Most states require caregivers to take a 4-hour training course with a pharmacist or registered nurse before allowing medication assistance.

Copyright © Mometrix Media. You have been licensed one copy of this document for personal use only. Any other reproduction or redistribution is strictly prohibited. All rights reserved. This content is provided for test preparation purposes only and does not imply an endorsement by Mometrix of any particular political, scientific, or religious point of view.

COMMON DRUG TYPES

Drug	Function	Examples
Analgesics	Acts as a minor pain reliever.	Aspirin, Tylenol, Advil, or Aleve
Anesthetic	Produces loss of sensation for painful procedures.	Local anesthetics: Procaine and lidocaine General anesthetics: Halothane, and methohexital
Antibiotics	There are 7 classes of antibiotics, all targeting different types of bacteria. The mode of action varies; some kill bacteria by impairing the cell membrane, others interfere with cell metabolism, leading to death of the cell.	Common classes: Penicillins, cephalosporins, aminoglycosides, carbapenems, fluoroquinolones, glycopeptides, macrolides, sulfonamides, and tetracyclines
Beta Blockers	Lower blood pressure by blocking adrenaline and slowing the heart	Inderal, Lopressor, and Tenormin
Cathartics	Encourages bowel movements (defecation) before x-rays of the colon or to treat poisoning	Sorbitol and senna
Diuretics	Increases the formation of urine to relieve edema (swelling) or high blood pressure	Hydrochlorothiazide, Furosemide (Lasix), and Triamterene
Expectorants	Helps expel mucous from the lungs through coughing by breaking down and mobilizing the secretions	Guaifenesin
Hypoglycemics (diabetic)	Oral medications help the body metabolize carbohydrates, decrease production of glucose (sugar) by the liver, or stimulate the pancreas to produce more insulin. Insulins (given by injection) replace natural insulin the pancreas can no longer produce to metabolize carbohydrates.	Oral: Sulfonylureas (glipizide), biguanides (Metformin) Insulin injection: Rapid-acting, Regular (short-acting), Intermediate-acting, Long-Acting, Ultra-long-acting
Sedatives	Makes insomniacs drowsy, relieves seizures, or calms anxious patients	Nembutal, Seconal, Ativan, Xanax, and Valium
SSRIs	Increase the level of serotonin (a neurotransmitter) to decrease depression	Prozac
Statins	Inhibit production of cholesterol in the liver and lower blood cholesterol levels	Atorvastatin (Lipitor), Simvastatin (Zocor)
Vaccines	Builds the patient's active immunity against a specific disease.	DPTP (diphtheria, polio, tetanus, and pertussis) and MMR (measles, mumps, and rubella)
Vasodilators	Relaxes smooth muscles in blood vessels to allow them to expand, decreases BP	ACE inhibitors, Hydralazine, and Minoxidil

Copyright © Mometrix Media. You have been licensed one copy of this document for personal use only. Any other reproduction or redistribution is strictly prohibited. All rights reserved.
This content is provided for test preparation purposes only and does not imply an endorsement by Mometrix of any particular political, scientific, or religious point of view.

CONTROLLED SUBSTANCES

Controlled substances are categorized under the *Controlled Substances Act of 1970*. There are five groups of controlled substances, categorized from Schedule I to Schedule V.

- **Schedule I substances** have a high potential for abuse and dependence and have NO accepted medical use in the United States. These drugs are not considered safe to use even under medical supervision. Schedule I substances are for research and instructional purposes only. Schedule I drugs include Ecstasy, Heroin, and LSD.
- **Schedule II substances** have a high potential for abuse, but have an accepted medical use. Use is severely restricted because severe psychological and/or physical dependence may develop. Schedule II drugs include PCP, Methamphetamine, Ritalin, and most narcotics.
- **Schedule III substances** have less potential for abuse than Schedule I and II substances, and have an accepted medical use in the United States. Abuse of these substances may lead to moderate or low physical dependence and/or high psychological dependence. Schedule III drugs include anabolic steroids for body building, like Winstrol, narcotics with less than 90 mg of codeine per dose, and buprenorphine (Suboxone).
- **Schedule IV drugs** have a low potential for abuse compared to substances in Schedule III. Schedule IV substances have an accepted medical use in the United States. Abuse of substances in this category may lead to limited physical and/or psychological dependence. Examples of Schedule IV drugs are Xanax, Librium, Valium, and the date rape drug Rohypnol.
- **Schedule V** substances have a low potential for abuse compared to Schedule IV drugs. Schedule V substances have an accepted medical use in the United States. Abuse of Schedule V drugs may lead to limited physical and/or psychological dependence compared to Schedule IV substances. Examples of Schedule V drugs are Robitussin A-C, Lomotil, and Pediacof.

COMPLICATIONS IN MEDICATION ADMINISTRATION AND USE

Various complications can arise from drug administration and the medical assistant must be aware of these risks for each specific drug type:

- **Side-effect**: An unwanted effect of a therapeutic dose of a drug. A side-effect may or may not cause the patient harm. An example is drowsiness for cold medications.
- **Adverse event (AE)**: A minor side-effect that may or may not be expected. For example, a patient may develop indigestion after using Aspirin for a headache.
- **Sentinel event (SE)**: An unexpected outcome causing serious physical or psychological harm, or even death. For example, a child may develop brain damage from Reyes Syndrome after taking Aspirin for influenza.
- **Substance abuse**: Excessive use of any substance, but usually drugs or alcohol, which impairs or distresses a patient for 12 months or more. Substance abuse is characterized by failure at school, work, or home due to frequent absences, neglect, or bizarre behavior. Substance abuse produces legal problems, such as arrests for disorderly conduct or driving while impaired. The abuser continues to crave the substance despite its physical hazards and social problems.

RESOURCES
PHYSICIANS' DESK REFERENCE (PDR)

The *Physicians' Desk Reference (PDR),* which is issued each year, contains a wealth of information about drugs, and is an invaluable resource for information about adverse effects, correct dosage,

Copyright © Mometrix Media. You have been licensed one copy of this document for personal use only. Any other reproduction or redistribution is strictly prohibited. All rights reserved. This content is provided for test preparation purposes only and does not imply an endorsement by Mometrix of any particular political, scientific, or religious point of view.

and administration. The PDR contains reference lists of telephone numbers for the FDA (such as medical product reporting programs), for poison control centers, and for drug information centers. The product information guide provides colored pictures of medications in actual size to help to identify unlabeled medications. Manufacturers provide information about the drugs that matches the package inserts, which are required by the FDA to provide indications, effects, dosages, routes, methods, frequency and duration of administration and any warning, hazards, contraindications, side effects, and precautions. The PDR is available in a print edition and also an online version (PDR.net) and includes a mobile version with safety alerts.

DRUG REFERENCE MANUALS

Common drug manuals for the medical office are the *American Drug Index*, *Compendium of Pharmaceuticals and Specialties*, Lippincott's *Nursing Drug Guide*, and Stoklosa and Ansel's *Pharmaceutical Calculations*. The definitive online drug reference is the *United States Pharmacopeia–National Formulary (USP–NF)*. When in doubt about a drug, always contact a pharmacist.

Medication Administration, Dosage, and Storage

ROUTES OF DRUG ADMINISTRATION

The route of administration is the manner by which a drug is introduced into the body. The routes of administration include the following:

- **Enteral** (oral, rectal, or by feeding tube)
- **Topical** (on the skin, in the eyes or nose, vaginal, or inhaled)
- **Parenteral** (IV, subcutaneous, intramuscular, intracardiac, intraosseous, intradermal, intrathecal, intraperitoneal, transdermal, transmucosal, intravitreal, and epidural)

The route of administration affects the way the medication is absorbed, distributed, and eliminated. The effect of a medication is local or systemic. There are many variations on these three basic routes of administration. The FDA acknowledges over 100 different routes of administration. When deciding on the route of administration, the doctor and pharmacist consider:

- How **fast** the patient requires the drug
- How **effective** it will be by a given route
- The likelihood of **toxicity**
- The **discomfort** it will cause
- How likely the patient is to **comply** with the route
- How likely the route is to play into the patient's **addictive habits**

SYRINGE PARTS

The syringe is used to inject medications, to irrigate wounds, and to obtain specimens. The barrel holds the medication or solution and the rubber stop keeps the fluid from leaking out. The plunger is inserted to inject the fluid, and the flanges allow the fingers to grasp the syringe. The needle is interchangeable so that different sizes can be attached to the tip by being inserted into the hub. A Luer lock or slip about the hub helps to secure the needle so that it doesn't inadvertently come loose.

Copyright © Mometrix Media. You have been licensed one copy of this document for personal use only. Any other reproduction or redistribution is strictly prohibited. All rights reserved. This content is provided for test preparation purposes only and does not imply an endorsement by Mometrix of any particular political, scientific, or religious point of view.

INJECTIONS
FORMS OF INJECTIONS

Common forms of injection include the following:

- **Subcutaneous Injection**: Delivers the drug under the skin using a 0.5" long, 24- or 25-gauge needle held at a 45° angle to reach the fat. The upper arm, abdomen, thigh, or lower back can be used as the site. The maximum volume of administration for a subcutaneous medication is 0.5 mL. An example is insulin for a patient with diabetes.
- **Intramuscular Injection**: Delivers the drug into the muscle with a 1" long, 20-gauge needle held at a 90° angle perpendicular to the muscle, to reach the deep tissue. For obese patients, use a 2" needle. In adults, intramuscular injection sites include the vastus lateralis (thigh) in volumes of 0.5-3.0 mL, the ventrogluteal region (hip) in volumes of 0.5-3.0 mL, the deltoid (upper arm) in volumes of 0.5-2.0 mL, or the dorsogluteal region (buttocks) in volumes of 1-3 mL.
- **Intravenous Injection:** Delivers the drug into a vein of the arm, hand, leg, foot, scalp, or neck with an Angiocath, butterfly, or Insyte Autoguard needle. The medication is infused via venous catheter by syringe or pump. The nurse sets the drip rate per minute by adjusting the clamp and monitoring the drip chamber. An example is Zoledronate that is given yearly to prevent bone fractures for individuals with osteoporosis.

Two less frequently used forms of injection are: Intradermal (into the skin) for Mantoux TB test, and intraosseous access (IO) into the bone, which an Emergency Response team uses for emergency cases when intravenous access is not available.

NEEDLE GAUGE AND LENGTH

The route, needle length and gauge, angle, site, and volume administered depends on the contents of the injection. On the syringe package, the first number indicates the **gauge** and the second number the **length** (e.g., 28-gauge, ½"). Gauge refers to the size of the borehole in the cannula (needle). The higher the gauge number, the thinner the needle and the smaller the borehole. Therefore, a 28-gauge cannula is thinner than a 25-gauge cannula. Thinner needles should be used for children and frequent injections.

Z-TRACK METHOD OF MEDICATION ADMINISTRATION

The Z-track method of medication administration is used to administer deep IM injections of substances that are irritating to the subcutaneous tissue. The procedure is as follows:

1. Draw up medication into syringe and then change the needle so no drug residue adheres to the needle.
2. Use a circular method with an alcohol wipe to cleanse the tissue of the dorsogluteal injection site.
3. Holding the syringe vertically with needle upward, draw 0.2-0.5 mL of air into the syringe.
4. With the fingers, pull the skin of the injection site 2-3 inches to the left and hold in place.
5. Rapidly insert the needle at a 90-degree angle to the skin and up to the hub (to ensure the aspirated air clears the needle), aspirate slightly, and (if no blood appears) inject slowly to prevent tissue damage. (If blood appears, remove needle.)
6. Rapidly remove needle and release the tissue so that it moves back into place and seals the drug into place.
7. Apply pressure to site with alcohol wipe but do not massage tissue.

Copyright © Mometrix Media. You have been licensed one copy of this document for personal use only. Any other reproduction or redistribution is strictly prohibited. All rights reserved. This content is provided for test preparation purposes only and does not imply an endorsement by Mometrix of any particular political, scientific, or religious point of view.

OPTIONS OF MEDICATION AVAILABILITY

Medication availability comes in the various options. Aseptic technique should be utilized when drawing up and administering medication regardless of its availability.

- **Single dose vials (SDV)**: Provides a single dose of a medication and is used only once within one hour after removal. Any remaining medication is discarded, as using leftover medication has proven to cause infection in patients.
- **Multiple-dose vials (MDV)**: Provide multiple doses but should be used for only one patient. Expires according to manufacturer's date or 28 days after first use. These vials are identified as multiple-use with an FDA label and contain preservatives to prevent the possibility of bacteria growth.
- **Ampules**: Glass ampules contains 1-10 mL of a single dose of medication. A gauze pad should be wrapped about the neck before breaking open. The medication is aspirated into a syringe using a special filter needle in case of glass residue. The needle must be replaced with a regular needle before injecting the medication.
- **Pre-filled cartridge-needle units**: Some cartridge-needle units are placed in special injection devices, for injection and contain a single dose of medication. Other prefilled cartridge-needle units are complete and do not require an injection device. Multi-dose cartridges (such as for insulin) require that a new needle be attached for each use.

HAZARD PREVENTION WITH PARENTERAL MEDICATIONS

Hazard prevention with parenteral medications includes preparing medications in a designated clean area; using appropriate and aseptic techniques when accessing drugs, such as in vials, ampules, and cartridges; and following the manufacturer's guidelines regarding safety. When withdrawing medications from a vial, only sterile needles should be utilized. Medications should not be prepared near a source of running water because the danger of water droplets contaminating the medication. Medications should be prepared immediately before use. Directions must be carefully followed when reconstituting powdered medications or diluting liquid medications to ensure that the appropriate dosage is prepared. Once a medication is reconstituted, the dosage must be carefully calculated to avoid overdose or underdose. The mode of administration (IM, SQ, ID, IV) should be verified to ensure adequate absorption and avoid tissue damage and the correct syringe, needle, and angle of injection utilized.

COMPLETING PRESCRIPTIONS AND AUTHORIZATION OF MEDICAL REFILLS

Requests for **prescriptions and refills** are often per telephone. In some cases, the physician may need to handle prescriptions and refills personally, but if these tasks are delegated to the medical assistant, the medical assistant should follow established protocol and should determine the identity of the caller (using their name, birthdate, or other identifier) and the telephone number. If the pharmacy is calling, the medical assistant may take a message that includes the name of the patient and the medication, and advise when the physician will respond or ask the pharmacy representative to hold while the patient's record is checked. If a patient/caregiver is calling, the medical assistant should ask the name of the medication and the pharmacy, and then check the patient's record. If the physician authorizes prescriptions/refills, the medical assistant should provide the record to the physician to review. If the medical assistant has been delegated to order refills, the medical assistant should check the original order to make sure that the physician has authorized refills.

Copyright © Mometrix Media. You have been licensed one copy of this document for personal use only. Any other reproduction or redistribution is strictly prohibited. All rights reserved.
This content is provided for test preparation purposes only and does not imply an endorsement by Mometrix of any particular political, scientific, or religious point of view.

CALCULATING DRUG DOSAGE

The medical assistant must weigh the patient accurately because the drug dosages are calculated by milligrams of medication per kilogram of patient's body weight. For example, if the drug reference manual states the general dosage is 20 mg/kg and the child patient weighs 25 kg (55 lb), then the patient receives 500 mg.

However, in pediatric medicine, some drugs have a maximum dosage that must not be exceeded within 24 hours, regardless of the patient's weight. Divide the maximum dosage by the general dosage to find out if a child gets an adult dose. For example, the maximum dose is 600 mg and the general dosage is 20 mg/kg. The child who weighs 31 kg (68 lb) gets an adult dose but the child who weighs 25 kg (55 lb) gets a pediatric dose.

Sometimes the doctor's prescription is different from the available dosage. For example, the pharmacist has 250 mg capsules of ampicillin in stock but the doctor's prescription calls for a dose of 500 mg. Divide the required dose by the available dose. This patient gets two 250 mg capsules to equal 500 mg.

STORAGE

STORING DRUGS

Correct storage maintains a drug's efficacy and safety. Store most drugs at room temperature (22-25 °C). Protect drugs from insects, dust, light, and humidity. Patients and visitors should not be able to see the automated dispensing cabinet or drug cupboard. Keep all drugs out of the reach of children, known drug addicts, and patients who may be suicidal. Some biologicals, especially ointments, hormones, and vaccines, require refrigeration.

Improper storage causes the drug to degrade before its expiration date. Most drugs last 2-5 years from their date of manufacture, provided they are kept in ideal conditions. However, some specialty preparations, such as eye drops, may only last a few hours, days, or weeks.

Controlled drugs are supervised by the Drug Enforcement Administration (DEA) and include human anesthetics, analgesics, sedatives, and drugs used to euthanize animals. Controlled drugs must be double locked in a wall cabinet and the key must not be kept nearby. Record use in a log. When the drug expires or the bottle is empty, return the log and bottle to Pharmacy.

Copyright © Mometrix Media. You have been licensed one copy of this document for personal use only. Any other reproduction or redistribution is strictly prohibited. All rights reserved.
This content is provided for test preparation purposes only and does not imply an endorsement by Mometrix of any particular political, scientific, or religious point of view.

STORING VACCINES

Vaccinations have various storage recommendations due to the delicate nature of their contents:

- **Flu, DTaP, Hib, HepB, PCV7, PPV23, and EIPV**: Protect vaccines from light. Never store a vaccine on the refrigerator door. Always keep open vials of vaccine on a tray in the main refrigerator compartment. Keep a liquid or mercury thermometer on the same shelf as the vaccine tray. Check and record the thermometer reading twice per day, when the shift starts and before leaving, and record it in a log. The refrigerator *should* be at 5 °C (41 °F), but *must* be 2-8 °C (36-46 °F).
- **Varicella and MMR** must be frozen, ideally at -18 °C (0 °F), but the freezer must be -15 °C (5 °F) or colder.
- Use a plug guard on the refrigerator and post a sign on it that reads "Biologicals" with a biohazard sign.
- NEVER store food or specimens in the same refrigerator as vaccines.
- Rotate stock weekly, so the oldest vaccine is used first. A vaccine marked only with month and year is viable until the last day of the month. Never use an expired vaccine.
- Never pre-draw a vaccine or leave it out of the refrigerator between uses.
- During transport, keep refrigerated vaccines in an insulated container on a cold gel pack and use dry ice for frozen vaccines.
- Report all accidents to the safety officer, and do not use compromised vaccines.
- If an unusual vaccine is encountered, read the product insert, refer to *The Red Book* if the insert is missing, or phone the manufacturer.

Copyright © Mometrix Media. You have been licensed one copy of this document for personal use only. Any other reproduction or redistribution is strictly prohibited. All rights reserved.
This content is provided for test preparation purposes only and does not imply an endorsement by Mometrix of any particular political, scientific, or religious point of view.

Immunizations

IMMUNIZATION VS. VACCINATION

Immunization refers to the body's buildup of defenses (antibodies) against specific diseases. It has an important role in preventing the spread of infection. Immunization prevents the patient from contracting a disease or lessens the severity of the disease, and can also prevent the complications (encephalitis, hearing loss, paralysis) associated with the infectious diseases. **Vaccination** is one method of creating immunity through the introduction of a small amount of the virus's or bacteria's antigen to the body, which then stimulates the body's creation of antibodies against that disease. Vaccination prevents the spread of infection to infants who are too young to have developed immunity and to those who are immunocompromised (cancer patients, transplantation recipients). Herd immunity results from a majority of the population being immune to a disease, therefore minimizing transmission. It is defined in terms of the percentage of the population that must be immunized in order to prevent outbreaks. This percentage may range from 80-85% for some disorders, but those that are highly contagious, such as measles, may require a herd immunity of 93-95%. Herd immunity can be obtained via widespread vaccination or widespread infection, though it is not recommended that individuals avoid immunization and rely on herd immunity for protection, as rates of immunization vary from one community to another.

VACCINATIONS PROGRAMS

Vaccination programs seek to promote health by preventing large-scale outbreaks of preventable disease. Public health has the responsibility of weighing the benefits and risks of a vaccine before recommending widespread vaccination for any given disease. Vaccines consist of an **antigen** in solution designed to stimulate the immune system of an individual to produce **antibodies** against the antigen to prevent disease from future exposure. The antigen may be alive or dead. The CDC periodically updates recommendations for all ages and has information concerning each vaccine's composition, contraindications, dosage, administration, and storage. Vaccines are recommended for adults who travel, have occupational risks of exposure, have chronic disease, or are immunocompromised. Some individuals may not receive certain vaccines due to allergies or the presence of certain diseases. Vaccines that are currently recommended for adults include tetanus, diphtheria, pneumococcal, Hepatitis A and B, measles, mumps, rubella, varicella, influenza, and meningococcal.

TYPES OF VACCINES

There are a number of different types of vaccines:

- **Conjugated forms:** An organism is altered and then joined (conjugated) with another substance, such as a protein, to potentiate immune response (such as conjugated Hib).
- **Killed virus vaccines:** The virus has been killed but can still cause an immune response (such as inactivated poliovirus).
- **Live virus vaccines:** The virus is live but in a weakened (attenuated) form so that it doesn't cause the disease but confers immunity (such as measles vaccine).
- **Recombinant forms:** The organism is genetically altered and, for example, may use proteins rather than the whole cell to stimulate immunity (such as Hepatitis B and acellular pertussis vaccine).
- **Toxoid**: A toxin (antigen) that has been weakened by the use of heat or chemicals so it is too weak to cause disease but stimulates antibodies.

Some vaccines are given shortly after birth; others begin at 2 months, 12 months, or 2 years and some later in childhood.

Copyright © Mometrix Media. You have been licensed one copy of this document for personal use only. Any other reproduction or redistribution is strictly prohibited. All rights reserved. This content is provided for test preparation purposes only and does not imply an endorsement by Mometrix of any particular political, scientific, or religious point of view.

HEPATITIS A VACCINE

Hepatitis A is a contagious virus that causes liver disease and can cause serious morbidity and death. It is spread through the feces of a person who is infected and often causes contamination of food and water. The **Hep A vaccine** is now recommended for all children at one year of age. It is not licensed for use in younger infants. Two doses are needed:

- 12 months (12-23 months)
- 18 months (or 6 months after previous dose)

Older children and teenagers may receive the two-injection series if they are considered at risk, depending upon lifestyle, such as young males having sex with other males or those using illegal drugs. It is also recommended if outbreaks occur. Adverse reactions are mild and include soreness, headache, anorexia, and malaise although severe allergic reactions can occur as with all vaccines.

HEPATITIS B VACCINE

Hepatitis B is transmitted through blood and body fluids, including during birth; therefore, it is now recommended for all newborns as well as all those <18 and those in high-risk groups >18. Hepatitis B can cause serious liver disease leading to liver cancer. Three injections of **monovalent HepB** are required to confer immunity:

- Birth (within 12 hours)
- At 1-2 months
- ≥24 weeks

Note: If combination vaccines are given after the birth dose, then a dose at 4 months can be given.

If the mother is Hepatitis B positive, the child should be given both the monovalent HepB vaccination as well as HepB immune globulin within 12 hours of birth. Adolescents (11-15) who have not been vaccinated require 2 doses, 4-6 months apart. Adverse reactions include local irritation and fever. Severe allergic reactions can occur to those allergic to baker's yeast.

ROTAVIRUS VACCINE

Rotavirus is a cause of significant morbidity and mortality in children, especially in developing countries. Most children, without vaccination, will suffer from severe diarrhea caused by rotavirus within the first 5 years of life. The new **rotavirus vaccine** is advised for all infants but should not be initiated after 12 weeks or administered after 32 weeks, so there is a narrow window of opportunity. Three doses are required:

- 2 months (between 6-12 weeks)
- 4 months
- 6 months

An earlier vaccine was withdrawn from the market because it was associated with an increase in intussusception, a disorder in which part of the intestine telescopes inside another. Rates of intussusception in those receiving the current (RotaTeq®) vaccine have been investigated and incidence of intussusception was within the range of normal occurrences with no evidence linking the occurrences to the vaccine.

DTAP AND TDAP VACCINES

Diphtheria and pertussis (whooping cough) are highly contagious bacterial diseases of the upper respiratory tract. Cases of diphtheria are now rare in the United States, although they still occur in

Copyright © Mometrix Media. You have been licensed one copy of this document for personal use only. Any other reproduction or redistribution is strictly prohibited. All rights reserved. This content is provided for test preparation purposes only and does not imply an endorsement by Mometrix of any particular political, scientific, or religious point of view.

some developing countries. There have, however, been recent outbreaks of pertussis in the United States. Tetanus is a bacterial infection contracted through cuts, wounds, and scratches. The **diphtheria, tetanus, and pertussis (DTaP) vaccine** is recommended for all children. DTaP is a newer and safer version of the older DTP vaccine, which is no longer used in the United States. **Tdap** is the DTaP booster shot meant to continue immunity to these diseases through adulthood, given every 10 years starting at age 11. DTaP requires 5 doses:

- 2 months
- 4 months
- 6 months
- 5-18 months
- 4-6 years (or at 11-12 years if booster missed between 4-6)

According to recent ACIP recommendations, DTap may now also be administered to children ages 7-9 as part of a catch-up series, but children will then require their routine Tdap dose at age 11-12. If DTap is administered to children ages 10-18 it can be counted as their adolescent Tdap booster. Adverse reactions can occur, but they are usually mild soreness, fever, and/or nausea. About 1 in 100 children will have high fever (>105 °F) and may develop seizures. Severe allergic responses can occur.

INACTIVATED POLIOVIRUS VACCINE

Poliomyelitis is a serious viral infection that can cause paralysis and death. Prior to introduction of a vaccine in 1955, there were >20,000 cases of polio in the United States each year. There have been no cases of polio caused by the poliovirus for >20 years in the United States, but it still occurs in some third world countries, so continuing vaccinations is very important. Oral polio vaccine (OPV) is no longer recommended in the United States because it carries a very slight risk of causing the disease (1:2.4 million). Children require 4 doses of injectable polio vaccine (IPV):

- 2 months
- 4 months
- 6-18 months
- 4-6 years (booster dose)

IPV is contraindicated for those who have had a severe reaction to neomycin, streptomycin, or polymyxin B. Rare allergic reactions can occur, but there are almost no serious problems caused by this vaccine.

VARICELLA VACCINE

Varicella (chickenpox) is a common infectious childhood disease caused by the varicella zoster virus, resulting in fever, rash, and itching, and it can also cause skin infections, pneumonia, and neurological damage. After infection, the virus retreats to the nerves by the spinal cord and can reactivate years later, causing herpes zoster (shingles), a significant cause of morbidity in adults. Infection with varicella conveys immunity, but because of associated problems, it is recommended that all children receive varicella vaccine. Two doses are needed:

- 12-15 months
- 4-6 years (or at least 3 months after 1st dose

Children ≥13 years and adults who have never had chickenpox or previously received the vaccine should receive 2 doses at least 28 days apart. Children should not receive the vaccine if they have

Copyright © Mometrix Media. You have been licensed one copy of this document for personal use only. Any other reproduction or redistribution is strictly prohibited. All rights reserved. This content is provided for test preparation purposes only and does not imply an endorsement by Mometrix of any particular political, scientific, or religious point of view.

had a serious allergic reaction to gelatin or neomycin. Most reactions are mild and include soreness, fever, and rash. About 1:1000 may experience febrile seizures. Pneumonia is a very rare reaction.

MMR VACCINE

Measles is a viral disease characterized by fever and rash but can cause pneumonia, seizures, severe neurological damage, and death. Mumps is a viral disease that causes fever and swollen glands but can cause deafness, meningitis, and swelling of the testicles. Rubella, also known as German measles) is also a viral disease that can cause rash, fever, and arthritis, but the biggest danger is that it can cause a woman who is pregnant to miscarry or deliver a child with serious birth defects. The **measles, mumps, and rubella (MMR) vaccine** is given in 2 doses:

- 12-15 months
- 4-6 years

Children can get the injections at any age if they have missed them, but there must be at least 28 days between injections. Children with severe allergic reactions to gelatin or neomycin should not get the injection. Severe adverse reactions are rare, but fever and mild rash are common. Teenagers may have pain and stiffness in joints. Occasional seizures (1:3000) and thrombocytopenia (1:30,000) occur.

HPV VACCINE

Human papillomavirus (HPV) comprises >100 viruses. About 40 are sexually transmitted and invade mucosal tissue, causing genital warts, which are low risk for cancer, or changes in the mucosa, which can lead to cervical cancer. Most HPVs cause little or no symptoms, but they are very common, especially in those 15-25. Over 99% of cervical cancers are caused by HPV and 70% are related to HPVs 16 and 18. The HPV vaccine, Gardasil®, protects against HPVs 6 and 11 (which cause genital warts), along with 16 and 18, which can cause cancer. Protection is only conveyed if the female has not yet been infected with these strains. The vaccine is currently recommended for females under 26 but studies have determined that those not adequately covered over the age of 26 and up to 45 can benefit. A series of 3 injections is required over a 6-month period:

- Initial dose 11-12 years (but may be given as young as 9 or ≥18)
- 2 months after 1st dose
- 6 months after 1st dose

PCV-7

Heptavalent pneumococcal conjugate vaccine (PCV-7) (Prevnar®) was released for use in the United States in 2001 for treatment of children under 2 years old. It provides immunity to 7 serotypes of *Streptococcus pneumoniae* to protect against invasive pneumococcal disease, such as pneumonia, otitis media, bacteremia, and meningitis. Because children are most at risk ≤1, vaccinations begin early:

Administration is in 4 doses:

- 1st dose: 6-8 weeks
- 2nd dose: 4 months
- 3rd dose: 6 months
- 4th dose: 12-18 months

Copyright © Mometrix Media. You have been licensed one copy of this document for personal use only. Any other reproduction or redistribution is strictly prohibited. All rights reserved. This content is provided for test preparation purposes only and does not imply an endorsement by Mometrix of any particular political, scientific, or religious point of view.

Although less effective for older children, PCV-7 has been approved for children between 2 and 5 years of age who are at high risk because of the following conditions:

- Chronic diseases: sickle cell disease, heart disease, lung disease, liver disease
- Damaged or missing spleen
- Immunosuppressive disorders: diabetes, cancer
- Drug therapy: chemotherapy, steroids

PCV-7 may also be considered for all children ≤ 5, especially those ≤3 and in group day care and in some ethnic groups (Native American, Alaska Natives, and African Americans).

PPV

Pneumococcal polysaccharide-23 vaccine (PPV) (Pneumovax® and Pnu-Immune®) is a vaccine that has been available since 1977 to protect against 23 types of pneumococcal bacteria. It is given to adults ≥65 and children ≥2 years in high-risk groups that include:

- Children with chronic heart, lung, sickle cell disease, diabetes, cirrhosis, alcoholism, and leaks of cerebrospinal fluid
- Children with lowered immunity from Hodgkin's disease, lymphoma, leukemia, kidney failure, multiple myeloma, nephrotic syndrome, HIV/AIDS, damaged or missing spleen, and organ transplant

Children ≤2 may not respond to this vaccine and should take PCV-7. Administration is as follows:

- One dose is usually all that is required although a second dose may be advised for children with some conditions, such as cancer or organ/bone marrow transplantations.
- If needed, a second dose is given 3 years after the first for children ≤10 and 5 years after the first for those ≥10.

MENINGOCOCCAL VACCINE

Meningitis is severe bacterial meningitis that can result in severe neurological compromise or death. A number of different serotypes of *meningococci* can cause meningitis and current vaccines protect against 4 types although not against subtype B, which causes about 65% of meningitis cases in children. However, the vaccines provide 85-100% protection against sub-types A, C, Y, and W-135. There are 2 types of vaccine:

- **Meningococcal polysaccharide vaccine (MPSV4)** is made from the outer capsule of the bacteria and is used for children 2-10.
  - One dose is given at 2 years, although those at high risk may receive 2 doses, 3 months apart.
  - Under special circumstances, children 3-24 months may receive 2 doses, 3 months apart.
- **Meningococcal conjugate vaccine (MCV4)** is used for children ≥11 (who have not received MPSV4). One dose is required:
  - Ages 11-12, all children should receive the vaccine.
  - If not previously vaccinated, high school and college freshmen should be vaccinated.
- Side effects are usually only local tenderness.

27

Copyright © Mometrix Media. You have been licensed one copy of this document for personal use only. Any other reproduction or redistribution is strictly prohibited. All rights reserved. This content is provided for test preparation purposes only and does not imply an endorsement by Mometrix of any particular political, scientific, or religious point of view.

HIB VACCINE

Haemophilus influenzae **type b (Hib) vaccine** (HibTITER® and PedvaxHIB®) protects against infection with *Haemophilus influenzae,* which can cause serious respiratory infections, pneumonia, meningitis, bacteremia, and pericarditis in children ≤5 years old. *Administration* is as follows:

- 1st dose: 2 months
- 2nd dose: 4 months
- 3rd dose: 6 months (may be required, depending upon the brand of vaccine)
- Last dose: 12-15 months (this booster dose must be given at least 2 months after the earlier doses for those who start at a later age than 2 months)

Children over age 6 usually do not require Hib, but it is recommended for older children and adults. Here are some conditions that place them at risk:

- Sickle cell disease
- HIV/AIDS
- Bone marrow transplant
- Chemotherapy for cancer
- Damaged or missing spleen

Some chemotherapy drugs, corticosteroids, and other immunosuppressive drugs may interact with the vaccine.

INFANT IMMUNIZATION SCHEDULE SUMMARY

The recommended schedule for immunizations for the infant is summarized below:

- All newborns receive **ophthalmic drops or ointment**, to prevent blindness from possible gonorrhea infection, and an injection of vitamin K to prevent hemorrhagic disease.
- Before discharge, newborns are tested for **phenylketonuria** and **hypothyroidism**, and will possibly have their **hematocrit** and **hemoglobin** checked.
- **Hepatitis B vaccine** is given at birth, 1-2 months, and 6-18 months.
- **Diphtheria/tetanus/pertussis vaccine** is administered at 2 months, 4 months, 6 months, and 15-18 months.
- **Hib (Haemophilus influenza type b) vaccine** is given at 2 months, 4 months, and 12 months or later.
- **Poliovirus vaccine** is given at 2 months, 4 months, and 6-18 months.
- **MMR vaccine** is given at 12-18 months.
- **Varicella (chickenpox) vaccine** can be given at 12 months.

REQUIRED IMMUNIZATION HISTORY FOR CHILDREN UP TO 6 YEARS OF AGE

According to the Centers for Disease Control and Prevention, by 6 years of age, children in the United States should receive a three-part series of hepatitis B, three doses of rotavirus prevention; four injections protecting against diphtheria, tetanus, and pertussis; four doses of *Haemophilus influenzae* type b; four doses of pneumococcal vaccine; four doses of polio vaccine; two injections that protect against measles, mumps, and rubella; two varicella vaccinations; one hepatitis A vaccination; and a yearly influenza prevention injection.

VACCINATION OF CHILDREN WITH UNCERTAIN IMMUNIZATION HISTORIES

Children who have uncertain immunization histories may need vaccinations to meet guidelines. The number of vaccinations needed depends on the child's history. For children who are not up-to-date

Copyright © Mometrix Media. You have been licensed one copy of this document for personal use only. Any other reproduction or redistribution is strictly prohibited. All rights reserved. This content is provided for test preparation purposes only and does not imply an endorsement by Mometrix of any particular political, scientific, or religious point of view.

on immunizations, the necessary injections must be determined. These vaccinations can then be given on a schedule so that the child can catch up. For children with no immunization history or uncertain status, such as refugees or internationally adopted children, restarting the immunization series may be necessary to ensure adequate coverage with all vaccines, particularly measles, mumps, and rubella; varicella; hepatitis B; *Haemophilus influenzae* type b; and polio.

IMPORTANT CONSIDERATIONS WHEN GIVING IMMUNIZATIONS

Every time a child comes into contact with the healthcare system, his **immunization status** should be assessed. Children are required, by all states, to be immunized before entering a licensed school or day care. Specific requirements will vary from state to state. Vaccines must be handled and stored according the manufacturers guidelines. Immunizations must be documented according to specific guidelines and parents must sign a consent form every time a vaccine is administered. Common illnesses such as colds, ear infections and diarrhea will not usually preclude giving vaccines. The MMR and varicella vaccines should not be given during pregnancy. There are two situations in which immunizations are contraindicated: a previous severe allergic reaction to a vaccine or one of its components and encephalopathy occurring within 7 days of giving a DTP or DTaP vaccine.

POSSIBLE SIDE EFFECTS

Immunization reactions can be minimized and the child made more comfortable by giving acetaminophen prior to the immunizations. Common reactions to immunizations include irritability, decrease in appetite, fever less than 102 °F, and swelling, redness and tenderness at injection site. These may last for the first 1-2 days and can be treated with acetaminophen every 4-6 hours for the first day. If more severe reactions occur, such as fever greater than 102 °F, severe prolonged irritability, or high-pitched crying, or the symptoms last more than 2 days, the parents should call the healthcare provider immediately.

THE ANTI-VACCINATION MOVEMENT

While **opposition to vaccination** is not a new concept, it is a movement that has gained momentum with the power of information sharing via social media. Opposers to vaccination, often referred to as "Anti-Vaxxers," believe that vaccinations can cause complications such as autism and SIDS, especially when administered in infancy and early childhood, and believe that these risks far outweigh the benefits. There are also those who oppose such medical interventions due to religious beliefs.

While the therapeutic effects of vaccinations have been supported by evidence for both individuals and communities, it is important that healthcare providers be equipped to respectfully inform and care for those that oppose vaccinations. The healthcare provider is responsible for educating the individual on evidence supporting vaccinations and the vaccinations required by law. For this reason, the CDC offers a wealth of resources for healthcare workers and for patients regarding vaccinations. The most notable resource is the CDC's Vaccine Information Statement, a living document that outlines the benefits and risks of vaccines, that healthcare workers can use to inform patients and parents. If, despite efforts to educate, the patient or caregiver still refuses vaccination, there are ICD codes that providers are required to use to document this refusal (for example, ICD-10-CM: Z28.82: Immunization not carried out because of caregiver refusal). The healthcare worker must also document that preventive medical counseling was provided.

Copyright © Mometrix Media. You have been licensed one copy of this document for personal use only. Any other reproduction or redistribution is strictly prohibited. All rights reserved. This content is provided for test preparation purposes only and does not imply an endorsement by Mometrix of any particular political, scientific, or religious point of view.

Clinical Medical Procedures

Infectious Diseases

VIRAL INFECTIONS

HERPES SIMPLEX VIRUS INFECTIONS

There are 2 types of the herpes simplex virus (HSV), human herpesvirus 1 and 2. **HSV-1** usually causes a **gingivostomatitis** (often referred to as "cold sores" or "fever blisters") and is transmitted through **close contact**. **HSV-2** usually causes painful **genital lesions** through **sexual contact**. Either may be found in other areas of the body.

- **Incubation** period is around 2-12 days.
- The primary infection is usually more severe (causes systemic **symptoms**) than the reactivated infection, but it may be asymptomatic. After the primary infection, the virus remains dormant in the nerve ganglia, and can be reactivated especially during times of stress, illness, immunosuppression, or sun exposure. While patients are most contagious during times of active lesions, the disease may be spread while asymptomatic. The frequency of the outbreaks usually decreases over time.
- HSV **lesions** are grouped vesicles with an erythematous base. They are usually painful, and a prodrome of tingling, pain, or burning sensations may be felt hours to a couple days before the eruption. Lesions last for approximately 2-3 weeks in primary infection (up to 4 weeks with genital HSV), and 1-2 weeks in recurrent infections.
- HSV is **diagnosed** clinically and confirmed with a + culture, PCR test, or HSV antibody tests (HSV-1 or HSV-2: IgM= active or recent infection; IgG= previous infection).
- Symptomatic **treatment**, proper wound care, and antivirals (acyclovir, valacyclovir, or famciclovir) may be given.
- **Complications** include perinatal infection, keratitis, herpetic whitlow, herpes gladiatorum, secondary infections, and encephalitis.

EPSTEIN-BARR INFECTION

Epstein-Barr virus (EBV) is a **herpesvirus** (human herpesvirus 4) and is responsible for causing **infectious mononucleosis**. After the initial infection, it remains latent in B cells and epithelial cells. It has been linked to certain epithelial and lymphatic neoplasms (e.g., nasopharyngeal carcinoma, Burkitt lymphoma, Hodgkin lymphoma).

- EBV is **transmitted** through **body fluids** like saliva, so it is sometimes referred to as the kissing disease. It is most common in teenagers and college-age young adults
- **Incubation** period is typically 30-50 days.
- **Symptoms** of EBV infection range from being asymptomatic to swollen painful lymph nodes, pharyngitis (can mimic strep pharyngitis), extreme fatigue, fever, and possibly hepatosplenomegaly. The WBC count is elevated (~10,000-20,000 cells/mL) with 10-30% atypical lymphocytes in the differential.
- Confirm **diagnosis** with a Mono Spot test or EBV antibody serology tests.

Copyright © Mometrix Media. You have been licensed one copy of this document for personal use only. Any other reproduction or redistribution is strictly prohibited. All rights reserved.
This content is provided for test preparation purposes only and does not imply an endorsement by Mometrix of any particular political, scientific, or religious point of view.

Mometrix

- **Treatment** is supportive, and antibiotics are not helpful in treating this viral infection. Therefore, avoid unnecessary antibiotics in those with EBV, especially since administration of ampicillin or amoxicillin is often associated with a pruritic, maculopapular rash. Analgesics, warm salt water gargles, increased fluid intake, and rest will help to relieve some of the symptoms. Symptoms may last for several weeks and fatigue may last even longer. Patients should avoid contact sports for up to 2 months.
- **Complications** include hepatitis, cytopenias (e.g., thrombocytopenia), Guillain Barré syndrome, and splenic rupture.

MEASLES, MUMPS, AND RUBELLA

Measles (rubeola) virus is highly contagious, is spread through **respiratory secretions** (incubation is 7-14 days), and peaks in late winter to spring. It causes a prodrome of high fever (4-7 days), cough, congestion, conjunctivitis; then Koplik spots (pathognomonic), and finally a maculopapular rash (spreads cephalocaudally). Report suspected cases immediately to the health dept. **Diagnose** with a + IgM antibody test (collected after 3 days of rash), viral culture, or PCR. **Treatment** is supportive.

Mumps (parotitis) is a viral infection that is spread via **saliva** (incubation is 12-24 days), and often occurs during winter and spring. It causes painful swelling of the salivary glands (parotid). Report to health dept. Supportive **treatment**. Complications include orchitis (infertility), pancreatitis, and meningitis.

Rubella (German measles) is a virus that spreads via **respiratory droplets** (incubation is 2-3 weeks), and peaks in the spring. There is a mild prodrome (fever, aches, sore throat, conjunctivitis, swollen nodes [esp. suboccipital, postauricular, & posterior cervical]), then a maculopapular rash (face 1st then down). Report to health dept. Confirm with rubella antibodies IgM or IgG. Symptomatic care.

INFLUENZA

Influenza is a highly contagious viral infection that affects the entire **respiratory system** from the nose to the lungs. There are 3 types of **influenza virus**: **A** (causes epidemics), **B** (only in humans), and **C**. Types A and B are seen most often and are the strains that the annual flu vaccine is most effective against; and type C is not as common and much less severe.

- Prevention is key and annual, age-appropriate influenza **vaccines** should be given to those ≥6 months; 2 vaccines are required in first-time vaccine patients if 6 mo. through 8-year-olds (separated by 28 days).
- **Incubation** period is 1-4 days and it is spread via respiratory droplets.
- Though **symptoms** can be very similar, the flu and the common cold differ in that the flu has a very sudden onset. Symptoms of influenza include a high fever (may last up to 5 days), headache, myalgias, dry cough, rhinorrhea, and fatigue. There may also be vomiting and diarrhea, although children are more prone to this.
- Clinical judgement, community patterns, and rapid influenza tests (high specificity, but lower sensitivity) aid in **diagnosis**, but RT-PCR or viral culture definitively confirm the diagnosis; pulse oximetry and CXR as needed for pulmonary issues.

Copyright © Mometrix Media. You have been licensed one copy of this document for personal use only. Any other reproduction or redistribution is strictly prohibited. All rights reserved.
This content is provided for test preparation purposes only and does not imply an endorsement by Mometrix of any particular political, scientific, or religious point of view.

- Antibiotic **treatment** is not effective unless there is a secondary bacterial infection (e.g., pneumonia). Look for signs of secondary infections (e.g., dyspnea, cyanosis, fever that goes away and returns, confusion/lethargy). Supportive treatment with rest, fluids, and analgesics. Antivirals should be considered in those who are at high risk (<5 years old, elderly, pregnant, chronic conditions). These are most effective if initiated within 24-48 hours of symptom onset. The neuraminidase inhibitors (oseltamivir, zanamivir) treat type A, type B, and avian H5N1. There is extensive resistance to the adamantanes (amantadine, rimantadine) so they are rarely used.
- **Complications** include pneumonia, ARDS, and death.

CORONAVIRUS

A coronavirus is a common virus that causes cold-like symptoms, including a cough, runny nose, sore throat, and congestion. Most cases of coronavirus are not dangerous and are often given little attention or go entirely unnoticed. However, specific coronavirus strains have led to two worldwide pandemics. The first, **severe acute respiratory syndrome (SARS)**, appeared in China in 2002 and quickly spread worldwide. Presenting symptoms of SARS were fever, cough, dyspnea, and general malaise. It was extremely virulent, spreading easily from person to person through close contact by way of contaminated droplets produced by coughing or sneezing. SARS was also very deadly, with a case fatality rate of nearly 10%. High rates of infection occurred in health care workers and others in contact with infected patients, so prompt diagnosis and proper isolation were essential. By 2004, there were no longer any documented active cases of SARS.

The most recent coronavirus outbreak was the **COVID-19** strain, which first appeared in December of 2019, in the Chinese city of Wuhan, and quickly became a global pandemic. Presentation of COVID-19 was similar to that of SARS, with the notable additional symptom of acute loss of taste/smell as a unique identifier. Much is still unknown about this strain, including exact transmission methods (though droplet transmission is suspected), effective treatment protocols, and long-term effects.

Precautions to take when treating patients with pandemic coronavirus include the following:

- Contact and droplet precautions, including eye protection and appropriate personal protection equipment.
- Airborne precautions (recommended by the CDC), especially with aerosol-producing procedures (ventilators, nebulizers, intubation).
- Immediate notification of public health authorities and institution of contact tracing.
- Activity restrictions of exposed health care workers planned in coordination with public health officials.

FIFTH DISEASE

Fifth disease, or **erythema infectiosum**, is a viral illness caused by parvovirus B19. It is most prevalent in the spring, with outbreaks in preschools, daycares, and elementary schools.

- The **incubation** period is 4-20 days, and it may be communicable for several days before the rash appears.
- **Transmission** occurs through oral and nasal secretions and possibly blood.
- **Symptoms** are possible fever, headache, nasal congestion, general unwell feeling, and rash starting on the cheeks (slapped cheek appearance). The rash typically spreads to the rest of the body as a lacy red rash that may come and go for up to a month.

Copyright © Mometrix Media. You have been licensed one copy of this document for personal use only. Any other reproduction or redistribution is strictly prohibited. All rights reserved. This content is provided for test preparation purposes only and does not imply an endorsement by Mometrix of any particular political, scientific, or religious point of view.

- Use over-the-counter fever medications as needed and provide **supportive care**.
- The virus can cause fetal death if contracted during pregnancy. There is no vaccine for fifth disease, and because it is a viral infection, it is not treated with antibiotics.

CHICKENPOX

Chickenpox (Varicella) is a viral infection, most prevalent in the late winter and early spring in children under 10 years of age.

- It has an **incubation** period of 10-21 days and is communicable from 1-2 days before the rash appears to after all lesions have dried up.
- **Transmission** is through direct contact and contact with respiratory droplets.
- **Symptoms** are low fever and feeling unwell, followed by the itchy rash (raised red bumps that develop vesicles which then ooze and crust over).
- The patient should be isolated until all lesions are dry. Aveeno baths and Benadryl help with the itching. Ibuprofen or acetaminophen can be used for the fever, and acyclovir is indicated in some cases. Encourage the patient not to scratch the lesions to prevent secondary infections. Provide supportive care as indicated.

ROSEOLA

Roseola is a viral illness, most prevalent in children 6-24 months of age.

- The **incubation** period is about 9 days.
- **Transmission** may be through oral and nasal.
- The illness begins with a high fever for 3-5 days; the patient appears well otherwise. The fever drops and then the rash appears. The rash is a light pink maculopapular rash which lasts 1-2 days.
- Parents should **treat the fever** as needed with anti-inflammatory medications.

POLIOMYELITIS

Poliomyelitis (commonly referred to as **polio**) is caused by an enterovirus and occurs most often in babies and young children.

- The **incubation** period is 3-14 days, and transmission occurs through direct contact with respiratory secretions and the oral-fecal route.
- The **symptoms** are slight fever, sore throat, general malaise, nausea and vomiting, headache, stomach ache, and constipation, but there can be severe pain, muscular weakness, and then paralysis.
- There are no drug therapies for polio. Observe for respiratory distress, provide general support measures, and provide for physical therapy.

CYTOMEGALOVIRUS

Cytomegalovirus (CMV) is a herpes virus, occurring in most people by the time they are adults.

- **Transmission** can occur through secretions during personal contact and from mother to baby before, during or after birth.
- Most cases have no **symptoms**, although a few infants will have fetal damage, such as jaundice, hepatitis, brain damage, or growth retardation.
- **Treatment** for those with severe infections is with ganciclovir, an antiviral drug.

Copyright © Mometrix Media. You have been licensed one copy of this document for personal use only. Any other reproduction or redistribution is strictly prohibited. All rights reserved. This content is provided for test preparation purposes only and does not imply an endorsement by Mometrix of any particular political, scientific, or religious point of view.

RESPIRATORY SYNCYTIAL VIRUS

Respiratory syncytial virus (RSV) is a virus that infects the respiratory tract, causing symptoms of nasal congestion, cough, sore throat, and headache. Severe cases can lead to high fever, breathing difficulties, severe cough, and cyanosis.

- Respiratory syncytial virus may **manifest** as a cold in adults and older children; however, there are some children who are more at risk of developing complications.
- **Transmission** is through contact with droplets from an infected person's nose or throat, generally through coughing and sneezing.
- Infants born prematurely, children with chronic lung disease, children with cystic fibrosis, and children who are in an immunocompromised state because of surgery or illness are at **high risk** of breathing difficulties, poor oxygenation, and even death from RSV.

ROTAVIRUS

Rotavirus is a viral illness that causes diarrhea, fever, and vomiting in children.

- It can be extremely **contagious** within groups where large numbers of children are present, such as in daycare centers, preschools, pediatric offices, clinics, and children's units in hospitals.
- Rotavirus can be prevented through **immunization** with a vaccine, as recommended by the American Academy of Pediatrics. Immunization can prevent up to 98% of severe cases of the illness.
- Children should wash their hands before eating and after using the bathroom to avoid spreading the disease. Caregivers should wash their hands before preparing food, after changing diapers, and after using the bathroom; they should avoid letting small children place toys or other items in their mouths and should disinfect surfaces after use.

BACTERIAL INFECTIONS

SCARLET FEVER

Scarlet fever, caused by **group A beta-hemolytic streptococci**, is most prevalent in school-age children during the fall, winter, and spring.

- The **incubation** period is 1-7 days, and transmission occurs through direct or indirect contact with oral and nasal secretions.
- The illness begins with a high fever, very sore throat, headache, malaise, chills and possibly vomiting and stomach pain. A rash appears in about 12 hours as sandpapery red pinpoints in creases of the skin, flushed face and then a strawberry tongue.
- Antibiotics will be prescribed, but patients should be isolated until taking the antibiotic for 24 hours. Analgesics are needed to bring down the fever and the patient should be encouraged to drink plenty of fluids.

DIPHTHERIA

Diphtheria, caused by *Corynebacterium diphtheriae*, is most prevalent in fall and winter.

- The **incubation** period is 2-7 days, possibly longer, and transmission is through direct contact with nasal, eye, and oral secretions.
- The **symptoms** are slight fever, nasal discharge, sore throat, feeling unwell, poor appetite, and swelling of the airway.

Copyright © Mometrix Media. You have been licensed one copy of this document for personal use only. Any other reproduction or redistribution is strictly prohibited. All rights reserved. This content is provided for test preparation purposes only and does not imply an endorsement by Mometrix of any particular political, scientific, or religious point of view.

- If the disease is severe, death can result. The patient requires isolation, bed rest, fluids, antibiotics, medication for fever, and an antitoxin. The patient may also require oxygen therapy and tracheostomy if the airway is obstructed.

WHOOPING COUGH

Whooping cough, caused by **Bordetella pertussis bacillus**, is most prevalent in infants and children who were not immunized.

- The **incubation** period is 6-20 days, and transmission occurs through direct contact with oral and nasal secretions.
- The **symptoms** are cold symptoms for 1-2 weeks, when the cough will worsen and progress to a whoop sound, usually occurring at night. Vomiting will usually follow an episode of intense coughing. As the patient recovers, the coughing will subside. In babies, a mucus plug or apnea can result in death by respiratory arrest. Hospitalization is usually required for infants less than 6 months of age and those with a severe case of pertussis.
- The patient needs isolation and bed rest, with a calm, quiet environment to limit coughing spells. Fluid intake needs to be monitored and humidified air will help.
- Watch for signs of respiratory distress and give antibiotic and pertussis immune globulin as prescribed.

TETANUS

Tetanus, caused by **Clostridium tetani**, occurs all over the world. The spores formed by the bacillus are present in soil, dust, and the GI tracts of animals and humans.

- The **incubation** period is 3-21 days.
- **Symptoms** start with headache, irritability, jaw muscle spasms, and inability to open the mouth. This is followed by severe back muscle spasms, seizures, incontinence, and fever.
- **Treatment** requires human tetanus immune globulin, penicillin G, Valium, and placement on a ventilator. The environment should be kept quiet because the spasms are initiated by stimuli.

IMPETIGO

Impetigo is a skin infection that is most commonly seen in preschool children or those in young childhood.

- Impetigo causes blister-like sores on skin areas that may already be compromised, such as under the nose, on the hands or neck, or in the diaper area. It is caused by a bacterial infection, most commonly *Staphylococcus aureus* or group A *Streptococcus*. The sores may itch or the patient may already have irritation at the site, such as a diaper rash.
- To **prevent the spread of infection**, children and caregivers should wash their hands frequently and avoid scratching the sores and then touching items. Isolation by staying home from school or daycare may be necessary until the sores have crusted over. Treating skin irritations, such as poison ivy or eczema, can also prevent infection from spreading to impetigo.

Copyright © Mometrix Media. You have been licensed one copy of this document for personal use only. Any other reproduction or redistribution is strictly prohibited. All rights reserved.
This content is provided for test preparation purposes only and does not imply an endorsement by Mometrix of any particular political, scientific, or religious point of view.

FUNGAL INFECTIONS

CRYPTOCOCCOSIS

Cryptococcosis is an infection resulting from inhaling the **fungus** *Cryptococcus neoformans,* which is found worldwide in soil (can be associated with bird droppings), or *Cryptococcus gattii,* which is associated with certain trees in the Northwest.

- Cryptococcosis is most often due to *C. neoformans*. It is often found among those with compromised immune systems and is an **AIDS-defining opportunistic infection**.
- Healthy patients may be asymptomatic and the only finding may be pulmonary lesions on CXR that resolve spontaneously. The fungus can disseminate and cause meningitis, encephalitis, cutaneous lesions, and affect long bones and other tissues. **Symptoms** are based on the area of involvement. Patients may experience cough, pleuritic chest pain, weight loss, and fever if there is pulmonary involvement; headache, double vision, light sensitivity, N/V, and confusion if CNS involvement; cutaneous lesions (papules, pustules, nodules, ulcers) if the skin is involved.
- **Diagnosis** includes microscopic analysis, culture (gold standard), or an antigen test (highly sensitive; good for detecting early infection) for *Cryptococcus* using CSF, tissue, sputum, blood, or urine. Check CSF by India ink (limited sensitivity) or culture so meningitis can be ruled out. Confirm that no mass lesion is present by CT or MRI before LP is performed.
- Mild cases may only require monitoring to ensure that the infection does not spread. In more advanced cases, the infection is treated with different antifungal medications (e.g., fluconazole for pulmonary infections, amphotericin B ± flucytosine for meningitis). The patient should also be monitored for CNS infection and medication side effects. AIDS patients may need lifelong antifungals.
- **Complications** include cryptococcal meningitis, neural deficits, optic nerve damage, and hydrocephalus.

HISTOPLASMOSIS

Histoplasmosis is an infection caused by inhalation of **spores** from the fungus *Histoplasma capsulatum* that is found in soil and is associated with bird and bat droppings (e.g., chicken coops, caves).

- Healthy patients are usually asymptomatic and those with symptoms are typically immunocompromised or those who've had a heavy exposure to spores. The primary **pulmonary infection** occurs 3-17 days after exposure and can present with flu-like symptoms. It is typically self-limited but may become chronic. Histoplasmosis can also spread through the **blood** and can cause progressive disseminated disease in the immunocompromised (high mortality rate); this is an **AIDS-defining illness**.
- **Diagnose** through antigen tests (urine, serum), histopathology, or cultures; order a CXR. Mild and even moderate acute pulmonary histoplasmosis may resolve on its own.
- If needed, **treat** mild to moderate infections with itraconazole and severe illness with amphotericin B.

Copyright © Mometrix Media. You have been licensed one copy of this document for personal use only. Any other reproduction or redistribution is strictly prohibited. All rights reserved. This content is provided for test preparation purposes only and does not imply an endorsement by Mometrix of any particular political, scientific, or religious point of view.

PNEUMOCYSTIS

Pneumocystis jiroveci is a **fungus** (previously known as *Pneumocystis* carinii) that causes **pneumonia** (PJP, previously PCP) in the immunocompromised. Most people have been exposed to this by the age of 3 or 4.

- **Symptoms** of PJP include a dry nonproductive cough, fever, dyspnea, and weight loss.
- CXR may show diffuse bilateral infiltrates or it may be normal; and pulse oximetry may be low, especially on exertion. **Diagnosis** is confirmed with sputum histopathology using sputum induction or bronchoalveolar lavage.
- **Treat** immediately with TMP-SMX (trimethoprim/sulfamethoxazole) for 21 days if HIV + and for 14 days in other cases. Steroids may be added for HIV patients with severe PJP. HIV/AIDS patients with CD4 counts <200/μL should receive PJP prophylaxis with TMP-SMX. Dapsone and pentamidine are alternatives.
- **Complications** include ARDS and death.

CANDIDAL INFECTIONS

Candida is a type of yeast that may cause a variety of infections:

- **Oral thrush** is commonly seen in diabetic patients and those who are immunosuppressed (HIV or underlying neoplasm). Patients often complain of burning on the tongue or in the mouth, associated with "curd-like" white patches that can be scraped away leaving reddish tissue underneath. Diagnosis is with KOH prep. Treatment is with oral or topical antifungals, including nystatin (swish and swallow or troches).
- **Candida esophagitis** also occurs in the immunosuppressed population, and patients may complain of dysphasia, odynophagia, and chest pain. This is diagnosed on EGD and may be treated with oral or IV antifungals (ketoconazole).
- **Candidal intertrigo**, or diaper rash, presents with beefy-red lesions at skin fold areas as well as satellite lesions. Treatment is with topical antifungals.
- **Candidemia** is diagnosed with fungal blood cultures and may lead to osteomyelitis, endocarditis, and other complications. Treatment is with IV antifungals.

RINGWORM

Ringworm is caused by an infection from the ***Tinea* fungus**, which produces patches on the skin that have normal centers, giving the appearance of a ring.

- The fungus can cause hair loss and patches of scaly skin that may develop blisters that ooze or crust.
- It is **transmitted** by touching the affected skin or through objects that have touched the affected skin.
- Ringworm may be **diagnosed** by viewing the skin section under a Wood's lamp. Skin cultures may also be taken for examination to identify the fungus. A potassium hydroxide (KOH) exam involves scraping the affected skin and placing the skin sample in KOH to test for the presence of the fungus.

VECTOR-BORNE AND PARASITIC INFECTIONS

MALARIA

Malaria is a **blood-borne disease** caused by a **parasite** from the genus *Plasmodium and* found in tropical areas. There are 4 known to cause disease in humans (*P. malariae*, *P. vivax*, *P. ovale*, and *P. falciparum*). These protozoa are transmitted by the **female *Anopheles* mosquito**. They travel to the **liver** where they multiply, are released, and then infect the RBCs, where they continue to multiply.

Copyright © Mometrix Media. You have been licensed one copy of this document for personal use only. Any other reproduction or redistribution is strictly prohibited. All rights reserved. This content is provided for test preparation purposes only and does not imply an endorsement by Mometrix of any particular political, scientific, or religious point of view.

Incubation time can be as little as 9 days or as much as multiple years depending on the species of the infecting parasite.

- **Signs and symptoms** include headache, high fever with shaking chills and sweating (rigors; occurs when merozoites, an immature form of the parasite, are released from RBCs), jaundice, anemia, and hepatosplenomegaly. Take a thorough history including recent travel.
- **Diagnose** with 3 thin and thick blood smears (gold standard) stained with Giemsa (preferred) and obtained 12-24 hours apart. Labs typically show elevated LDH, thrombocytopenia, and atypical lymphocytes. Rapid antigen tests are also available as well as PCR.
- **Treat** with chloroquine. If travelling, chemoprophylaxis depends on the area of travel due to species and resistance patterns, and may include chloroquine, primaquine, mefloquine, Malarone®, or doxycycline. Report infections to your local or state health department.
- **Complications** include severe anemia and hemolysis, organ failure (liver, spleen, kidneys), cerebral malaria, ARDS, and death.

LYME DISEASE

Lyme disease occurs from a bite from a **deer tick** (blacklegged tick) infected with the **spirochete bacterium** *Borrelia burgdorferi*. It is the most common tick-borne disease in the U.S. and is more prevalent in heavily wooded areas. Adult ticks are more active during colder times whereas the nymphs (<2 mm in size) are more active in the warm, spring or summer months. Once the tick bites, it stays attached; however, it takes about 36-48 hours for nymphs and about 48-72 hours for adult ticks before the spirochete is transmitted to the person. **Incubation** period is 3-30 days. There are 3 stages to this disease: early localized, early disseminated, and chronic disseminated.

- At **Stage 1**, 75% have the characteristic expanding red rash (erythema migrans; can be large, ~30cm) which can progress to have central clearing (bull's eye), headache, fever, chills, myalgias, and fatigue.
- **Stage 2** occurs weeks to months after initial infection and involves systemic symptoms (flu-like), neck stiffness, headaches, migrating pain in muscles and joints, rashes, paresthesias, Bell's palsy, confusion, fatigue, myocarditis, and heart palpitations.
- **Stage 3** occurs months to years after initial infection and involves neurologic (e.g., encephalitis) and rheumatologic issues, especially arthritis of large joints (e.g., knee).

DIAGNOSIS AND TREATMENT OF LYME DISEASE

Diagnose Lyme disease using 2-tiered testing: antibodies (IgM, IgG), then Western blot. Antibiotic treatment for localized Lyme disease involves 2-3 weeks of doxycycline, amoxicillin, or cefuroxime axetil is started immediately after diagnosis. IV antibiotics may be needed for severe disease (e.g., IV ceftriaxone). Prevention is key by wearing clothes covering the skin, using tick repellents, showering soon after being outdoors in tick-prone areas, and thoroughly checking for ticks (especially in hard to see areas by using a mirror). The Lyme vaccine is no longer available and previous vaccine recipients are still at risk of contracting the disease as protection decreases over time. Complications are prevalent with untreated Lyme disease and include chronic arthritis, fatigue, chronic musculoskeletal issues, acrodermatitis chronica atrophicans, and memory and concentration issues. Report cases to the local health dept.

Copyright © Mometrix Media. You have been licensed one copy of this document for personal use only. Any other reproduction or redistribution is strictly prohibited. All rights reserved.
This content is provided for test preparation purposes only and does not imply an endorsement by Mometrix of any particular political, scientific, or religious point of view.

ROCKY MOUNTAIN SPOTTED FEVER

Rocky Mountain spotted fever is a tick-borne illness caused by **Rickettsia rickettsii**. It tends to occur in spring and summer throughout the United States.

- **Incubation** period is about one week.
- **Symptoms** include headache, fever, nausea, vomiting, loss of appetite, muscle pain, and rash on the ankles and wrists.
- **Treatment** requires an antibiotic, usually Vibramycin.

ZIKA VIRUS IN PREGNANT WOMEN

Zika virus is a **flavivirus** that is transmitted by the *Aedes* mosquito and through sexual contact. This virus can be passed on to an unborn baby causing severe congenital defects while causing mild or no disease in the mother. It is advised that all pregnant women avoid traveling to areas with the Zika virus (e.g., Central and South America, Mexico, Caribbean, Africa).

- **Incubation** period is 3-14 days and symptoms may last 4-7 days. The virus has been found to remain longer in semen than in other body fluids.
- If **symptoms** are present, they may include fever, headache, myalgias, arthralgias, a maculopapular rash, and conjunctivitis. Congenital defects include severe microcephaly, severe brain abnormalities, macular scarring, hearing loss, motor disabilities (e.g., hypertonia), and contractures. Women should be screened for Zika exposure at each prenatal visit.
- **Diagnostic** testing is recommended for all asymptomatic pregnant women who have continued exposure to Zika and for all symptomatic pregnant women who have possibly been exposed to the Zika virus. Testing includes RNA NAT testing on serum and urine, and serum IgM Zika antibody testing. Prenatal ultrasound helps determine if the effects of Zika are present. Report cases to the state health department; and the CDC can be consulted.
- There is **no treatment** or cure for the Zika virus.

HELMINTH INFESTATIONS

Helminth infestations (worms) include **roundworms** [nematodes: *Ascaris*, hookworms (cause anemia), **filariae** (cause elephantiasis)] and **flatworms** [tapeworms (cause weight loss); **flukes** (intestinal or liver)]. **Pinworms** are a type of roundworm that cause enterobiasis and is the most common helminth infestation. Pinworms are more prevalent in warmer areas of the country and infestations occur more frequently in children. The worms lay eggs within the digestive tract and then travel to the anal area where they are usually found. Pinworms are highly contagious. As a patient itches the anal area where the eggs are located, the eggs cling to the fingers and can easily be transmitted to other people either directly or through food or surfaces. The eggs can survive for 2-3 weeks on inanimate objects.

- Patients may be asymptomatic or have intense anal itching that is usually worse at night and can cause insomnia. Abdominal pain, nausea, and vomiting can also occur.
- **Diagnose** with the "tape test" which involves pressing cellophane tape over the perianal area to pick up eggs or worms and examine under the microscope. Most other helminth infestations can be diagnosed with a stool sample for ova and parasites; filariasis requires a blood smear or antigen test.
- Anthelmintic medications are given in a single dose and repeated in 2 weeks to kill the pinworms and their larvae (mebendazole, albendazole, or pyrantel pamoate). The entire family and close contacts should be treated simultaneously since pinworms are so contagious.

Copyright © Mometrix Media. You have been licensed one copy of this document for personal use only. Any other reproduction or redistribution is strictly prohibited. All rights reserved. This content is provided for test preparation purposes only and does not imply an endorsement by Mometrix of any particular political, scientific, or religious point of view.

GIARDIA LAMBLIA

Giardia lamblia is a **protozoan** that infects water supplies and spreads to children through the fecal-oral route. It is the most common cause of non-bacterial diarrhea in the United States, causing about 20,000 cases of infection each year in all ages.

- Children often become infected after swallowing recreational waters (pools, lakes) while swimming or putting contaminated items into the mouth. *Giardia* live and multiply within the small intestine where cysts develop.
- **Symptoms** occur 7-14 days after ingestion of 1 or more cysts and include diarrhea with greasy floating stools (rarely bloody), stomach cramps, nausea, and flatulence, lasting 2-6 weeks. A chronic infection may develop that can last for months or years.
- **Treatment** includes Furazolidone 5-8 mg/kg/day in 4 doses for 7-10 days or Metronidazole 40 mg/kg/day in 3 doses for 7-10 days. Chronic infections are often very resistant to treatment.

TOXOPLASMOSIS

Toxoplasmosis is an infection caused by the **parasite *Toxoplasma gondii***, which is commonly found in soil. It is widespread and transmitted through cat feces; however, it also may be contracted by eating undercooked meat (especially pork, lamb, or venison) or poorly washed vegetables. Toxoplasmosis can cause serious disease and can affect various organs; and immunocompromised and pregnant women and their unborn babies are especially likely to have side effects of the disease (the "T" in congenital TORCH infections).

- Healthy patients are usually asymptomatic; however, once infected the parasite can remain latent until the patient becomes immunocompromised and the parasite is reactivated causing **symptoms**. The disease can cause a flu-like illness with fever, myalgias, and lymphadenopathy. More serious effects include retinochoroiditis, brain lesions, and encephalitis. Congenital toxoplasmosis may cause retinochoroiditis, microcephaly, hydrocephalus, intellectual disability, and possibly miscarriage or stillbirth.
- **Diagnose** with serology for *Toxoplasma* antibodies IgM and IgG. Also, PCR may be used to test amniotic fluid, CSF, or tissue.
- **Treat** with pyrimethamine (preferred) plus folinic acid or sulfadiazine plus folinic acid. Pregnant women should avoid high-risk practices like changing the cat litter and should avoid sand boxes.

40

Copyright © Mometrix Media. You have been licensed one copy of this document for personal use only. Any other reproduction or redistribution is strictly prohibited. All rights reserved. This content is provided for test preparation purposes only and does not imply an endorsement by Mometrix of any particular political, scientific, or religious point of view.

Asepsis

MODES OF INFECTION TRANSMISSION

Modes of infection transmission include the following (with possible infectious diseases in parenthesis):

- **Direct contact**: Direct touching, kissing (mononucleosis) and sexual intercourse (gonorrhea, syphilis, chlamydia, HIV). Vertical transmission involves mother to infant during pregnancy, delivery, or breastfeeding (HIV, hepatitis B, gonorrhea, herpes).
- **Indirect contact**: A contaminated fomite (inanimate object), such as a doorknob, syringe, or catheter, spreads infection (*Clostridium difficile*).
- **Airborne**: Particles less than 5 μm in size inhaled from cough, sneeze, or exhalation. Particles stay suspended in the air and travel large distances (tuberculosis, measles, COVID-19).
- **Droplet**: Particles greater than 5 μm in size are inhaled from a cough, sneeze, or exhalation (influenza, mumps, meningitis, pertussis, pneumonia, rubella). Droplets travel less than 3 feet and do not stay suspended, therefore are less contagious than airborne particles.
- **Vehicle**: Contact with contaminated water, air, or food (*E. coli* diarrhea, Cryptosporidiosis, hepatitis A).
- **Vector (mechanical)**: Contact with an animal, insect, or device that carries infection from one host to another (such as a fly carrying bacteria from feces of an infected host to food [dysentery]).
- **Vector (biological)**: Infected biological vector (such as a tick or flea) transmits infection directly to another host (Chagas disease, malaria, West Nile virus, Lyme disease).

CHAIN OF INFECTION AND NATURAL BARRIERS TO INFECTION

There are six components to the chain of infection:

- **Infectious microorganisms**: Bacteria, viruses, fungi, parasites
- **Reservoir**: The place the microorganism lives and reproduces (water, feces, body fluids, toilet seats, door knobs, blood)
- **Portal of exit**: The place where the microorganism leaves the reservoir (nose, mouth, rectum, blood, sputum)
- **Transmission mode**: The method (direct or indirect) by which a microorganism travels from one host to another
- **Portal of entry**: The site at which a microorganism enters a host (wounds, mucous membranes, feeding tubes, urinary catheter, ventilation tube, IV)
- **Susceptible host**: The host at risk of developing the infection

Copyright © Mometrix Media. You have been licensed one copy of this document for personal use only. Any other reproduction or redistribution is strictly prohibited. All rights reserved.
This content is provided for test preparation purposes only and does not imply an endorsement by Mometrix of any particular political, scientific, or religious point of view.

Natural barriers to infection include an effective immune system, intact skin, adequate cough reflex and air filtering (nose and lungs), digestive acids and enzymes (destroy some pathogens), healthy mucous membranes (prevent infections), blood components (white blood cells), inflammation response (walls off infection), urethra (provides protection of urinary system), and fever (increases body defense system).

INFECTION CONTROL PRECAUTIONS

Various levels of infection control precautions exist to aid in the prevention of the spread of infection amongst health care workers and facilities:

- **Standard or universal precautions** are means through which healthcare workers control the spread of disease by assuming every patient's samples are infectious, and following the OSHA standards for proper hand washing, wearing gloves and other personal protective equipment (PPE), bagging specimens in biohazard bags, and disposing of needles and lancets in a sharps container.
- **Contact precautions** prevent direct and indirect contact transmission of infectious pathogens such as those found with herpes simplex, infected wounds, and infectious diarrhea. PPE includes wearing gloves and gown upon room entry and properly discarding before exiting the patient room.
- **Droplet precautions** are used to prevent the transmission of pathogens transmitted by respiratory droplets from coughing, sneezing, or talking. PPE includes a mask for the patient when being transported outside patient room, and a mask for medical personnel when entering the patient room.
- **Airborne precautions** are used for airborne transmission microbes such as tuberculosis, which require a negative pressure private room and a HEPA or fit-tested N95 mask.

Isolating infectious patients is essential to reduce the risk of infection.

- **Strict isolation** segregates infectious patients to one room, and visitors are restricted.
- **Modified isolation** attempts to limit infection with protective techniques, like donning gloves, gowns, and masks when handling the patient's body fluids.
- **Reverse isolation** protects a patient from others in a clean room, as after kidney transplant.

Antisepsis is reducing the flora and transient microorganisms on the skin for minor procedures like venipuncture. Clean gloves are worn. It requires a short-acting antiseptic like 70% isopropyl alcohol that can denature proteins.

Asepsis prevents the spread of infection by reducing pathogens. There are two types of asepsis: medical asepsis and surgical asepsis. Some procedures require surgical asepsis while others only require medical asepsis.

Copyright © Mometrix Media. You have been licensed one copy of this document for personal use only. Any other reproduction or redistribution is strictly prohibited. All rights reserved. This content is provided for test preparation purposes only and does not imply an endorsement by Mometrix of any particular political, scientific, or religious point of view.

MEDICAL ASEPSIS

Medical asepsis is defined as the absence of disease-causing microorganisms and is often referred to as **clean**. Medical asepsis is used to prevent the spread of hospital-acquired (nosocomial) disease and cross-infections (different pathogens passed between two patients):

- Wash hands using proper hand hygiene whenever visibly soiled, before and after any contact with patients, and after gloves are removed.
- Disinfect patient care materials before use with the proper chemical agent, according to the manufacturer's specifications.
- Maintain a clean patient care environment, with adequate space, ventilation, sunlight, and cool temperature.
- Dispose of infectious material as soon as soiling is discovered in the proper bin (concurrent cleaning).
- Disinfect patient care materials after a patient leaves the office, dies, or is transferred to another floor or facility (terminal cleaning).
- Use clean and dirty utility rooms to separate unused equipment from used equipment and prevent contamination.
- Store clean linen separate from used linen, and limit access to the clean linen room to authorized personnel only.

SURGICAL ASEPSIS

Surgical asepsis is defined as the absence of all microorganisms and is often referred to as **sterile**. Surgical asepsis is used in the sterilization of instruments, sutures, drapes, sponges, and other surgical equipment and storing them safely, so they do not become reinfected. The principles of surgical asepsis are used when the skin is not intact and when internal areas of the body are being entered, cared for, or treated. This includes wound care, surgical procedures, invasive procedures such as endoscopy, and insertion of internally placed tubes such as an indwelling urinary catheter or central IV line. Sterility is not required for instruments introduced into the vagina, ear canal, or mouth; a vaginal speculum, otoscope, or tongue depressor can be clean (disinfected), rather than sterile.

Appropriate technique for setting up sterile field and maintaining asepsis:

- Sterile gowns, gloves, and masks are worn by staff setting up or working with a sterile field.
- Only sterile items are placed on the sterile field.
- NEVER lean over a sterile field or turn your back to a sterile field.
- NEVER have the sterile field below waist level.
- Maintain a one-inch border around the sterile field that is not sterile. Sterile items are put inside of this one-inch border.
- Sterile field must remain dry. Coughing or sneezing over the sterile field contaminates the sterile field.
- Sterile liquids must be poured carefully into sterile containers on the sterile field without the solution running over.

If the sterile field is not maintained continuously throughout the procedure, the entire sterile field and its contents are discarded and the entire setup must be redone.

Copyright © Mometrix Media. You have been licensed one copy of this document for personal use only. Any other reproduction or redistribution is strictly prohibited. All rights reserved. This content is provided for test preparation purposes only and does not imply an endorsement by Mometrix of any particular political, scientific, or religious point of view.

HAND-WASHING TECHNIQUE

Handwashing is the most effective way to prevent the spread of infection when done properly. To **wash hands correctly**, wet the hands with clean running water and apply soap. Lather hands by rubbing them together with soap, scrubbing the backs of hands, between fingers, and under nails for at least 20 seconds. Note any cuts, rashes, broken or long nails that need treatment before resuming work. Rinse well under clean running water and dry hands with paper towels, not a blow dryer. Use a clean paper towel to turn off the taps and to open the exit door.

If there is no sink nearby, a 60% alcohol-based hand sanitizer can be used. Rub gel over all the surfaces of hands and fingers until hands are dry, about 20 seconds. Although hand sanitizers are effective against most pathogenic microorganisms, they are not effective against Clostridium difficile.

Hands should be washed before and after each client contact, anytime they are visibly soiled, and before and after donning and removing gloves. Change gloves frequently by turning them inside out from the wrists.

Copyright © Mometrix Media. You have been licensed one copy of this document for personal use only. Any other reproduction or redistribution is strictly prohibited. All rights reserved.
This content is provided for test preparation purposes only and does not imply an endorsement by Mometrix of any particular political, scientific, or religious point of view.

Instrument Sterilization

SANITIZATION, DISINFECTION, AND STERILIZATION

Sanitization is the decontamination process that is intended to reduce the number of pathogenic organisms to a number that is no longer considered harmful, although some viruses and spores are resistant to sanitization. Sanitizing agents include sodium hypochlorite, chlorine gas, and calcium hypochlorite.

Disinfection is a decontamination process that is intended to greatly reduce pathogenic microorganisms from inanimate objects, including surfaces, most often through the use of chemical disinfectants, such as hydrogen peroxide, peroxyacetic acid, and isopropanol.

Sterilization is a process that is intended to kill or deactivate all microorganisms, including viruses, bacteria, fungi, spores, and unicellular eukaryotic organisms, rendering the items sterile. Methods of sterilizations include heat (dry, steam incineration), irradiation (non-ionizing, ionizing), filtration, and high pressure as well as the application of chemicals (ethylene oxide, glutaraldehyde, formaldehyde, peracetic acid).

SPALDING CLASSIFICATION SYSTEM OF DISINFECTION

Earle H. Spalding developed a 3-category classification system for different levels of **sterilization/disinfection** based on the type of item (instrument and/or equipment) and its use. While not applicable in all situations, this system is often used for reference:

- **Critical items** are items or pieces of equipment entering the vascular system or sterile tissue, including breaching the mucosal barrier. These include surgical instruments, probes, and urinary catheters and must be sterilized before use. Many of these items are purchased as already sterilized; others are sterilized with steam sterilization or high-level chemical sterilants, such as 7.5% stabilized hydrogen peroxide.
- **Semicritical items** are those items that contact mucous membranes or non-intact skin, including respiratory and anesthesia equipment and manometry probes and catheters. These devices require high-level disinfectants, such as glutaraldehyde and hydrogen peroxide, in accordance with FDA guidelines.
- **Noncritical items** are those items that come in contact with skin that is intact, such as bedpans and blood pressure cuffs. These devices require low-level disinfectants, such as alcohol or diluted bleach.

Copyright © Mometrix Media. You have been licensed one copy of this document for personal use only. Any other reproduction or redistribution is strictly prohibited. All rights reserved.
This content is provided for test preparation purposes only and does not imply an endorsement by Mometrix of any particular political, scientific, or religious point of view.

SANITIZATION OF EQUIPMENT, EXAM ROOM SURFACES, AND INSTRUMENTS

Sanitization of equipment, surfaces in the exam room, and instruments should first begin with cleaning to remove all organic and other residue so that the sanitization process can make direct contact. Guidelines vary depending on the sanitizing agent utilized, but manufacturing guidelines should be carefully followed in order to achieve reduction of 99.9% of microorganisms within 30 seconds of application:

- **Equipment**: Must be cleaned according to manufacturer's guidelines with special attention to any knobs or switches.
- **Surfaces**: High-touch surfaces, such as doorknobs, handles, light switches, and telephones, must be cleaned frequently following manufacturer's guidelines and regulations (government, CDC, OSHA). Other surfaces (floors, walls) require periodic sanitization.
- **Instruments**: Should be cleaned thoroughly with soap and water before sterilization, and cleaning must take place in a special "dirty" area. The process for sanitation depends on the classification of the instrument.

CARE AND HANDLING OF LOCAL ANESTHETIC SETUP

When sanitizing the **local anesthetic setup**, sanitize the harpoon of a stainless-steel reusable aspirating syringe after each use, and then autoclave the entire syringe. From time to time, lubricate parts or the harpoon may require replacement. Discard plastic syringes in a biohazard container. Discard the cannula into a sharps container after normal use if there is any evidence of a broken seal or if tissue penetration occurs more than four times. Anesthetic cartridges come in sterilized, sealed blister packs and should be stored at room temperature in a dark area. Inspect the cartridge before use. Discard a cartridge that has expired or has large bubbles, rust, corrosion, or extruded stoppers. Dispose of a used cartridge in a tamper-proof container approved by the pharmacist. Be aware that addicts scavenge garbage for residual drugs.

GAS AND CHEMICAL STERILIZATION METHODS

Gas sterilization methods have been developed because many of the synthetic materials in use are not heat tolerant; however, many gases are highly toxic.

- **Ethylene oxide** is an effective sterilizer but is toxic and combustible, so specialized equipment is necessary to ensure safety.
- **Hydrogen peroxide plasma gas** provides low temperature, low moisture sterilization of medical devices. Because there is no heat involved in the process, the items can be removed as soon as the process completes.

Chemical sterilization may be used for heat sensitive critical and semi-critical items that can be immersed in a liquid. The duration of time required varies. In some cases, the difference between chemical sterilization and disinfection relates to the length of time the process takes. For example, many chemicals require 10–20 minutes (and some up to 12 hours) for effectiveness. Chemical sterilants include glutaraldehyde, hydrogen peroxide, and peracetic acid, sometimes in combination.

Copyright © Mometrix Media. You have been licensed one copy of this document for personal use only. Any other reproduction or redistribution is strictly prohibited. All rights reserved. This content is provided for test preparation purposes only and does not imply an endorsement by Mometrix of any particular political, scientific, or religious point of view.

PREPARING A TRAY FOR THE AUTOCLAVE

An **autoclave oven** sterilizes instruments. The medical assistant cleans instruments promptly after use by immersion in an ultrasonic bath or instrument washer. Instruments that cannot be cleaned immediately are presoaked in disinfectant temporarily. Use a scrub brush for stubborn debris. Separate the blades of all instruments. Ultrasonic solution should cover all the instrument parts. Instruments that have hinges (e.g., scissors and forceps) should be sanitized first and later sterilized in the open position. Remove instruments from the ultrasonic bath, hold them under running water, dry, and then wrap them for the autoclave. Seal the pack with pressure-sensitive striped tape, which turns color when the correct temperature has been reached. Set the autoclave thermostat to:

- Dry heat at 170 °C (340 °F) for 1 hour for powders and swabs that deteriorate when wet
- Steam at 121 °C (250 °F) and 15 psi for 30 minutes for most metal and glass

Dry the instruments well prior to storage. If the doctor requests an instrument that is not on the autoclaved tray prepared, then use a flash pre-vacuum sterilizer at 134 °C (275 °F) for 4 minutes to sterilize the instrument.

RECORDS OF STERILIZED INSTRUMENTS

Records of sterilized instruments must be kept in case there is a recall that requires the items to be traced, retrieved, and re-sterilized. All sterilization records must include the following:

- Date, sterilizer number, and load number
- Lot number and general contents of load
- Exposure time, temperature, and pressure
- Operator's name or initials
- Chemical indicator results
- Biological indicator results
- Bowie-Dick test results for steam vacuums

A record of every sterilizer's performance must also be kept for accreditation. It should show the model and serial number, service dates, reason for the service request, services performed by the technician, and parts replaced.

Copyright © Mometrix Media. You have been licensed one copy of this document for personal use only. Any other reproduction or redistribution is strictly prohibited. All rights reserved. This content is provided for test preparation purposes only and does not imply an endorsement by Mometrix of any particular political, scientific, or religious point of view.

Hazard Management

SAFETY DATA SHEETS (SDSs)

Safety Data Sheets (SDSs), formerly known as Material Safety Data Sheets (MSDSs), explain how to handle caustic substances in the event of an accident or injury and provide pertinent information on the composition and toxic effects of the chemicals in the lab. SDSs outline proper storage of chemicals, procedures for cleanup, and dumping of caustic substances as well as procedures in the event of a chemical spill or injury and proper locations in the facility for clean-up. The SDSs should also contain information indicating which substances may cause allergic effects or asthma from contact or inhalation. The medical assistant should obtain SDSs for common chemicals and products being used as a safety measure so that the information is readily available. Manufacturers and suppliers should have SDSs on file and can be contacted for copies. OSHA/EPA Occupational Chemical Database provides links for SDSs for some products. SDSs are available from various other sources, including Toxicology Data Network (TOXNET), Pathogen Safety Data Sheets (biological hazards), and Poison Control centers.

OSHA's REQUIREMENT TO GLOVE FOR SPECIMEN COLLECTION

OSHA recommends all health care workers wear gloves during specimen collection due to the heightened risk of contact with the patient's blood during this procedure. Gloves should be changed between each patient. If the medical assistant does not change gloves between each patient, he or she runs the risk of contaminating patients with infectious body fluids. Remove the gloves after collection by turning them inside out from the wrist, not by pulling on the fingers. Wash hands after removing gloves. Hand hygiene should also be performed on the following occasions, at the very least:

- Before donning gloves
- Before and after washroom breaks and meals
- Before leaving the collection area
- Whenever gloves are punctured or torn
- Whenever gloves are soiled
- At the end of a shift

DISPOSAL OF BIOHAZARDOUS MATERIAL

Biohazardous material must be appropriately disposed of to protect staff and patients from possible infectious diseases. Wear a gown, gloves, and mask when handling all tissue. Post biohazard signs on walls and containers. Properly label all containers. Ventilate biohazardous areas very well and consult the Safety Officer regarding fume hoods and filters. Avoid using aerosols, especially for quick freezing tissue, because they increase the risk of exposure to infectious material. Dispose of all soft waste material in red or yellow biohazard bags, and disposable blades in red or yellow sharps containers. Disinfect non-disposable objects, such as tables. The CDC and EPA recommend steam sterilization and incineration for all waste except pathological waste, which only needs incineration. Dispose of blood in the sink with adequately running water. If the medical assistant or a co-worker is exposed to hazardous materials, start decontamination procedures immediately. Familiarize oneself with the written procedures in the policy and procedures manual (P&P). By law, P&Ps must be readily available to all staff, and the employer must train staff fully to use them.

Copyright © Mometrix Media. You have been licensed one copy of this document for personal use only. Any other reproduction or redistribution is strictly prohibited. All rights reserved. This content is provided for test preparation purposes only and does not imply an endorsement by Mometrix of any particular political, scientific, or religious point of view.

PROTOCOLS FOR EXPOSURE/CONTAMINATION VIA EYE SPLASH

Protocols for exposure/contamination from an eye splash should be made known to all staff. If any body fluids are sprayed or accidentally splashed into the eyes, the medical assistant must immediately flush the eyes with water for at least 20 minutes at an eye station if one is available or under a faucet. If possible, water should be lukewarm for comfort. It's important to leave contact lenses in for the initial flushing as they may provide some protection, but they should be removed at the end if they have not washed out. Avoid rubbing or bandaging the eyes. Report the splash and seek medical attention.

Copyright © Mometrix Media. You have been licensed one copy of this document for personal use only. Any other reproduction or redistribution is strictly prohibited. All rights reserved.
This content is provided for test preparation purposes only and does not imply an endorsement by Mometrix of any particular political, scientific, or religious point of view.

Emergency Preparedness and Management

TRIAGE

Triage refers to the dividing of casualties/emergencies into one of three groups: immediate, delayed, or non-transport. The triage officer commands, and should be the most qualified individual, regardless of rank and seniority.

Primary triage is conducted at the scene of the incident. The triage group sorts patients according to the severity of their injuries with a color-coding system:

- Red tag: first priority patient
- Yellow tag: second priority patient
- Green tag: delayed priority patient
- Black tag: the patient is deceased

Colored ribbon, tape, or labels are also appropriate.

Secondary triage is conducted in the treatment area to prioritize medical care and transportation to hospital. The treatment group arranges the medical care for patients after they have been triaged. The supply group obtains necessary resources and distributes these as needed. The transportation officer contacts the receiving hospital about the incoming casualties. The staging group directs incoming ambulances. The extrication group frees trapped patients. Minimal documentation is required for triage because treatment is top priority. Complete documentation after attending to the casualties.

START SYSTEM OF TRIAGING CASUALTIES

START is a triage system used at multi-casualty incidents. The acronym stands for **S**imple **T**riage **A**nd **R**apid **T**reatment. START assesses patients using three parameters: Respiration, perfusion, and mentation **(RPM)**. The assessment of a patient using START takes no more than 30 seconds. Patients are triaged using START according to:

- The patient's ability to walk away from the incident site
- Whether respiratory rate is under or over 30 respirations per minute
- Whether capillary refill is over or under 2 seconds and whether the patient has a radial pulse
- Whether the patient is able to follow basic commands

The medical assistant should ensure the safety of oneself, the safety of the general public, and the safety of the patient, in that order. Don appropriate personal protective equipment (PPE) before approaching a contaminated patient. Identifying a hazardous substance should not take precedence over the health and safety of the patient. Fire department officials or a Haz-Mat team are better able to identify the hazard. Medical assistants are not generally responsible for securing or controlling the scene of the emergency; that is a police function.

BEING SECONDED DURING A NATURAL DISASTER

When a natural disaster strikes a community, the **Multi-Agency Coordination System (MACS)** responds. EMS (police, fire department, and ambulance), Red Cross, and military search and rescue teams conduct rescue efforts. Healthcare facilities and community agencies, such as public health agencies, the CDC, and community care nurses, are second-line responders. Mass casualties require the assistance of private doctors and allied health personnel, so the medical assistant may be **seconded** to help away from their usual post. Public buildings such as schools, sports arenas, and

50

Copyright © Mometrix Media. You have been licensed one copy of this document for personal use only. Any other reproduction or redistribution is strictly prohibited. All rights reserved. This content is provided for test preparation purposes only and does not imply an endorsement by Mometrix of any particular political, scientific, or religious point of view.

churches are used as shelters. Extra medical supplies, food, clean water, and morgues are secured by deputies in case of looting. U.S. states and Canadian provinces follow the **Standardized Emergency Management System (SEMS)** for natural disaster preparedness, mitigation, response, and recovery. The facility's manager helps to set up the **Incident Command System (ICS)** for the healthcare facility. The Administrator On-Call liaises with community leaders and designates a spokesperson for the healthcare facility.

EMERGENCY PREPAREDNESS INFORMATION AND TRAINING

The CDC provides free tools for **emergency preparedness** at emergency.cdc.gov/preparedness/. The Safety Officer and facility's Incident Management System (IMS) must ensure that the facility has proper emergency training and equipment.

Medical assistants must recertify in CPR with the American Red Cross or the American Heart Association every two years at the Healthcare Provider Level. All staff must attend emergency preparedness training. This includes fire, natural disasters, severe weather, and CBRN (chemical, biological, radiation, and nuclear training against terrorism). The role of each person in the medical office during an emergency must be clearly identified in the job description. For example:

- The front desk receptionist phones EMS, notifies the doctor, directs traffic, and reschedules patients.
- The medical assistant obtains the crash cart, provides first aid, and assists the doctor with life support.
- The nurse administers drugs, first aid, and contacts the patient's next-of-kin and physician.
- The doctor leads two-person CPR and administers resuscitation drugs.

The medical assistant must rehearse and cross-train. Long-term inpatients and outpatients who are on the premises for extended periods (e.g., dialysis) and are capable of understanding and participating are required to have evacuation training.

Copyright © Mometrix Media. You have been licensed one copy of this document for personal use only. Any other reproduction or redistribution is strictly prohibited. All rights reserved. This content is provided for test preparation purposes only and does not imply an endorsement by Mometrix of any particular political, scientific, or religious point of view.

Quality Assurance and Office Safety

QA MANAGER AND SAFETY OFFICER

Every facility must comply with The Joint Commission's Standards Improvement Initiative to obtain accreditation. If a facility treats Medicare patients, then it must also comply with the federal Healthcare Quality Improvement Program (HCQIP), Quality Improvement Organization (QIO) projects, and Quality Improvement System for Managed Care (QISMC). The facility may want the prestige associated with the International Standards Organization (ISO) standard for quality management (9001:2015).

The **quality assurance (QA) manager** ensures that the facility follows best practices required by these standards. The QA manager uses tracer methodology to ensure the quality of patient care is excellent. Help the QA manager with data collection when asked.

The **safety officer** arranges for safety training at the employer's expense and informs the staff of pertinent changes OSHA makes. The safety officer checks waste disposal of radioactive, infectious, and chemically contaminated items. The safety officer devises a computerized error reporting system, focused on processes rather than individuals and punitive actions, and reviews errors to find trends and patterns. The safety officer establishes rapid response teams and investigates adverse incidents.

OSHA BULLETINS

The US Department of Labor's Occupational Health and Safety Administration has a website that provides important **bulletins** that medical assistants are required to adopt as part of their standards of practice. The safety officer must check the site regularly, notify staff of any pertinent changes, and arrange for training at the employer's expense. Medical assistants need to check the site themselves in the following circumstances:

- Whenever they need a refresher about established safe practices, such as bloodborne pathogens
- Whenever a serious new threat develops, like an influenza pandemic
- When equipment or supplies change in the laboratory to make sure the current best practices for infection control and hazardous chemicals cover the change
- When contemplating a grievance against an employer for allowing unsafe practices to verify the correct standards before registering a complaint

CREATING SAFE WORKPLACE ENVIRONMENTS

The medical assistant should take an active role in creating a safe workplace environment and preventing accidents:

- **Slips**: Most slips occur when the floor is wet or lacks adequate traction. Common causes include spills (water, urine, soap), oily substances (leaking oil), loose rugs and mats, and excessive floor waxing. Slips are especially a risk during wet weather as people may track water or snow in from outside. Floors should be checked and kept clean and dry.
- **Trips**: Most trips occur when the foot encounters obstacles (wrinkled rugs, cables, cords, clutter), view/walkway is obstructed, or lighting is poor. Traffic areas should be kept clear of clutter and lighting checked. Uneven steps should have warning signs.
- **Falls**: Many falls result from slipping or tripping, but some occur from a height, such as from a ladder or stairs. Patients who are unstable should always be assisted when walking and assisted at an appropriate pace.

52

Copyright © Mometrix Media. You have been licensed one copy of this document for personal use only. Any other reproduction or redistribution is strictly prohibited. All rights reserved. This content is provided for test preparation purposes only and does not imply an endorsement by Mometrix of any particular political, scientific, or religious point of view.

NEEDLE STICK INJURY

Most medical assistants perform phlebotomy (blood collection from a vein). Rarely does the phlebotomist contract bacterial, viral, or fungal infections, but it is possible. Keep immunizations up to date, particularly for Hepatitis B and tetanus, and follow OSHA bloodborne pathogens standards. If a **needle stick injury occurs,** follow these procedures:

1. Let the wound bleed freely.
2. Wash the wound immediately with povidone iodine.
3. Report the injury within 24 hours to the employer. The medical assistant is entitled to a confidential medical evaluation and follow up.
4. Fill out Workers' Compensation forms and keep copies.
5. If breastfeeding, stop until the doctor advises otherwise.
6. Request prophylactic Hepatitis B immune globulin (HBIG) to boost antibodies. This may help even if one's immunization did not include Hepatitis B.
7. Request disclosure of the disease status of the patient in contact with the sharp in question. If it is possible, the employer is legally obligated to determine whether the source was infected with hepatitis B or HIV. The medical assistant is also entitled to precautionary blood screening.
8. If the patient is HIV+, consider taking AZT and getting antibody tests at baseline, three months, and six months after exposure. There are health and insurance risks associated with this decision, so consult a doctor first.

REPORTING UNSAFE ACTIVITIES AND BEHAVIORS IN THE WORKPLACE

Each organization should have protocols in place for the **reporting of unsafe activities and behaviors**. In most cases, reports are made to the medical assistant's immediate supervisor. Unsafe activities and behaviors include:

- **Failure to follow standard procedures**: Taking shortcuts to save time often increases risk to staff and patients.
- **Lack of understanding/information**: Carrying out tasks without completely understanding what is expected or needed can result in doing the task incorrectly. Overconfidence can lead to attempting activities for which the person is not adequately trained.
- **Inadequate housekeeping**: Improper cleaning can lead to risk of falls (from clutter) and infection (from improper disinfection).
- **Noncompliance with safety protocols**: Ignoring safety rules (oxygen storage, smoke alarms) can put everyone at risk.
- **Distractions**: Emotional upset, pain, and illness can all increase risk of errors.
- **Inadequate planning**: Last minute assignments, constantly changing assignments and duties, and inadequate preparation all can lead to unsafe behaviors.

DISCLOSURE OF ERRORS IN PATIENT CARE

Each healthcare facility/office should have established protocols for **disclosure of errors in patient care**, and the medical assistant must always immediately report any error to a supervising nurse or physician so that steps can be taken to prevent further problems or injury to the patient involved. An incident report should be filled out to document the error, initiated by the person involved or closest to the patient when the incident occurred. The report should be detailed, listing the date, time, and exact sequence of events as well as any witnesses. The report should be reviewed by a supervisor. If the patient is aware of the error (such as when a medical assistant accidentally strikes a patient), the medical assistant should immediately apologize and ensure that the patient is examined by a nurse or physician. For more serious errors or those for which the patient may be unaware, risk management may have protocols in place that preclude discussing the error for liability reasons.

Copyright © Mometrix Media. You have been licensed one copy of this document for personal use only. Any other reproduction or redistribution is strictly prohibited. All rights reserved.
This content is provided for test preparation purposes only and does not imply an endorsement by Mometrix of any particular political, scientific, or religious point of view.

Medical Terminology

REFERENCE SOURCES FOR MEDICAL TERMINOLOGY

Reliable sources to check spelling, selection, and use of medical terminology include the following:

- **Abbreviations**: Use safe terms and definitions from The American Society for Testing and Materials' (ASTM). Obtain a list of dangerous abbreviations to be avoided from the Institute for Safe Medication Practices.
- **Style guides**: Provide guidelines for format and presentation in documents. Use the *American Medical Association Manual of Style: A Guide for Authors and Editors* for an overview.
- **Anatomy and physiology texts**: Contain essential information regarding body structure, function of body parts, disease processes, and common health disorders. *Grey's Anatomy* is one classic example.
- **Specialty texts**: Assist with specialty transcriptions. Try Sloan's *Medical Word Book*, Tessier's *Surgical Word Book*, and Pagana's *Laboratory and Diagnostic Tests*.
- **English dictionary**: Helps with spelling, definitions, and pronunciation. *Cambridge Dictionary of American English* is one example.

ORIGIN OF MEDICAL TERMINOLOGY USED IN THE U.S.

Most medical terms are derived from Greek or Latin. If the Greek or Latin word is broken into its root, prefix and suffix, unfamiliar terminology can be understood. To avoid awkward pronunciation when there is no vowel between the root word and suffix, add an "o" to the combining form. For instance, adding the suffix "metry" (meaning the measure of) to the root word for eye, "opt," creates the word "optometry".

There also are a few English-, French-, and German-originating medical terms:

- Examples of **English terminology** include: Epstein-Barr virus, HIV-positive, 100-mL sample, oxygen-dependent, or self-image. English words use a dash instead of a joining vowel.
- An example of **French terminology** is *grand mal* (the big sickness) for epileptic seizures (although they are now referred to as a generalized or tonic-clonic seizures).
- An example of **German terminology** is *mittelschmerz* (middle pain) for the discomfort of ovulation. French and German do not have convenient combining forms, so they must be memorized.

PREFIX, ROOT, AND SUFFIX

Medical terms have three parts:

- **Root** containing the basic meaning
- **Prefix** before the root that modifies the meaning
- **Suffix** after the root that modifies the meaning

Copyright © Mometrix Media. You have been licensed one copy of this document for personal use only. Any other reproduction or redistribution is strictly prohibited. All rights reserved.
This content is provided for test preparation purposes only and does not imply an endorsement by Mometrix of any particular political, scientific, or religious point of view.

Examples:

- Menorrhagia is excessive bleeding during menstruation and at irregular intervals. The prefix is meno-, meaning menstruation and the suffix is -rrhagia, meaning a flow that bursts forth.
- Rhinoplasty is a "nose job." The root is rhino, meaning nose. The suffix is -plasty, meaning reconstructive surgery.
- Antecubitum is the bend of the arm where blood is often drawn. The root is cubitum, meaning elbow. The prefix is ante-, meaning forward or before.

When confronted with an unfamiliar term, break it into its root, prefix, and suffix to understand its meaning.

COMMON PREFIXES

Common prefixes that the medical assistant must be familiar with include the following:

Prefix	Meaning	Example
Ab-	from, not here, off the norm	Abnormal
Ad-	toward, in the direction of	Adduct
Ante-	prior to, in front of, previously	Antecedent
Anti-	hostile to, against, contradictory	Antisocial
Be-	make, aligned with, greatly	Benign
Bi-	two, occurring twice	Bipolar
De-	away, versus, reduce	Deduct
Dia-	transverse, across	Diameter
Dis-	contradictory, disparate, away	Disjointed
En-	create, put in or on, surround	Engulf
Syn-	by means of, together, same	Synthesis
Trans-	across, far away, go through	Transvaginal
Ultra-	extreme, beyond in space	Ultrasound
Un-	opposing, antithetical, not	Uncooperative

COMMON SUFFIXES

Common suffixes that the medical assistant must be familiar with include the following:

Suffix	Meaning	Example
-fication/-ation	manner or process	classification
-gram	written down or illustrated	cardiogram
-graph	a machine or instrument that records data	cardiograph
-graphy	the process of recording of data	cardiography
-ics	science or skill of	synthetics
-itis	red, inflamed, swollen	bursitis
-meter	means of measure	thermometer
-metry	action of measuring	telemetry
-ology/-ogy	the study of	biology
-phore	bearer or maker	semaphore
-phobia	intense, irrational fear	arachnophobia
-scope	instrument used for visualizing data	microscope
-scopy	visualize or examine	bronchoscopy

Copyright © Mometrix Media. You have been licensed one copy of this document for personal use only. Any other reproduction or redistribution is strictly prohibited. All rights reserved. This content is provided for test preparation purposes only and does not imply an endorsement by Mometrix of any particular political, scientific, or religious point of view.

PLURALIZING MEDICAL TERMS

Most medical laboratory terms derive from Latin and Greek. Most Latinate terms originated from the Greek. The basic **rules for pluralizing medical terms** are as follows:

Rule	Examples
-a changes to -ata	Stigma to stigmata Condyloma to condylomata
-on changes to -a	Criterion to criteria Phenomenon to phenomena
-s changes to -des	Iris to irides Arthritis to arthritides
Feminine -a ending changes to -ae	Ulna to ulnae Concha to conchae
Masculine ending -us changes to -i	Radius to radii Musculus to musculi
Neutral ending -um changes to -a	Bacterium to bacteria Treponeum to Treponea
-osis changes to -oses	Diagnosis to diagnoses Anastomosis to anastomoses
-x changes to -ces or -ges	Phalanx to phalanges Varix to varices

STANDARDIZED TERMINOLOGY AND ABBREVIATIONS

Standardized terminology and abbreviations are vital for patient safety. Use abbreviations to save time and space only when there is no potential for confusion over the meaning of the message. Avoid Latin if there is an accepted English equivalency. The Medical Records manager decides acceptable terminology and forbidden abbreviations. If working in a small office and the medical assistant is in charge of Medical Records, use the list of safe terms from The American Society for Testing and Materials' (ASTM) and the list of dangerous abbreviations from the Institute for Safe Medication Practices (ISMP). The Joint Commission also has a "Do Not Use" List for medical abbreviations and symbols that are included on the ISMP's more comprehensive list. Post them throughout the office. Use one type of units only. For example, do not use SI units (International System of Measurement) for Lab and Imperial units for Pharmacy without listing equivalencies. Adopt the U.S. Postal Service database's two-letter abbreviations for states.

FORMS OF ABBREVIATIONS

Health professionals use abbreviations to save time when charting or to be discreet when speaking around a patient. Abbreviations take these forms:

- **Brief form** means shortening a common term or difficult to pronounce term (e.g., *telephone* into *phone* and *Papanicolaou smear* into *Pap smear*).
- **Acronym** means making a new word from the first letter of each word in a phrase, pronounced as a word (e.g., laser for light amplification by stimulated emission of radiation).
- **Initialism** means referring to a phrase by its initials, pronounced as a series of letters (e.g., MRI for magnetic resonance imaging or HIV for human immunodeficiency virus).
- **Eponym** means naming a test or sign for its discoverer (e.g., Coombs' test and McBurney's sign).

Copyright © Mometrix Media. You have been licensed one copy of this document for personal use only. Any other reproduction or redistribution is strictly prohibited. All rights reserved. This content is provided for test preparation purposes only and does not imply an endorsement by Mometrix of any particular political, scientific, or religious point of view.

COMMON ABBREVIATIONS FOUND IN DOCTOR'S NOTES

Common abbreviations found in doctor's notes include the following:

Term	Meaning
a.d.	right ear, auris dextra*
a.s.	left ear, auris sinistra*
a.u.	both ears, auris utraque*
o.d.	right eye, oculus dexter* [NOTE: Do not confuse with OD (once daily)]
o.s.	left eye, oculus sinister*
o.u.	both eyes, oculus uterque*
a.c.	before meals
p.c.	after meals
h.s.	hour of sleep, bedtime
ad lib	freely or whenever desired
p.r.n.	as needed
q.4h.	every four hours
q.d. or OD	once daily* [NOTE: Do not confuse with o.d. (right eye)]
b.i.d.	twice a day
t.i.d	three times a day
q.i.d.	four times a day*

*These terms are on ISMP's list of error prone abbreviations.

USE OF MEDICAL SLANG

Medical staff should not write slang terms in written reports because they may:

- Be vague and not give the precise meaning required in a subpoenable medical document
- Make the report seem condescending or disparaging to the patient, portraying the author as prejudiced, offensive, or unprofessional
- Leave the report open to interpretation, which could be used against the author in a court of law

58

Copyright © Mometrix Media. You have been licensed one copy of this document for personal use only. Any other reproduction or redistribution is strictly prohibited. All rights reserved. This content is provided for test preparation purposes only and does not imply an endorsement by Mometrix of any particular political, scientific, or religious point of view.

Brief forms are contractions of words that can be found in a medical dictionary, which have been accepted and recognized as suitable for court documents through common usage. They include exam, lab, Pap smear, and prepped. The following jargon can be safely used when talking privately with medical colleagues:

- Appy: Appendectomy
- BP: Blood pressure
- Cath: Catheter (generally referring to urinary catheters)
- Chem: Blood test (CBC)
- Coag: Blood test (coagulation profile)
- D/C: Dilation and curettage
- Dig: Digoxin
- Echo: Echocardiogram
- Lytes: Electrolytes
- Meds: Medications
- Nitro: Nitroglycerin
- Peds: Pediatrics
- ROMI: Rule-out myocardial infarction
- Script: Prescription
- Temp: Temperature
- tib-fib: Tibia fibula (generally relating to a fracture)
- Trach: Tracheostomy
- URI: Upper respiratory infection
- UTI: Urinary tract infection
- V-tach or V-fib: Ventricular tachycardia or ventricular fibrillation

The rule for charting is: "When in doubt, write it out."

NAMING OF COMMON MEDICAL AND SURGICAL SPECIALTIES

The suffix -ology means "the study of" and the suffix –iatrics means "medical treatment." Add the body system root to obtain the name of the **specialty**:

- Anesthesiology: Study of pain relief
- Bariatrics: Treatment of obesity
- Cardiology: Study of the heart
- Dermatology: Study of the skin
- Endocrinology: Study of the hormone system
- Gastroenterology: Study of the digestive system
- Geriatrics: Treatment of the elderly
- Hematology: Study of the blood
- Neurology: Study of the nervous system
- Obstetrics: Treatment of pregnant women
- Pediatrics: Treatment of children
- Psychiatry: Treatment of the mind
- Radiology: Study of radiation (for medical imaging)
- Rheumatology: Study of rheumatoid diseases, like arthritis
- Toxicology: Study of poisons
- Urology: Study of the urinary system

Copyright © Mometrix Media. You have been licensed one copy of this document for personal use only. Any other reproduction or redistribution is strictly prohibited. All rights reserved.
This content is provided for test preparation purposes only and does not imply an endorsement by Mometrix of any particular political, scientific, or religious point of view.

COMMON SURGICAL PROCEDURES

Common surgical procedures that the medical assistant should be familiar with include the following:

Appendectomy	Removal of the vermiform appendix
Breast Biopsy	Removal of suspicious tissue to detect cancer
Cesarean Section	Birth through the mother's abdomen
Cholecystectomy	Gall bladder removal
Coronary Artery Bypass Graft	CABG grafts a vessel from the aorta to the coronary artery to relieve angina or blockage
Debridement	Removal of foreign matter and dead or damaged skin from a wound
Free Skin Graft	Detach skin from one body part to repair another
Hemorrhoidectomy	Removal of swollen veins in the anus
Hysterectomy	Removal of the uterus
Inguinal Hernia Repair	Pulling a loop of bowel that protrudes through the groin back into place
Mastectomy	Removal of the breast
Partial Colectomy	Removal of part of the large intestine
Prostatectomy	Removal of the prostate gland
Release of Peritoneal Adhesions	Removal of the peritoneum membrane from abdominal organs to which it is sticking
Tonsillectomy	Removal of lymphatic tissue at the back of the throat

ANATOMICAL POSITION

The anatomical position is the medical standard used when describing the orientation and location of the parts of the human body. A patient in the anatomical position stands with the feet facing to the front. The hips and shoulders are square and level. The feet are placed slightly apart. The arms are held straight at the sides of the body with the palms of the hands facing forward. The little fingers are therefore nearest the body, and the thumbs point away from the body. The arms do not touch the trunk but are held close to it. The head faces forward, as do the eyes.

ABDOMINAL QUADRANTS

The four abdominal quadrants are:

- Right Upper Quadrant (**RUQ**)
- Left Upper Quadrant (**LUQ**)
- Right Lower Quadrant (**RLQ**)
- Left Lower Quadrant (**LLQ**)

Copyright © Mometrix Media. You have been licensed one copy of this document for personal use only. Any other reproduction or redistribution is strictly prohibited. All rights reserved.
This content is provided for test preparation purposes only and does not imply an endorsement by Mometrix of any particular political, scientific, or religious point of view.

BODY PLANES

The six body planes are:

- **Transverse plane** divides the patient's body into imaginary upper (superior) and lower (inferior or caudal) halves.
- **Sagittal plane** divides the body, or any body part, vertically into right and left sections. The sagittal plane runs parallel to the midline of the body.
- Equal halves are the **midsagittal plane.**
- **Median plane** divides the body into right and left halves. The median plane runs vertically through the midline of the body, or any body structure. The median plane is a type of sagittal plane.
- **Coronal plane** divides the body, or any body structure, into front and back (anterior and posterior sections). The coronal plane runs vertically through the body at right angles to the midline. The coronal plane is also called anterior or frontal plane.
- **Posterior plane** is the back, also called dorsal or ventral.

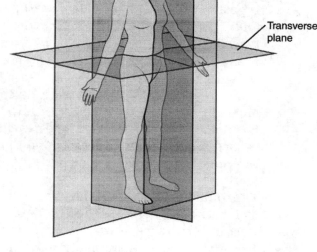

BODY TISSUE

The four major types of body tissue are:

- **Connective tissue** (e.g., bones, tendons, and ligaments) joins and protects the organs and keeps them in their proper position.
- **Muscle tissue** contracts and expands to allow movement and pump blood, lymph, and other fluids.
- **Nerve tissue** transmits messages from the brain and spinal cord to all of the peripheral parts of the body.
- **Epithelial tissue**, the most common type of tissue, is the skin (integument) covering the body and the lining inside organs and tracts.

Body tissue is 55-78% water, depending on the patient's age and sex. Infants contain the most water. Adult women contain the least. If tissue has too little water, the patient is dehydrated. If tissue is oversaturated with water, the patient has edema (swelling).

Copyright © Mometrix Media. You have been licensed one copy of this document for personal use only. Any other reproduction or redistribution is strictly prohibited. All rights reserved. This content is provided for test preparation purposes only and does not imply an endorsement by Mometrix of any particular political, scientific, or religious point of view.

Anatomy and Physiology

BODY SYSTEMS

Functions of the human body can be divided into the following body systems:

- **Cardiovascular**: Pumps blood throughout the body via the heart and blood vessels
- **Digestive**: Transforms food into energy and eliminates solid waste
- **Endocrine**: Releases hormones into the bloodstream to control metabolism, growth, and reproduction
- **Immune**: Defends against all foreign substances
- **Integumentary**: Skin prevents moisture loss, regulates temperature, protects from sunburn, and senses pain, pressure, touch, hot and cold
- **Musculoskeletal**: Skeletal muscles move the body, smooth muscles control the physical functioning of internal organs, and cardiac muscle pumps blood. The skeleton supports and shapes, protects internal organs, stores minerals, and produces blood cells
- **Nervous**: Controls movement, memory, and senses and communicates with the outside world
- **Reproductive**: Allows continuation of the human species through reproduction and childbearing and differentiates the sexes
- **Respiratory**: Regulates gas exchange (oxygen intake and carbon dioxide expulsion)
- **Urinary**: Removes waste and toxins from the blood and expels them from the body through urine

CARDIOVASCULAR SYSTEM

The cardiovascular system controls blood flow throughout the body and to the tissues, controls gas exchange (carbon dioxide and oxygen) by transporting oxygenated blood from the lungs, serves as a reservoir for blood, maintains blood pH through a buffer system, responds to infections, and facilitates coagulation (blood clotting). The cardiovascular system has the following components:

- **Heart**: The heart has four chambers, two upper (right atrium, left atrium) and two lower (right ventricle and left ventricle). The heart muscle receives blood from four major coronary arteries (right, left main, left anterior descending, and left circumflex) and their branches, and then distributes blood via the aorta and pulmonary arteries.
- **Vessels**: The venous system includes veins, venules, and venous capillaries and returns blood back to the heart via the inferior and superior vena cava. The arterial system, (including the coronary arteries) branches from the aorta after it leaves the heart and includes arteries, arterioles, and arterial capillaries.
- **Blood**: Blood consists of red blood cells (erythrocytes), white blood cells (leukocytes including monocytes, lymphocytes, basophils, neutrophils, and eosinophils), platelets (thrombocytes), and plasma, the liquid portion of the blood (which contains clotting factors). Blood carries oxygen from the lungs and distributes it to the rest of the body.

The cardiovascular system is responsible for oxygenation of cells, perfusion (carrying of blood with oxygen, glucose, and nutrients to cells) and removing waste products, such as carbon dioxide.

> **Review Video: Circulatory System**
> Visit mometrix.com/academy and enter code: 376581

Copyright © Mometrix Media. You have been licensed one copy of this document for personal use only. Any other reproduction or redistribution is strictly prohibited. All rights reserved. This content is provided for test preparation purposes only and does not imply an endorsement by Mometrix of any particular political, scientific, or religious point of view.

ANATOMY OF THE HEART

The human heart is about the size of a fist and weighs 7–15 ounces. It is located in the middle of the chest, behind the sternum, and leans slightly left. The heart is covered by a double-layered membrane called the **pericardium**. The outer layer, called the parietal pericardium, is fibrous and surrounds the roots of the major blood vessels of the heart. The inner layer, called the visceral pericardium, is attached to and covers the heart muscle. The two layers of membrane are separated by fluid. The heart itself has **four connecting chambers**. The two upper chambers are the **right atria and left atria**; the lower chambers are the **left ventricle and right ventricle**. The left and right atria and the left and right ventricle are separated by a muscular structure called the septum.

Review Video: <u>Heart Anatomy and Physiology</u>
Visit mometrix.com/academy and enter code: 569724

HEART'S CONDUCTION SYSTEM

The **sinoatrial node (SA)** is referred to as the pacemaker of the heart because electrical impulses normally originate in the SA, within the wall of the right atrium. The SA produces electrical impulses that are transmitted to the **atrioventricular node (AV)** by specialized conducting tissue. The AV node is found between the atria and ventricles. From here, the electrical impulse is relayed down the conducting tissue called the Bundle of His. The **Bundle of His** splits into a right bundle branch (RBB) and a left bundle branch (LBB), which serve the right and left ventricles, respectively, through both sides of the intraventricular septum. The bundle branches then split to form the **Purkinje fibers**, which transmit electrical impulses to the myocardium.

Review Video: <u>Electrical Conduction System of the Heart</u>
Visit mometrix.com/academy and enter code: 624557

A **normal sinus rhythm** on an EKG (the expected result in a healthy individual) denotes that the electrical impulses start in the sinoatrial node (SA) first. The intrinsic rate of the SA node is 60–100

Copyright © Mometrix Media. You have been licensed one copy of this document for personal use only. Any other reproduction or redistribution is strictly prohibited. All rights reserved.
This content is provided for test preparation purposes only and does not imply an endorsement by Mometrix of any particular political, scientific, or religious point of view.

beats per minute (bpm), which reflects the normal range for an adult's pulse rate. If the SA node does not initiate the electrical impulse, the atrioventricular node (AV) can do so. However, the AV node is not as capable of increasing the heart rate, with an intrinsic rate of only 40-60 beats per minute. The patient may require a pacemaker to address the slow heart rate. All of the cells of the heart are capable of generating the electrical impulses necessary to trigger a heartbeat (automaticity). Signal conduction problems (block) can occur at any site along the conduction pathway, causing alterations in the normal rhythm (arrhythmia).

HEART VALVES AND BLOOD FLOW

Four heart valves regulate the flow of blood through the heart.

- The **tricuspid valve** controls the flow of deoxygenated blood from the right atrium to the right ventricle.
- The **pulmonary semilunar valve** controls the flow of blood from the right ventricle to the pulmonary artery. The pulmonary artery carries the blood into the lungs where it is oxygenated.
- The blood then flows through the pulmonary vein back to the heart, and the **mitral valve** controls the flow of the now oxygenated blood from the left atrium to the left ventricle.
- The **aortic semilunar valve** regulates blood flow from the left ventricle to the aorta. From the aorta, the oxygenated blood is conducted to the rest of the body. The deoxygenated blood travels through the venules, then the veins, and then the inferior vena cava and superior vena cava back to the right atrium.

Review Video: <u>Heart Blood Flow</u>
Visit mometrix.com/academy and enter code: 783139

Copyright © Mometrix Media. You have been licensed one copy of this document for personal use only. Any other reproduction or redistribution is strictly prohibited. All rights reserved.
This content is provided for test preparation purposes only and does not imply an endorsement by Mometrix of any particular political, scientific, or religious point of view.

CARDIOVASCULAR DISORDERS

Cardiovascular disorders include the following:

- **Atherosclerosis**: Atherosclerosis is characterized by fatty deposits that build up inside of arteries, resulting in decreased blood flow because of narrowing and stiffening of the arteries, which in turn leads to high blood pressure and increased risk of thrombi (blood clots) and emboli (moving clots).
- **Edema**: Edema is swelling from fluid retention. Edema may occur because of heart failure (weakness of the heart muscle) that causes fluid to build up in the legs and feet and/or in the lungs (causing shortness of breath). Edema (often involving the whole body) may also occur with kidney disease and severe allergic (anaphylactic) reaction.
- **Thrombophlebitis**: Thrombophlebitis is inflammation of a vein that occurs as the result of a thrombus (blood clot) forming in the vein. The vein appears red, swollen, and tender and is at increased risk of spreading emboli to other areas of the body, such as the brain (stroke) and heart (heart attack).
- **Heart failure**: Heart failure is cardiac disease that includes disorders of contractions (systolic dysfunction) or filling (diastolic dysfunction) or both and may include pulmonary, peripheral, or systemic edema. The most common causes are coronary artery disease, systemic or pulmonary hypertension, cardiomyopathy, and valvular disorders. The incidence of chronic heart failure correlates with age. Heart failure progresses through Class I to Class IV, involving congestion in the lungs, limitations of activity, and discomfort. Uncontrolled heart failure leads to death.
- **Myocardial infarction with ST-elevation (STEMI)**: STEMI is the more severe type of MI that involves complete blockage of one or more coronary arteries with myocardial damage, resulting in ST elevation on the EKG. Symptoms are those of an acute MI (crushing pain substernally, radiating down the left arm or both arms, though less obvious in women and the elderly). As necrosis occurs, Q waves often develop, indicating irreversible myocardial damage, which may result in death, so treatment involves immediate reperfusion before necrosis can occur.

Review Video: Myocardial Infarction
Visit mometrix.com/academy and enter code: 148923

Copyright © Mometrix Media. You have been licensed one copy of this document for personal use only. Any other reproduction or redistribution is strictly prohibited. All rights reserved. This content is provided for test preparation purposes only and does not imply an endorsement by Mometrix of any particular political, scientific, or religious point of view.

ENDOCRINE SYSTEM

The major glands that comprise the endocrine system, the hormones they secrete, and diseases resulting from their dysfunction include the following:

Gland	Hormones	Disease
Adrenal Cortex	Aldosterone Cortisol Androgens	Addison's Disease Cushing's Disease
Adrenal Medulla	Epinephrine Norepinephrine	Anxiety Attacks Depression
Anterior Pituitary	Adrenocorticotropic hormone (ACTH) Follicle-stimulating hormone (FSH) Gonadotropic hormones Growth hormone (GH) Luteinizing hormone (LH) Prolactin Thyroid Stimulating Hormone (TSH)	Dwarfism Gigantism
Hypothalamus/ Posterior Pituitary	Inhibiting hormones (stop the release of other hormones) Antidiuretic hormone (ADH) Oxytocin Releasing hormones (trigger the release of other hormones)	Diabetes Insipidus
Kidneys	Calcitriol Erythropoietin	Hypertension
Ovaries	Estrogen Progesterone	Endometriosis Menometrorrhagia
Pancreas	Insulin Glucagon	Diabetes Mellitus
Parathyroid	Parathyroid hormone	Tetany Renal calculi
Pineal	Melatonin	Alzheimer's Disease
Testes	Testosterone	Gynecomastia Klinefelter Syndrome
Thymus	Thymic factor (TF) Thymosin Thymic humoral factor (THF) Thymopoietin	DiGeorge Syndrome
Thyroid	Calcitonin Thyroxine (T4) Triiodothyronine (T3)	Cretinism Hypo/Hyperthyroidism Goiter Myxedema
Digestive tract	Gastrin Cholecystokinin Secretin Ghrelin Motilin	Gastritis Gastroesophageal reflux

Copyright © Mometrix Media. You have been licensed one copy of this document for personal use only. Any other reproduction or redistribution is strictly prohibited. All rights reserved.
This content is provided for test preparation purposes only and does not imply an endorsement by Mometrix of any particular political, scientific, or religious point of view.

MAJOR ENDOCRINE GLANDS

MALE   FEMALE

PITUITARY GLAND — ... — PINEAL GLAND

THYROID GLAND —

THYMUS

ADRENAL GLANDS —

PANCREAS

OVARY

TESTIS

> **Review Video: Endocrine System**
> Visit mometrix.com/academy and enter code: 678939

GASTROINTESTINAL SYSTEM
DIGESTIVE TRACT

The gastrointestinal tract (GI tract) is divided into upper and lower sections:

- The **upper GI tract** consists of the mouth (buccal mucosa, tongue, and teeth), pharynx, esophagus, and stomach.
- The **lower GI tract** is comprised of the small intestine (duodenum, jejunum, ileum, and ileocecal valve) and the large intestine (ascending, transverse, and descending colon, sigmoid flexure, rectum, and anus).

The vermiform appendix is attached to the cecum, the first section of the ascending colon, closest to the ileocecal valve. The sigmoid flexure leads into the rectum, which terminates in the anus. An internal and external sphincter control the anus. The liver, gall bladder, and pancreas secrete digestive enzymes into the GI tract through various ducts that aide in the breaking down of food and absorption of nutrients.

67

Copyright © Mometrix Media. You have been licensed one copy of this document for personal use only. Any other reproduction or redistribution is strictly prohibited. All rights reserved. This content is provided for test preparation purposes only and does not imply an endorsement by Mometrix of any particular political, scientific, or religious point of view.

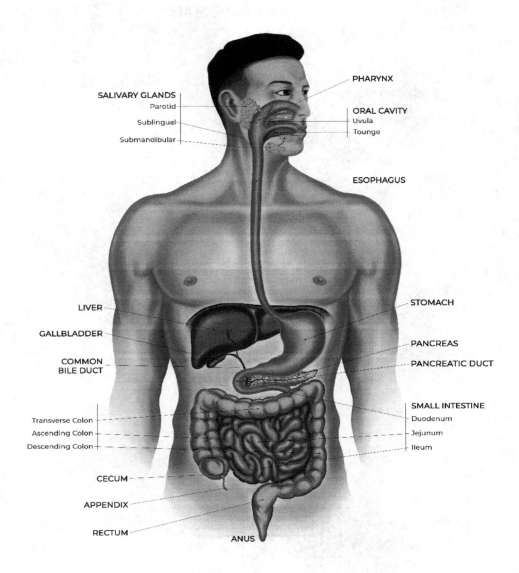

Review Video: <u>Gastrointestinal System</u>
Visit mometrix.com/academy and enter code: 378740

FUNCTIONS

The gastrointestinal tract is a system of organs responsible for the:

- Ingestion of food
- Digestion of food
- Absorption of nutrients and medications
- Production of Vitamins B_{12} and K
- Elimination of waste products

The process begins at the mouth with ingestion and ends at the anus with excretion. The GI tract breaks down and reabsorbs nutrients using ptyalin in the mouth, hydrochloric acid in the stomach,

68

Copyright © Mometrix Media. You have been licensed one copy of this document for personal use only. Any other reproduction or redistribution is strictly prohibited. All rights reserved.
This content is provided for test preparation purposes only and does not imply an endorsement by Mometrix of any particular political, scientific, or religious point of view.

bile from the gall bladder, and insulin, glucagon, amylase, lipase, and other chemicals from the pancreas. Food is digested into slurry in the stomach, where B_{12} is manufactured to prevent anemia. The small intestine absorbs nutrients. The large intestine (colon) reabsorbs water and salts and turns semi-liquid waste matter into firm, formed stools. Bacteria, normally found in the large intestine, produce Vitamin K, necessary for blood clotting. Fecal waste matter is held temporarily in the rectum and expelled by the anus.

ACCESSORY ORGANS OF DIGESTION

The accessory organs of digestion include the liver, the gallbladder, and the pancreas. The liver produces bile as a by-product of breaking down old red blood cells. The liver excretes bile into the small intestine to break up fatty foods by way of the biliary system. The gallbladder's only function is to store and concentrate bile, so if painful stones form in it, the gallbladder can be safely removed. The pancreas secretes hormones and excretes digestive enzymes, so it is both an endocrine and an exocrine gland. As an exocrine gland, the pancreas releases an isosmotic fluid into the small intestine containing the enzymes trypsin, chymotrypsin, lipase, pancreatic amylase, deoxyribonuclease, and ribonuclease. These enzymes break down proteins, fats, and starches. The pancreatic duct makes bicarbonate to decrease the acidity of the food slurry (chyle and chyme). As an endocrine gland, the pancreas regulates blood sugar with the hormone insulin, and the pancreas and liver regulate blood sugar with glucagon. The liver also metabolizes most drugs.

PASSAGE OF FOOD

The main parts of the digestive system in order of how food passes through them are as follows:

1. Digestion starts in the **mouth** with the action of saliva containing amylase to start starch digestion. The mouth also contains the hard and the soft palates.
2. The 20 primary or 32 permanent **teeth** are used for mastication of food.
3. The **tongue** holds the taste buds and moves the food towards the esophagus.
4. The **pharynx** connects the mouth to the esophagus. The **epiglottis** keeps food from entering the trachea. The pharynx is about 5" long.
5. The **esophagus** is a 12" tube leading to the stomach. Peristaltic waves start here and move food into the stomach.
6. The **stomach** sac is controlled by the lower esophageal sphincter (at the top) and the pyloric sphincter (at the bottom). Food mixes with hydrochloric acid in the stomach to make chyme. Food stays in the stomach for 2–4 hours.
7. The **small intestine** contains the duodenum (10"), jejunum (8'), and ileum (12'). The majority of digestion takes place in the duodenum. The small intestine receives bile, produced by the liver and stored in the gall bladder, to digest fats, and amylase and insulin from the pancreas to break down starches and sugars. Digestion in the small intestine can take between 3 and 10 hours.
8. The **large intestine** absorbs water and salts. The large intestine consists of the cecum (with vermiform appendix), ascending, transverse, descending, and sigmoid colon, the rectum, and anus for defecation. The ileocecal valve prevents food from reentering the small intestine.

Total digestion can take between 24 hours and 3 days.

Copyright © Mometrix Media. You have been licensed one copy of this document for personal use only. Any other reproduction or redistribution is strictly prohibited. All rights reserved. This content is provided for test preparation purposes only and does not imply an endorsement by Mometrix of any particular political, scientific, or religious point of view.

HEMATOLOGIC SYSTEM

COMPONENTS

Blood is the liquid that moves through the circulatory system. The average adult has about 5 liters of blood. Bone marrow produces red blood cells (RBC or erythrocytes), white blood cells (WBC or leukocytes), and platelets (thrombocytes).

- **Red blood cells** transport oxygen and carbon dioxide, **white blood cells** fight infection, and **platelets** clot blood after an injury. These blood cells travel through the circulatory system suspended in plasma: 55% of blood is yellow, liquid plasma, and 45% is cells. **Blood plasma** carries nutrients, proteins, hormones, and waste products.
- White blood cells that absorb Wright stain are classified as **granulocytes**, because there are granules in the cytoplasm, and agranulocytes, with no granules present. There are three different kinds of granulocytes: neutrophils, basophils, and eosinophils. The **agranulocytes** include lymphocytes (T and B cells) and monocytes. Each type of WBC proliferates to combat a different type of pathogen. For example, increased eosinophils (eosinophilia) can indicate allergies, whereas increased monocytes (monocytosis) can indicate tuberculosis (TB).

RED BLOOD CELLS

A red blood cell **(erythrocyte, RBC)** is a doughnut-shaped raft that transports oxygen to cells through hemoglobin. The RBC offloads its oxygen, takes on carbon dioxide from the cells, and changes color, turning a bluish-purple. The RBC then returns to the lungs, where it takes on oxygen again during gas exchange. Red blood cells typically have a life span of 120 days and require the nutrients iron, protein, B_{12}, and folate. If a patient has too few erythrocytes from heavy bleeding or lacks the nutrients, then he or she is considered anemic.

PLATELETS

Platelets **(thrombocytes)** clot the blood when a vessel is damaged by converging on the area to seal the leak. Platelets have a life span of nine days and work in conjunction with clotting factors in the blood, the proteins that work with platelets to produce a clot. If a patient lacks a clotting factor, then the platelets alone are unable to seal an injury adequately. This occurs in hemophiliacs, who lack Factor VIII. This disease and others that lead to decreased platelets put individuals at high risk for bleeding. Bone marrow produces red blood cells and platelets daily to replace dead or lost circulating cells.

IMMUNE SYSTEM

The immune system is the body's main defender against disease. The immune system is comprised of the spleen, thymus, bone marrow, and a series of transparent tubes that run throughout the body, parallel to the blood vessels. The tubes are lymph vessels, and carry 4 liters of clear lymphatic fluid, or lymph. Lymph circulates throughout the body in the same manner as blood, with valves opening and closing to move the liquid along. There are hundreds of small glands, called lymph nodes, stationed at intervals along the lymphatic vessels. The lymphatic fluid carries invaders to the nodes to be destroyed by lymphocytes, a type of white blood cell. Antibodies are also found in lymphatic fluid. Nodes swell during infections. Plasma from the blood vessels seeps out of the capillaries, immerses body tissues, and then drains off into the lymph vessels. Once in the lymphatic system, the plasma is called lymph. Lymph travels through the lymphatic vessels until it reaches the thoracic duct, the largest lymph vessel, extending from L2 to the neck. The lymph drains from the

Copyright © Mometrix Media. You have been licensed one copy of this document for personal use only. Any other reproduction or redistribution is strictly prohibited. All rights reserved. This content is provided for test preparation purposes only and does not imply an endorsement by Mometrix of any particular political, scientific, or religious point of view.

thoracic duct into the blood and is then carried to the kidneys and liver by the cardiovascular system where the waste is removed.

Review Video: Immune System
Visit mometrix.com/academy and enter code: 622899

THE COMPLEMENT SYSTEM

The complement system consists of proteins produced by the liver that work with an individual's antibodies to clear the body of pathogens. Complement proteins are a part of the immune system that burst (lyze) pathogens and alert the phagocytes that the dead pathogen must be removed. If the patient is hypersensitive, the complement system may work against its own body. An exaggerated inflammatory response may occur, called a cytokine storm. Young people are most prone to cytokine storm if they have pandemic influenza, rheumatoid arthritis, sepsis, bronchitis, bird flu, or pneumonia. Complications from the COVID-19 pandemic also included the overreaction of the immune system, leading to excessive fluid accumulation in the lungs and excessive clotting. In a cytokine storm, the complement system calls too many immune cells to defend the site of infection, which can cause the blockage of small arteries with clumped white cells (aggregate). The inflammatory response may be so extreme that gangrene develops in the fingers and toes or the patient dies from the cytokine storm.

WHITE BLOOD CELLS

The white blood cells of the immune system include the following:

WBC	Type	% of WBCs	Causes of Increase	Causes of Decrease
Basophils (black or purple)	Granulocyte	1%	Asthma, chronic myelocytic leukemia, Crohn's disease, dermatitis, estrogen, hemolytic anemia, Hodgkin's disease, hypothyroidism, polycythemia vera, and viruses	Allergies, corticosteroids, hyperthyroidism, pregnancy, and stress.
Eosinophils (orange-red, double-lobed nucleus)	Granulocyte	1-3%	Allergy, asthma, or parasitic infestation	Cushing's disease or glucocorticoids use
Lymphocytes (dark, large nucleus surrounded by thin cytoplasm rim)	Agranulocyte	15-40%	Antigens or chronic irritation	AIDS
Monocytes (lavender)	Agranulocyte	2-8%	Myeloproliferative process, like an inflammatory response or chronic myelomonocytic leukemia (CMML)	Hairy cell leukemia
Neutrophils (pink cytoplasm, dark nucleus)	Granulocyte	50-70%	Burns, kidney failure, heart attack, cancer, hemolytic anemia	Leukemia and abscess

Copyright © Mometrix Media. You have been licensed one copy of this document for personal use only. Any other reproduction or redistribution is strictly prohibited. All rights reserved.
This content is provided for test preparation purposes only and does not imply an endorsement by Mometrix of any particular political, scientific, or religious point of view.

Lymphocytes make proteins for immunoglobulins and cytokine production. Small B and T cells secrete antibodies and regulate the immune system. Large Natural Killer cells lyze tumors and virus-infected cells. Children, aged four months to four years, normally have inverted differential (relative neutropenia and increased lymphocytes). **Neutrophils** are phagocytic. A segmented nucleus (seg) indicates a mature cell. A banded nucleus (band) indicates an immature cell.

INTEGUMENTARY SYSTEM

The largest organ of the body is the skin, which forms the **integumentary system**, along with cutaneous glands, hair, and nails. It has three layers: epidermis, dermis, and hypodermis (subcutaneous or superficial fascia). The functions of the integumentary system are to:

- Excrete salts and nitrogenous wastes
- Metabolize vitamin D
- Prevent bacteria, parasites, and other invaders from entering the body
- Protect the body from chemicals
- Produce melanin as sunscreen
- Protect the body from water loss
- Regulate body temperature through perspiration, fat storage, and radiating heat from capillaries
- Serve as a sensory communication tool through temperature, touch, pain, and pressure receptors

Skin can be damaged by chemicals, sharp or blunt instruments, heat, friction, pressure and radiation. Among the injuries that can happen to the skin are abrasions, burns, contusions, crushing injuries, decubitus ulcers (bedsores), gunshots, hematomas, incisions, lacerations, and punctures.

STRATUM CORNEUM
STRATUM LUCIDUM
STRATUM GRANULOSUM
STRATUM SPINOSUM
STRATUM BASALE
BASEMENT MEMBRANE
DERMIS

Review Video: Integumentary System
Visit mometrix.com/academy and enter code: 655980

Copyright © Mometrix Media. You have been licensed one copy of this document for personal use only. Any other reproduction or redistribution is strictly prohibited. All rights reserved.
This content is provided for test preparation purposes only and does not imply an endorsement by Mometrix of any particular political, scientific, or religious point of view.

MUSCULOSKELETAL SYSTEM
BONES AND JOINTS

The bones of the musculoskeletal system include the following:

- **Head**: The cranium includes frontal (forehead), parietal (back), temporal (side), mandibular (lower jaw), maxillary (upper jaw), nasal conchae and septum (nose), and zygomatic (cheek) bones; the ear includes the malleus (hammer), incus (anvil) and stapes (stirrup) bones.
- **Spine**: Comprised of seven cervical (neck), 12 thoracic (upper back), and five lumbar (lower back) vertebrae, the sacrum, and the coccyx (tail bone).

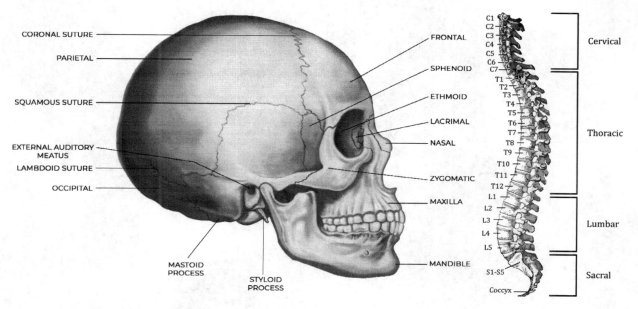

- **Chest**: Ribs, scapula (shoulder blade), and clavicle (collar bone).
- **Pelvis**: Ilium (upper), ischium (lower), and pubis (front).
- **Arms**: Humerus (upper), radius and ulna (forearm), carpals (wrist), metacarpals (hand), and phalanges (fingers).
- **Legs**: Femur (thigh), patella (knee), tibia and fibula (calf), tarsals (ankle), metatarsals (front foot), calcaneus (heel), and phalanges (toes).
- **Diarthrotic articulations**: Moveable joints with synovial fluid and cartilage cushions that are held together by ligaments, like the limbs.
- **Synarthrotic articulations**: Immovable joints, such as the spine and skull.

Copyright © Mometrix Media. You have been licensed one copy of this document for personal use only. Any other reproduction or redistribution is strictly prohibited. All rights reserved. This content is provided for test preparation purposes only and does not imply an endorsement by Mometrix of any particular political, scientific, or religious point of view.

SKULL

CLAVICLE

SCAPULA (SHOULDER BLADE)

STERNUM

HUMERUS

RIBS

VERTEBRAE

PELVIS

ULNA

RADIUS

PHALANGES (FINGERS)

FEMUR

PATELLA

TIBIA

FIBULA

CALCANEUS (HEEL)

PHALANGES (TOES)

Review Video: Skeletal System
Visit mometrix.com/academy and enter code: 256447

74

Copyright © Mometrix Media. You have been licensed one copy of this document for personal use only. Any other reproduction or redistribution is strictly prohibited. All rights reserved.
This content is provided for test preparation purposes only and does not imply an endorsement by Mometrix of any particular political, scientific, or religious point of view.

CARTILAGE AND LIGAMENTS

Cartilage is a dense connective tissue composed of collagen and/or elastin fibers on the end of bones, which provides a smooth surface for articulation by reducing friction.

- **Hyaline cartilage** contains chondrocytes that make it look glassy and is found in the nose, larynx, trachea, ribs, and sternum. Hyaline cartilage makes an embryo's skeleton.
- **Elastic cartilage** contains elastin, which makes it yellow, and is found in the outer ear (pinna) and epiglottis.
- **Fibrocartilage** is composed of strands of fibers that function to help limit movement and prevent bones from rubbing together. Fibrocartilage is found in the knee, the pubic bones in the pelvic region and between the vertebrae in the spine.

A **ligament** is a fibrous band composed of connective tissue stretching from one bone to another in a joint to provide lateral stability. Ligaments also connect cartilages and other structures. Injuries to ligaments are sprains, which are slow to heal and may require physiotherapy and surgery.

TENDONS

A tendon is also called a **sinew**, and connects muscle to bone. Tendons grow into the bone and make mineralized connections with the bone. Tendons transform muscle contraction into joint movement. Tendons can withstand great pressure, but tendons that tear do not heal well. A complete tear requires surgical repair. Damage to a tendon and its muscle in a joint is a strain. Tendonitis is inflammation of the tendon.

> **Review Video: Muscular System**
> Visit mometrix.com/academy and enter code: 967216

MUSCULOSKELETAL ABNORMALITIES

Musculoskeletal abnormalities include:

- **Atony**: Atony is the lack of tone and muscle weakness that impairs functioning, especially of organs that must contract, such as bladder atony and atonic colon.
- **Atrophy**: Atrophy is the wasting away of muscle because of poor nourishment, lack of use, impaired nerves, or poor circulation, such as may occur with paralysis after a stroke.
- **Hypertrophy**: Hypertrophy is the enlargement or overgrowth of muscle tissue, such as may occur with cardiac hypertrophy in which the heart muscle enlarges and weakens.
- **Fibrositis**: Fibrositis is inflammation of white fibrous tissue with hyperplasia (enlargement caused by cell overgrowth) found in connective tissue muscles, and muscle sheaths, such as may occur with tendonitis and fibromyalgia.
- **Myositis**: Myositis is inflammation of the muscle, such as may occur with autoimmune disorders in which the immune system attacks the muscle cells, with adverse effects of drugs, and with infection. Disorders include polymyositis, dermatomyositis, and infectious myositis.

MUSCULOSKELETAL DISEASES

Osteoporosis is a condition with thin porous bones that break easily because of low bone mass and structural deterioration, with more bone lost than gained. Osteoporosis is most common in post-menopausal women, although men >65 lose bone at the same rate as women. Osteoporosis is one of the leading causes for vertebral fractures and femur (hip) fractures in older adults, often associated with falls that break the brittle bones.

Copyright © Mometrix Media. You have been licensed one copy of this document for personal use only. Any other reproduction or redistribution is strictly prohibited. All rights reserved. This content is provided for test preparation purposes only and does not imply an endorsement by Mometrix of any particular political, scientific, or religious point of view.

Osteoarthritis is a degenerative joint disease in which joints become inflamed, stiff, and painful as cartilage (which covers bone ends) deteriorates. Osteoarthritis may affect any joint and often results from a previous injury to a joint, so it may affect only one joint. Joints most commonly affected include the knees, hips, neck, and lumbar (lower) back as well as finger joints. Osteoarthritis usually has a slow onset with symptoms appearing after age 60. Pain tends to increase with weight bearing. Osteoarthritis is the primary reason for joint replacement surgery.

GAIT DISORDERS

Functional movement disorders are defined as an involuntary, abnormal movement of part of the body in which pathophysiology is not fully understood. Functional tremors are the most frequent type of functional movement disorder. Dystonia, myoclonus, and Parkinsonism are other types of functional movement disorders. Functional gait disorders are another type of functional movement disorder and are common in the elderly. Gait disorders can manifest as a dragging gait, knee buckling, small slow steps or "walking on ice," swaying gait, fluctuating gait, hesitant gait, and hyperkinetic gait in which there is excessive movement of the arms, trunks and legs when ambulating. Patients with gait disorders are at an increased risk of falling. Gait disorders are diagnosed by a thorough clinical examination (including a neurologic assessment) and health history. Treatment for functional gait disorders includes strength and balance training. Assistive devices such as walkers and canes may also be utilized.

NERVOUS SYSTEM

The human nervous system is divided into the central nervous system (CNS) and the peripheral nervous system (PNS).

- The **CNS** is composed of the brain and spinal cord and is located in the dorsal cavity. The brain is protected by the skull, while the spinal cord is protected by the vertebrae.
- The **PNS** is made of those structures of the nervous system not contained in the dorsal cavity, such as long nerves (neuron axons). The PNS is divided into the somatic nervous system and the autonomic nervous system. The autonomic nervous system is further divided into the sympathetic nervous system and the parasympathetic nervous system.

> **Review Video: Nervous System**
> Visit mometrix.com/academy and enter code: 708428

SOMATIC NERVOUS SYSTEM

The somatic division of the peripheral nervous system is involved in the coordination of body movements. It is comprised of peripheral nerve fibers that receive sensory information and carry this information into the spinal cord. It also contains motor nerve fibers that connect to skeletal muscle. The somatic system employs an afferent nerve network to carry sensory information to the brain and an efferent nerve network with motor nerves that transmit information from the brain to the skeletal muscles. The somatic nervous system regulates activities that are under the individual's conscious control, processes sensory information, and executes voluntary movements. The somatic nervous system does not control reflex arcs.

AUTONOMIC NERVOUS SYSTEM

The **sympathetic division** of the peripheral nervous system is involved in the "fight-or-flight" response and is activated in times of danger or stress. Signs and symptoms of sympathetic stimulation are an increased heart rate (tachycardia), vasoconstriction and rise in blood pressure, dilation of the pupils (mydriasis), goose bumps on the skin (piloerection or cutis anserine),

Copyright © Mometrix Media. You have been licensed one copy of this document for personal use only. Any other reproduction or redistribution is strictly prohibited. All rights reserved. This content is provided for test preparation purposes only and does not imply an endorsement by Mometrix of any particular political, scientific, or religious point of view.

increased sweat secretion (diaphoresis), and feelings of excitement. These reactions are due to the release of adrenaline (epinephrine).

The **parasympathetic nervous system** is in charge when the individual feels relaxed or is resting. The parasympathetic system is responsible for constriction of the pupil, slowing of the heart rate, dilation of blood vessels, and stimulation of the digestive tract and genitourinary system. The neurotransmitter at work is acetylcholine.

DORSAL CAVITY

The dorsal cavity contains the brain and spinal cord, which are the organs of the central nervous system (CNS). Like the ventral cavity, the dorsal cavity is divided into two smaller cavities: the cranial cavity and the spinal cavity. The cranial cavity contains the brain, eyes, and ears, while the spinal cavity holds the spinal cord. The brain and spinal cord are covered by three layers of connective tissue called the meninges. The outermost layer is the dura mater; the middle layer is the arachnoid mater; and the innermost layer is the pia mater. The space between the arachnoid mater and the pia mater is filled with cerebrospinal fluid (CSF), which flows throughout the CNS. If an injured patient has clear yellow fluid leaking from the ears, nose, eyes, or mouth, it is probably CSF and indicates a skull fracture.

NEURONS

Neurons are nerve cells that transmit nerve impulses throughout the central and peripheral nervous systems. The basic structure of a neuron includes the cell body, the dendrites, and the axons. The **cell body**, also called the soma, contains the nucleus. The nucleus contains the chromosomes. The **dendrite** of the neuron extends from the cell body and resembles the branches of a tree. The dendrite receives chemical messages from other cells across the synapse, a small gap. The **axon** is a thread-like extension of the cell body, which varies in length, up to 3 feet in the case of spinal nerves. The axon transmits an electro-chemical message along its length to another cell. Peripheral nervous system (PNS) neurons that deal with muscles are myelinated with fatty Schwann cell insulation to speed up the transmission of messages. Gaps between the Schwann cells that expose the axon are **nodes of Ranvier** and increase the speed of the transmission of nerve impulses along the axon. Neurons in the PNS that deal with pain are unmyelinated because transmission does not have to be as fast. Some neurons in the central nervous system (CNS) are

Copyright © Mometrix Media. You have been licensed one copy of this document for personal use only. Any other reproduction or redistribution is strictly prohibited. All rights reserved. This content is provided for test preparation purposes only and does not imply an endorsement by Mometrix of any particular political, scientific, or religious point of view.

myelinated by oligodendrocytes. If the myelin in the CNS oligodendrocytes breaks down, the patient develops multiple sclerosis (MS).

The three **categories of neurons** are as follows:

- **Afferent neurons** carry sensory impulses from the environment to the brain and spinal cord and are also called sensory neurons or receptor neurons. Afferent neurons are found in the skin, muscles, joints, and sensory organs. They permit the perception of pressure, pain, temperature, taste, odor, sound, and visual stimuli.
- **Efferent neurons** transmit motor impulses from the brain and spinal cord to effectors, such as muscles and glands. Efferent neurons are involved in motor control and stimulate movement throughout the body.
- **Interneurons** connect sensory and motor neurons. Also called connection neurons or relay neurons, interneurons are located in the CNS; sensory and motor neurons are found in both the CNS and PNS.

NERVOUS SYSTEM DISEASES

Epilepsy is a seizure disorders with sudden involuntary abnormal electrical disturbances in the brain that can manifest as alterations of consciousness, spastic tonic and clonic movements, convulsions, and loss of consciousness. Following seizures, patients may have confusion, disorientation, and impairment of motor activity, speech, and vision for several hours and headache, nausea, and vomiting may occur. During the seizure, the patient should be turned to the

Copyright © Mometrix Media. You have been licensed one copy of this document for personal use only. Any other reproduction or redistribution is strictly prohibited. All rights reserved.
This content is provided for test preparation purposes only and does not imply an endorsement by Mometrix of any particular political, scientific, or religious point of view.

side and the head and body protected from injury, but no attempt should be made to insert anything into the mouth or restrain the person.

Parkinson's disease (PD) is a movement motor system disorder caused by loss of brain cells that produce dopamine. Typical symptoms include tremor of face and extremities, rigidity, bradykinesia (abnormal slowness of movement), akinesia (absence of or extremely limited movement), poor posture, and lack of balance and coordination, causing increasing problems with mobility, talking, and swallowing. Some may suffer depression, mood changes, and dementia.

REPRODUCTIVE SYSTEM
MALE

The functions of the male reproductive system are to produce, maintain, and transfer **sperm** and **semen** into the female reproductive tract and to produce and secrete **male hormones**.

The external structure includes the penis, scrotum, and testes. The **penis**, which contains the **urethra**, can fill with blood and become erect, enabling the deposition of semen and sperm into the female reproductive tract during sexual intercourse. The **scrotum** is a sack of skin and smooth muscle that houses the testes and keeps the testes outside the body wall at a cooler, proper temperature for **spermatogenesis**. The **testes**, or testicles, are the male gonads, which produce sperm and testosterone.

The internal structure includes the epididymis, vas deferens, ejaculatory ducts, urethra, seminal vesicles, prostate gland, and bulbourethral glands. The **epididymis** stores the sperm as it matures. Mature sperm moves from the epididymis through the **vas deferens** to the **ejaculatory duct**. The **seminal vesicles** secrete alkaline fluids with proteins and mucus into the ejaculatory duct also. The **prostate gland** secretes a milky white fluid with proteins and enzymes as part of the semen. The **bulbourethral**, or Cowper's, glands secrete a fluid into the urethra to neutralize the acidity in the urethra, which would damage sperm.

Additionally, the hormones associated with the male reproductive system include **follicle-stimulating hormone (FSH)**, which stimulates spermatogenesis; **luteinizing hormone (LH)**, which stimulates testosterone production; and **testosterone**, which is responsible for the male sex characteristics. FSH and LH are gonadotropins, which stimulate the gonads.

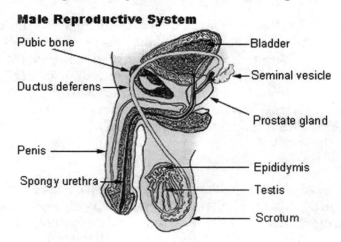

Male Reproductive System

79

Copyright © Mometrix Media. You have been licensed one copy of this document for personal use only. Any other reproduction or redistribution is strictly prohibited. All rights reserved. This content is provided for test preparation purposes only and does not imply an endorsement by Mometrix of any particular political, scientific, or religious point of view.

FEMALE

The functions of the female reproductive system are to produce **ova** (oocytes or egg cells), transfer the ova to the **fallopian tubes** for fertilization, receive the sperm from the male, and provide a protective, nourishing environment for the developing **embryo**.

The external portion of the female reproductive system includes the labia majora, labia minora, Bartholin's glands, and clitoris. The **labia majora** and the **labia minora** enclose and protect the vagina. The **Bartholin's glands** secrete a lubricating fluid. The **clitoris** contains erectile tissue and nerve endings for sensual pleasure.

The internal portion of the female reproductive system includes the ovaries, fallopian tubes, uterus, and vagina. The **ovaries**, which are the female gonads, produce the ova and secrete **estrogen** and **progesterone**. The **fallopian tubes** carry the mature egg toward the uterus. Fertilization typically occurs in the fallopian tubes. If fertilized, the egg travels to the **uterus**, where it implants in the uterine wall. The uterus protects and nourishes the developing embryo until birth. The **vagina** is a muscular tube that extends from the **cervix** of the uterus to the outside of the body. The vagina receives the semen and sperm during sexual intercourse and provides a birth canal when needed.

REPRODUCTIVE CYCLE

The female reproductive cycle is characterized by changes in both the ovaries and the uterine lining (endometrium).

The ovarian cycle has three phases: the follicular phase, ovulation, and the luteal phase. During the **follicular phase**, FSH stimulates the maturation of the follicle, which then secretes estrogen. Estrogen helps to regenerate the uterine lining that was shed during menstruation. **Ovulation**, the release of a secondary oocyte from the ovary, is induced by a surge in LH. The **luteal phase** begins with the formation of the corpus luteum from the remnants of the follicle. The corpus luteum secretes progesterone and estrogen, which inhibit FSH and LH. Progesterone also maintains the thickness of the endometrium. Without the implantation of a fertilized egg, the corpus luteum begins to regress, and the levels of estrogen and progesterone drop. FSH and LH are no longer inhibited, and the cycle renews.

The uterine cycle also consists of three phases: the proliferative phase, secretory phase, and menstrual phase. The **proliferative phase** is characterized by the regeneration of the uterine lining. During the **secretory phase**, the endometrium becomes increasingly vascular, and nutrients are secreted to prepare for implantation. Without implantation, the endometrium is shed during **menstruation**.

Copyright © Mometrix Media. You have been licensed one copy of this document for personal use only. Any other reproduction or redistribution is strictly prohibited. All rights reserved. This content is provided for test preparation purposes only and does not imply an endorsement by Mometrix of any particular political, scientific, or religious point of view.

RESPIRATORY SYSTEM

The respiratory system is made up of the nasal cavity, pharynx, larynx, trachea, right and left bronchi, and lungs, which branch into bronchioles and alveoli. The respiratory system has two divisions. The upper respiratory tract is comprised of the nasal cavity and pharynx and their associated structures. The lower respiratory tract consists of the larynx, trachea, bronchi, and lungs.

The diaphragm and muscles of the thoracic wall are responsible for the bellows movements necessary for breathing. The process of external respiration (breathing) involves the inspiration of oxygen and the exhalation of carbon dioxide. Normally, respiration occurs through the nasal cavity. Patients who are congested or under exertion breathe through their mouths. Those with airway blockages are neck-breathers with stomas.

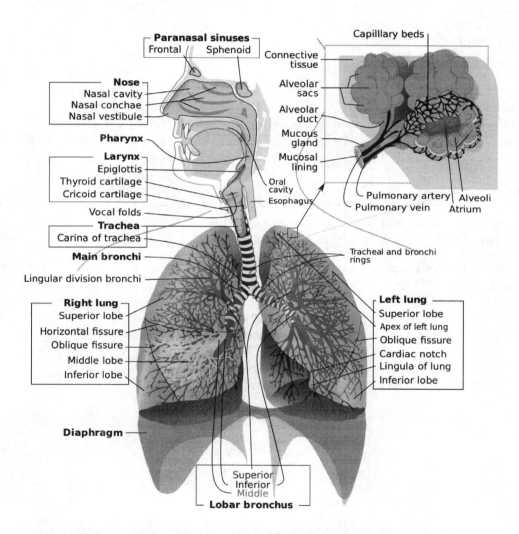

Review Video: Respiratory System
Visit mometrix.com/academy and enter code: 783075

CONTROL OF RESPIRATION

Respiratory neurons in the medulla, pons, and brainstem control the speed and depth of respiration and are responsible for maintaining its normal rhythm. The normal respiration rate in

Copyright © Mometrix Media. You have been licensed one copy of this document for personal use only. Any other reproduction or redistribution is strictly prohibited. All rights reserved.
This content is provided for test preparation purposes only and does not imply an endorsement by Mometrix of any particular political, scientific, or religious point of view.

adults is 12-20 breaths per minute. Infants breathe faster; the newborn rate is 44 breaths per minute. The respiratory neurons stimulate motor neurons in the spinal cord to cause the contraction of the muscular diaphragm and intercostal muscles. The respiratory neurons also receive information from receptors about the levels of carbon dioxide (CO_2), oxygen (O_2), and hydrogen (H) in the body, as well as the degree of stretch present in the lungs and chest. Chemoreceptors in the carotid arteries inform the respiratory neurons when the concentration of oxygen falls; chemoreceptors located in the medulla, carotid arteries, and aorta keep track of the levels of carbon dioxide and hydrogen. Breathing can be controlled consciously to a certain extent but is basically an autonomic function.

MECHANICS OF RESPIRATION

Respiration occurs when the air pressure within the alveoli differs from the air pressure external to the body. The air pressure in the lungs is altered by changes in the size of the thoracic cavity, which occur as a result of the contraction and relaxation of the muscular diaphragm and intercostal muscles. The muscular diaphragm is primarily responsible for allowing respiration. Inhalation is brought about by two actions that increase the size of the thoracic cavity. The contraction of the diaphragm causes it to flatten, lengthening the thoracic cavity, and the contraction of the intercostal muscles pulls the rib cage upward, widening it. With the enlargement of the thoracic cavity, the pressure within decreases and air enters the lungs. Air is then pushed out of the lungs as the muscular diaphragm and intercostal muscles relax and the volume of the thoracic cavity decreases.

INTERNAL AND EXTERNAL RESPIRATION

Internal respiration refers to the exchange of oxygen, carbon dioxide, and trace gases at the cellular level. **External respiration** refers to the exchange of oxygen, carbon dioxide, and other gases between the lungs and blood, commonly known as breathing. The passage of gases through the respiratory system can be traced as follows:

1. **Inspiratory neurons** in the respiratory center of the medulla oblongata (brain stem) tell the body to inhale.
2. **Nostrils** and **mouth** warm inhaled air by moving it over nasal conchae and sinuses.
3. Air passes through the **pharynx** to the **larynx** (voice box).
4. The **epiglottis** flips to cover the esophagus.
5. Air passes into the **trachea** (windpipe).
6. **Diaphragm** contracts and flattens to raise the ribs as breathing occurs.
7. **Intercostal muscles** between the ribs pull the ribs up enabling the chest to expand and air to pull inward.
8. Trachea splits into the left and right **bronchi** that connect to the **lungs**. The bronchi split into fine branches called **bronchioles**.
9. Bronchioles end in thin-walled, grape-like **alveoli** where the red blood cells absorb oxygen (O_2) from the inhaled air and give off carbon dioxide (CO_2).
10. **Expiratory neurons** in the brain stem tell the diaphragm and ribs to relax and exhale carbon dioxide into the atmosphere.

> **Review Video: Pulmonary Circuit**
> Visit mometrix.com/academy and enter code: 955608

NASAL CAVITY

The inside of the nose is the nasal cavity. The external nares (nostrils) are its outside openings; the internal nares (conchae) are its posterior openings; and the vestibule refers to the front (anterior) portion. Air is taken in through the external nares, warmed, humidified, and filtered by the conchae.

Copyright © Mometrix Media. You have been licensed one copy of this document for personal use only. Any other reproduction or redistribution is strictly prohibited. All rights reserved. This content is provided for test preparation purposes only and does not imply an endorsement by Mometrix of any particular political, scientific, or religious point of view.

The posterior part of the septum is made of bone, and the anterior part is cartilage. The nasal cavity is divided into left and right halves by the nasal septum (vomer). The hard palate forms the cavity floor. The nasal cavity is lined with mucous membrane. The goblet cells of the mucous membrane secrete mucus to trap particles of dust and debris. Ciliated cells wave hairs to stop large particles from advancing any further into the respiratory tract.

PHARYNX

The internal nares lead to the pharynx. Mucous is swept back in the nasal cavity to the pharynx, where it is swallowed and excreted through the digestive tract. Air is humidified and warmed in the nasal cavity before passing into the pharynx to prevent damage to the lining of the deeper respiratory passages. The pharynx is the common opening from the nasal cavity to the rest of the respiratory tract, as well as the digestive tract. It is split into three regions: the nasopharynx, oropharynx, and laryngopharynx. The nasopharynx is the upper (superior) part of the pharynx; it extends from the internal nares down to the uvula and contains the pharyngeal tonsil. The oropharynx runs between the uvula and epiglottis. The laryngopharynx lies below the upper edge of the epiglottis and opens to the esophagus.

LARYNX

The larynx is comprised of a cartilaginous skeleton, muscles, ligaments, and mucosal lining. The cartilages making up the larynx are the thyroid, cricoid, and arytenoid. The largest and most superior of these is the thyroid cartilage, or Adam's apple. The cricoid cartilage is the most inferior of the cartilages. If the patient's airway is closed by trauma, foreign body obstruction, or edema from anaphylaxis, the cricoid can be punctured to permit breathing (cricothyrotomy). The arytenoid cartilage lies between the cricoid and thyroid cartilages. The thyroid cartilage is attached to the epiglottis. It covers the opening of the larynx during swallowing to prevent food and fluid from entering the larynx. The vallecula is a depression that lies anterior to the epiglottis. The larynx contains the vocal folds (vocal cords) for speech and provides an entrance to the lower respiratory passages. The movement of the intrinsic muscles of the larynx alters the shape and tension of the vocal cords, adjusting voice pitch.

TRACHEA

Also called the windpipe, the trachea is a tube comprised of connective tissue, cartilage, and smooth muscle. Its lateral sides are made of cartilage, which protects the trachea and keeps the structure

Copyright © Mometrix Media. You have been licensed one copy of this document for personal use only. Any other reproduction or redistribution is strictly prohibited. All rights reserved. This content is provided for test preparation purposes only and does not imply an endorsement by Mometrix of any particular political, scientific, or religious point of view.

open for the passage of air. The posterior position of the trachea consists of ligamentous membrane and smooth muscle. The smooth muscle can alter the trachea's shape. The esophagus is positioned posterior to the trachea's back wall. Cilia in the trachea push mucus and particles of foreign matter toward the larynx. Their movement allows the mucus and foreign matter to enter the esophagus, where it can be swallowed. The trachea splits into the right and left mainstream bronchi at the carina.

PRIMARY BRONCHI

The primary bronchi (extrapulmonary bronchi) are large passageways that conduct air into the lungs; no gas exchange takes place. They form where the trachea splits at the carina and run from the mediastinum down into the lungs. The two primary bronchi are different shapes. The right bronchus is shorter, wider, and positioned more vertically than the left bronchus. If a patient has an obstructed bronchus, it is more likely the right one. The primary bronchi are supported by C-shaped cartilage rings and split into the secondary bronchi as they enter the lungs. This site, where the bronchi, vessels, and nerves enter the lungs, is called the hilus.

BRONCHIAL TREE

The primary bronchi split to form the **secondary bronchi**, and the secondary bronchi divide to form the **tertiary bronchi**. The tertiary bronchi reach into the lobules of the lungs and continue to branch into the bronchioles. The bronchioles divide many times to form the terminal bronchioles, which split into respiratory bronchioles. Each individual respiratory bronchiole also divides and becomes an alveolar duct. The alveolar ducts terminate in the alveoli, clusters of air sacs that resemble clusters of grapes. A single alveolus is 0.1-0.2 mm in diameter. Each one is surrounded by capillaries. It is here in the alveoli where the exchange of respiratory gases (oxygen for carbon dioxide) occurs.

LUNGS

The lungs (pulmones) are the main organs of respiration. They are light enough to float in water, elastic, smooth, shiny, and spongy. When touched, the tiny, grape-like alveoli crackle. The lungs are covered in a double-walled sac called the pleura. The base of each lung rests on the diaphragm, which raises and lowers the lungs. The right lung is the larger of the two lungs, comprised of three lobes, versus two lobes in the left lung. The lung's lobes are separated by fissures on the surface of the organs. Each lobe of the lung is split into lobules that are separated by connective tissue. Major blood vessels and bronchi do not pass through the connective tissue, so surgeons can remove diseased lobules fairly easily. The right lung contains 10 lobules, and the left lung holds nine. As the primary bronchi enter the lungs, they split into secondary bronchi.

> **Review Video: Lung Sounds**
> Visit mometrix.com/academy and enter code: 765616

PLEURA

The pleura is the thin membrane that protects the lungs. The parietal pleura lines the inside of the chest cavity; the visceral pleura covers the lungs. The space between the two is called the pleural space. The visceral pleura lubricates the surfaces of the lungs by secreting small amounts of fluid. The lungs expand and contract during respiration, and pleural fluid allows the different lung surfaces to glide smoothly across each other. Pleurisy is a painful condition in which the pleura become inflamed as a result of fluid collecting in the pleural space (wet pleurisy) or the two membranes rubbing together (dry pleurisy). A pleural rub may be audible with a stethoscope (auscultation) if the patient has pleurisy, pleural effusion, pneumonia, pulmonary infarction, neoplasm, lupus, or asbestosis.

Copyright © Mometrix Media. You have been licensed one copy of this document for personal use only. Any other reproduction or redistribution is strictly prohibited. All rights reserved. This content is provided for test preparation purposes only and does not imply an endorsement by Mometrix of any particular political, scientific, or religious point of view.

DYSPNEA, HYPERPNEA, BRADYPNEA, AND ORTHOPNEA

Dyspnea is characterized by difficulty breathing, such as shortness of breath (SOB) or painful breathing. **Hyperpnea** is rapid breathing. **Bradypnea** is abnormally slow breathing. **Orthopnea** causes difficulty breathing unless the patient is sitting upright or standing, as in congestive heart failure (CHF).

REGULATING THE ACID-BASE BALANCE

The lungs control blood pH by releasing **carbon dioxide**, a slightly acidic waste product of oxygen metabolism. The carbon dioxide is excreted by cells into the blood, carried into the lungs by red blood cells, and exhaled. As the level of carbon dioxide builds up in the blood, the blood pH decreases. The amount of carbon dioxide exhaled is controlled by the respiration rate. The normal respiration rate for seated adults is 12-20 breaths per minute. As the rate increases and breathing becomes deeper, the amount of carbon dioxide exhaled increases. As a consequence, the pH of the blood also increases. To decrease pH, the brain slows the speed and depth of breathing.

RESPIRATORY ALKALOSIS

Respiratory alkalosis is characterized by lower-than-normal levels of carbon dioxide in the blood, causing an increase in blood pH. Respiratory alkalosis disrupts the acid-base balance, with a decrease in PCO_2 (hypocapnia). Respiratory alkalosis can result from any heart or lung disease that causes fever, anxiety, shortness of breath, or hyperventilation from exhaling too much carbon dioxide. Drugs like progesterone, nicotine, salicylates, catecholamines, and methylxanthines can cause hypocapnia. Pregnant women have naturally increased progesterone and so are prone to this condition. If the patient rebreathes through a paper bag, it may help. However, patients with brain and spinal cord problems, who already have a low pH in their cerebrospinal fluid (CSF), may become worse if they use a paper bag. Signs and symptoms of respiratory alkalosis include agitation; dizziness; numbness in the hands, feet, and around the mouth; fainting (syncope); and in extremely rare cases, seizures. Respiratory alkalosis is rarely life threatening.

RESPIRATORY ACIDOSIS

Respiratory acidosis is a disturbance of the body's acid-base balance, which occurs when the lungs are unable to get rid of all their carbon dioxide. Respiratory acidosis decreases blood pH, and the body becomes too acidic. $PaCO_2$ increases (hypercapnia). Any disease, which makes the body less efficient at expelling carbon dioxide, weakens the chest muscles, or interferes with the nerve signals that inflate and deflate the lungs, can cause respiratory acidosis. Asthma, COPD, myasthenia gravis, Lou Gehrig's disease, Pickwickian syndrome of obesity, muscular dystrophy, and Guillain-Barré syndrome all cause respiratory acidosis. Signs and symptoms of respiratory acidosis include confusion, lethargy, sleepiness, fatigue, disturbed organ function, respiratory failure, and shock. Severe respiratory acidosis constitutes a medical emergency.

Copyright © Mometrix Media. You have been licensed one copy of this document for personal use only. Any other reproduction or redistribution is strictly prohibited. All rights reserved. This content is provided for test preparation purposes only and does not imply an endorsement by Mometrix of any particular political, scientific, or religious point of view.

ADDITIONAL RESPIRATORY DISEASES AND INFECTIONS

Common respiratory diseases and infections include the following:

Asthma	Condition characterized by recurrent attacks of severe wheezing, coughing, and shortness of breath because of spasms and contraction of the bronchi, limiting airflow. May be triggered by allergies, temperature variations, or exercise.
Bronchitis	Bacterial or viral infection of one or both bronchi resulting in severe cough, shortness of breath, and thick usually purulent sputum production. Bronchitis may be acute or chronic (recurrent).
Pneumonia	Bacterial, viral, or fungal infection of air sacs in the lungs, resulting in cough, fever, chills, malaise, difficulty breathing, and chest pain.
Diphtheria	Contagious bacterial (*Corynebacterium diphtheria*) infection of the mucous membranes of the nose and throat resulting in difficulty speaking, swallowing, and breathing. Most people in US are vaccinated against diphtheria.
Tuberculosis	Contagious bacterial (*Mycobacterium tuberculosis*) infection of the lungs resulting in weakness, weight loss, cough, fever, night sweats, chest pain, and bloody sputum.
Measles	Highly contagious viral infection that results in generalized rash, cough, high fever, sore throat, and runny nose. Usually resolves in 1–2 weeks but some may develop pneumonia or encephalitis. Prevention is through vaccination.

URINARY SYSTEM

The urinary system is comprised of two kidneys (which are located in the right and left flank areas), which filter the blood of toxins and excess fluid, creating urine. Ureters carry the urine to the bladder, and a urethra carries the urine to the external meatus (opening) during urination. The

Copyright © Mometrix Media. You have been licensed one copy of this document for personal use only. Any other reproduction or redistribution is strictly prohibited. All rights reserved. This content is provided for test preparation purposes only and does not imply an endorsement by Mometrix of any particular political, scientific, or religious point of view.

urethra of the female is about 0.5-1.5 cm long, and the male urethra is about 15-29 cm long, so the female is more at risk for ascending infections.

RIGHT KIDNEY

LEFT KIDNEY

URETER

BLADDER

SPHINCTER

URETHRA

Review Video: Urinary System
Visit mometrix.com/academy and enter code: 601053

KIDNEYS

Two kidneys are located in the retroperitoneal space, in the posterior abdomen, one on each side of the spinal column. They are bean-shaped and concave on their medial aspects. The concave area contains an opening called the hilum, the point of entrance for the renal artery, renal vein, nerves, and ureter. The kidney controls blood pressure through the renal artery with the hormone renin.

The kidney is surrounded by a capsule of fibrous and connective tissue. The renal cortex is the outer part of the organ, lying underneath this capsule. Inside the cortex is the renal medulla, split into 10–20 renal pyramids. A renal pyramid and the overlying cortex associated with it form a renal lobe. The tip of a renal pyramid is called a papilla. Each papilla drains into a minor calyx. A number of minor calyces act together to drain into a major calyx. The major calyces, in turn, drain into the renal pelvis, from which urine then drains from through the ureter into the urinary bladder.

Copyright © Mometrix Media. You have been licensed one copy of this document for personal use only. Any other reproduction or redistribution is strictly prohibited. All rights reserved.
This content is provided for test preparation purposes only and does not imply an endorsement by Mometrix of any particular political, scientific, or religious point of view.

Path of Blood and Urine

The path of blood through the kidney and the subsequent path of urine is as follows:

1. Unfiltered blood enters the **nephron** through the afferent arteriole and flows into the **renal corpuscle.**
2. Minerals and some fluid filter out of the blood in the **glomerulus**, a tuft of blood vessels.
3. Filtrate enters **Bowman's capsule**, a shell around the glomerulus, where the majority of filtration takes place.
4. Blood leaves the glomerulus through the efferent tubule and enters the **peritubular network**.
5. Water and salt get reabsorbed in the **proximal convoluted tubule** (PCT), and return to the bloodstream.
6. Filtrate flows into the **descending loop of Henle**.
7. Blood continues through the peritubular network and out of the nephron through a venule.
8. Filtrate flows into the **ascending loop of Henle**, and into the **distal convoluted tubule (DCT)** in the cortex.
9. Hormones fine tune the filtrate to reabsorb only what amino acids, glucose, and salts the body needs.
10. **Filtrate** is now urine, and flows into the **collecting duct**, where ADH controls its concentration.
11. Urine passes from the kidney to the **ureters, bladder, urethra, and meatus** for micturition (urination).

Kidney Function

The kidneys produce 2-3 liters of urine daily. Waste products excreted in the urine include urea from protein catabolism, uric acid from nucleic acid metabolism, creatinine, excess water, and some drugs and toxins. Necessary minerals are reabsorbed. The kidneys maintain the acid-base balance, regulate electrolyte concentrations, control the volume of blood, and govern blood pressure. The entire blood supply is filtered 20-25 times per day through the 1.4 million nephrons of a healthy kidney cortex. If the number of nephrons decreases to 700,000, the patient develops hypertension. The kidneys help maintain the body's homeostasis (balance) by communicating with other organs using three hormones: erythropoietin (EPO), renin, and calcitriol. EPO signals the bone marrow to produce red blood cells while the lack of it causes anemia, renin regulates blood pressure, and calcitriol is the active form of Vitamin D. Calcitriol aids in the maintenance of calcium, needed for bones, teeth, and normal chemical balance, particularly in the heart.

Regulation of pH

The pH of the blood is determined by the blood levels of carbon dioxide and bicarbonate. The kidneys work in conjunction with the lungs to modify these levels and regulate acid-base homeostasis. Acid-base balance is achieved by controlling the blood levels of carbon dioxide and bicarbonate. The lungs help to regulate carbon dioxide balance, while the kidneys control the levels of bicarbonate through the secretion and reabsorption of bicarbonate and hydrogen ions. The kidneys prevent and respond to acidosis by secreting hydrogen ions and reabsorbing bicarbonate ions. They correct alkalosis in the opposite way, releasing bicarbonate ions and reabsorbing hydrogen ions. Because the body normally contains 20 times more bicarbonate than carbonic acid, it is better able to correct acidosis than alkalosis.

RAS

The **renin-angiotensin system** (RAS), also referred as the renin-angiotensin-aldosterone system (RAAS), regulates blood pressure. Renin in the distal convoluted tubule reacts to sodium depletion

88

(e.g., through sweating) and blood pressure drops (e.g., due to blood loss) by converting angiotensinogen, a blood protein, to angiotensin I. Angiotensin I is converted into angiotensin II in the lung capillaries via the angiotensin-converting enzyme (ACE). Angiotensin II stimulates the adrenal cortex to secrete aldosterone, which acts on the renal tubules. Aldosterone balances salt and water levels by increasing the reabsorption of sodium ions in the distal convoluted tubules and water in the loop of Henle. Retaining water and salt causes blood volume to increase, which raises blood pressure.

URINARY TRACT INFECTIONS

Urinary tract infections include the following:

- **Cystitis** (bladder infection): Cystitis is especially common in females. It causes burning, frequency, urgency, pelvic pain, and discolored urine and is treated with oral antibiotics.
- **Urethritis** (urethral infection): Urethritis is caused by bacteria from fecal residue infect the urethra or from sexually-transmitted infection. It causes pain and swelling and can be treated with oral antibiotics.
- **Pyelonephritis**: Pyelonephritis is an infection that spreads from the bladder upward to infect the body of the kidney and the collecting tubules. It causes flank or back pain, nausea, vomiting, fever, chills, painful urination, and dark foul-smelling urine. Pyelonephritis can be treated with IV and oral antibiotics.

THE EYES

The main **parts of the eye** and their functions are as follows:

- **Aqueous humor** is watery fluid that maintains eye pressure.
- The **bony orbit** is the socket protecting the eye.
- **Cranial nerves** that help with the function of the eye such as movement or vision include the optic nerve (cranial nerve II), oculomotor (III), trochlear (IV), trigeminal (V), abducens (VI), and vagus (X) nerves.
- **Eyelashes and lids** protect the eye and sweep out particles.
- **Extrinsic muscles** focus the eye.
- The **lacrimal glands** are tear ducts to moisten the eye.
- The **lens** refracts light.
- The **optic disc** is the blind spot.
- The **pupil** regulates light entry.
- The **retina** has rods for black and white imaging and cones for color imaging, and helps trigger the optic nerve to send impulses to the brain.
- The **macula** is at the retinal center that is very sensitive to light. The black spot in the center is called the fovea which provides the sharpest vision.
- The **choroid** is a black layer behind the retina that absorbs light and nourishes the retina.
- The **cornea** is the window at the front of the eye that helps with focus.
- The **iris** regulates light entry.
- The **sclera** is tough, white fibrous connective tissue holding nerves and vessels that acts as protection for the eye.
- The **suspensory ligament** connects the lens to the ciliary muscles of the iris.
- The **vitreous humor** is jelly that maintains the eye's shape and refracts images.

Copyright © Mometrix Media. You have been licensed one copy of this document for personal use only. Any other reproduction or redistribution is strictly prohibited. All rights reserved. This content is provided for test preparation purposes only and does not imply an endorsement by Mometrix of any particular political, scientific, or religious point of view.

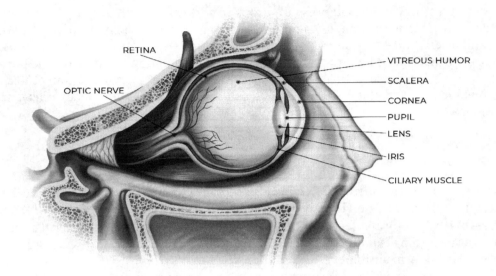

EYE DISEASES

The following eye diseases are common:

- **Astigmatism** results from faulty curvature and focusing errors, also called refractive error. Normal eyes are spheres, but eyes with astigmatism are football- or spoon-shaped. Patients with astigmatism require corrective eyeglasses to prevent headaches, blurred vision, and eye fatigue.
- **Cataracts** are clouded lenses, a problem common among the aged, diabetics, steroid users, head-injured patients, and workers exposed to radiation.
- **Conjunctivitis** is a red, inflamed conjunctiva due to chemicals or infection.
- **Glaucoma** sufferers have blocked aqueous humor between the lens and iris, which can cause blindness. Open-angle glaucoma is chronic; closed-angle glaucoma is acute. The condition affects people with a family history and is most prevalent in African Americans.
- **Hyperopia** results in farsightedness.
- **Myopia** is nearsightedness.
- **Presbyopia** is the inability to focus due to an aged, inelastic lens and requires reading glasses.
- **Strabismus** patients are cross-eyed.

Copyright © Mometrix Media. You have been licensed one copy of this document for personal use only. Any other reproduction or redistribution is strictly prohibited. All rights reserved. This content is provided for test preparation purposes only and does not imply an endorsement by Mometrix of any particular political, scientific, or religious point of view.

Patient Interview and Documentation

PATIENT HISTORY

A patient history is a written record gathered from a patient interview, listing past and present health, family information, and personal information pertinent to health, such as occupation.

- A **History and Physical Examination Report (H&P)** is a single report with two segments. It is usually dictated and transcribed, but can also be a form. The Joint Commission requires an H&P within 24 hours of admission for acute care patients and within 30 days prior to admission for chronic care patients. This must then be updated within 24 hours after the patient is admitted.
- A **Medical History and Review of Systems** forms the basis for the provisional diagnosis and treatment plan. The doctor collects information from the patient, guardian, or a reliable source (e.g., ambulance attendant or personal support worker). The headings are as follows:
  - Chief Complaint
  - Symptoms
  - History of Present Illness
  - Medical History
  - Family History
  - Social History
  - Health Maintenance
  - Review of Systems
- The Joint Commission requires **minors** to have a **developmental age evaluation** and educational needs assessment, also.

DATA COLLECTED IN PATIENT ADMISSION/ASSESSMENT

Objective data is that which can be directly measured or observed. Objective data may include blood pressure, pulse rate, respiratory rate, height, weight, size of wound, ECG tracings, gender, oxygen saturation, and description (brown hair, blue eyes, ambulatory). Objective data should be easily verified by other observers.

Subjective data, on the other hand, is not measurable or observable but is reported or assumed. Subjective data includes almost anything that the patient reports, including reports of symptoms (headache, diarrhea, pain, dizziness) or anything associated with feelings or assumptions (patient appears tired, angry, upset, anxious). For example, if a patient reports he had been coughing up thick yellow sputum the day prior, this information is subjective. If, however, the patient is observed coughing up thick yellow sputum into a sputum cup, this information is objective.

Copyright © Mometrix Media. You have been licensed one copy of this document for personal use only. Any other reproduction or redistribution is strictly prohibited. All rights reserved. This content is provided for test preparation purposes only and does not imply an endorsement by Mometrix of any particular political, scientific, or religious point of view.

CHARTING TECHNIQUES
FACT SYSTEM
All entries in a patient's chart must follow the FACT system and be:

- **Factual**: Patient complaints should be clearly described; for instance, a report of pain should include its specific location, quality (sharp and stabbing or dull ache), duration, and medications taken to relieve it.
- **Accurate**: Information reflects the patient's condition and is not assumed. Information is documented and signed off by the individual who conducted the assessment. In paper charts, entries are legible and in ink. Never use correction fluid or an eraser. Draw a single line through mistakes. The provider should write "error" beside mistakes along with his or her name and title or initials, according to unit policy.
- **Complete**: All fields should be completed to the best of the health care provider's ability. If unable to assess, the field should be marked as such. In paper charting, never leave lines completely or partially blank. Place a single line through the space to prevent someone else from adding to the line.
- **Timely**: Include a time stamp on all entries. This is automatic in electronic charting, but should be written out in paper charting.

HIPAA requires healthcare providers to maintain confidentially of all patient records. Release information on a need-to-know basis only. Never leave a paper chart or computer screen open to prying eyes. Report to the head nurse, IT, and security if approached by the press, an insurance company, or suspicious persons. Keep passwords secure and log off all sessions.

SOAP NOTE
The SOAP note format for composing chart notes is a reliable method of organizing and documenting information from the patient assessment. Do not transcribe in the chronological order in which the doctor dictates, but put the applicable parts of his or her dictation under these headings in this order:

- **S**: The **subjective** portion of the report is the chief complaint the patient or guardian makes.
- **O**: The **objective** portion includes all of the definite findings and observations dictated by the physician or nurse practitioner.
- **A**: The **assessment** portion of the report is where the physician reports the diagnosis.
- **P**: The **plan** section is where the physician prescribes the treatment program.

> **Review Video: SOAP**
> Visit mometrix.com/academy and enter code: 543158

ROLES OF THE PATIENT CHART
The patient's chart is a legal document of the events and procedures carried out during a treatment. It can be subpoenaed in court as a way to explain what care the patient did or did not receive. Charting is a method of communication between staff members about the patient, and it provides continuity of care from shift to shift. The chart is a diagnostic aid and the foundation upon which decisions are made concerning changes in medical therapy. The patient's chart also provides data for infection control, risk management, and quality control purposes and is subject to inspection by various regulating bodies, such as Medicare.

Copyright © Mometrix Media. You have been licensed one copy of this document for personal use only. Any other reproduction or redistribution is strictly prohibited. All rights reserved. This content is provided for test preparation purposes only and does not imply an endorsement by Mometrix of any particular political, scientific, or religious point of view.

Health and Wellness

LIFESTYLE CHOICES THAT INFLUENCE WELLNESS

Lifestyle choices that influence wellness include:

- **Exercise**: Children should exercise at least 3 times weekly for 30 minutes and adults at least 30 minutes daily or 150 minutes per week. Daily exercise is an important component of health but should be age- and condition-appropriate.
- **Smoking**: All those smoking should be encouraged to begin smoking cessation as smoking increases risks of cardiopulmonary disease, bladder cancer, and other disorders.
- **Substance abuse**: Users need to stop use or participate in rehabilitation programs. Substance abuse may lead to serious health problems, such as heart attack, overdose, stroke, and death.
- **Nutrition**: Diet must provide adequate nutrients to promote growth and development.
- **Weight control**: Obesity is a risk factor for cardiac disease, diabetes, hypertension, and hypercholesteremia, so dietary management and strategies to reduce weight are especially important.

NUTRITIONAL ELEMENTS THAT INFLUENCE WELLNESS

The nutritional elements that influence wellness include:

- **Fats**: 9 calories per gram. Fat provides the slowest but most efficient form of energy (taking 5 hours to metabolize). Fat should comprise 30% of the diet (with saturated fats no more than 10% of the diet).
- **Carbohydrates**: 4 calories per gram. Simple carbohydrates (sugars, fruits, dairy products) are the fastest source of energy (30 minutes). Complex carbohydrates (whole grains, vegetables) convert more slowly to energy (2 hours). Should comprise about 55% of the diet.
- **Proteins**: 4 calories per gram. Protein (meat, fish, dairy products, eggs, tofu), metabolizes more slowly (3 hours) and provides a long-lasting source of energy. Protein should provide about 15% of the diet.
- **Vitamins**: Organic compounds comprised of carbon, oxygen, hydrogen, nitrogen, and other elements. Vitamins are utilized for cellular biochemical reactions and include both fat soluble (A, D, E, and K) and water-soluble forms (thiamine [B_1], riboflavin [B_2], Niacin [B_3], pyridoxine [B_6], folate [B_{12}], pantothenic acid, biotin, and vitamin C).
- **Minerals**: Include calcium, phosphorus, potassium sulfur, sodium, chloride, iron, copper, zinc, magnesium, fluoride, selenium, chromium, and molybdenum. Minerals are needed for many bodily functions, including fluid balance, nerve transmission, muscle contraction, blood clotting, and BP regulation.

Copyright © Mometrix Media. You have been licensed one copy of this document for personal use only. Any other reproduction or redistribution is strictly prohibited. All rights reserved.
This content is provided for test preparation purposes only and does not imply an endorsement by Mometrix of any particular political, scientific, or religious point of view.

COMMON SCREENING MEASURES AND PREVENTIVE CARE

Common screening measures performed in the comprehensive assessment of an adult include the following:

Breast cancer	Manual exam, mammogram, ultrasound, MRI
Cervical cancer	Pap smear, pelvic exam
Skin cancer	Skin evaluation, encourage use of sunscreen
Lung cancer	Assess history of smoking (pack years), chest x-ray, encourage smoking cessation
Colorectal cancer	Fecal occult blood test, stool DNA test (Cologuard®), sigmoidoscopy, double-contrast barium enema, standard colonoscopy, or virtual colonoscopy
Testicular cancer	Manual exam, ultrasound
Prostate cancer	Manual exam, PSA
Osteoporosis	History, physical exam, and bone density scan, encourage exercise and adequate calcium and vitamin D in diet.
Sexually-transmitted diseases	History, testing for those having unprotected sex, campaign to encourage the use of condoms and safe sex practices
Domestic violence	Ask all patients in privacy (not with a partner or other person present) if they are victims of abuse in non-judgmental manner, discussing confidentiality and mandatory reporting requirements.

SMOKING RISKS AND CESSATION METHODS

Smoking damages the lining of the respiratory tract and the blood vessels, resulting in risk of respiratory disease (COPD, asthma attack) and heart disease (hypertension, heart attack). Smoking causes 90% of lung cancers and increases risk of coronary heart disease and stroke by 2-4 times, and is a factor in developing rheumatoid arthritis. Chemicals from smoking are filtered into the urine and increase risk of bladder cancer. Smoking increases the risk of preterm delivery and stillbirth and impairs male fertility. **Cessation methods** include:

- **Planned cessation**: Set a date, tell friends and family, remove smoking paraphernalia, list reasons, identify triggers, develop strategies for coping, establish a support system, and provide incentive rewards for compliance.
- **Support groups**: Online and in person support groups may help the patient cope with withdrawal and cravings.
- **Cold-turkey**: This approach is only successful if the patient is very motivated.
- **Medication-assisted**: Nicotine gum, nicotine patches, oral medications (varenicline) can help to control and manage cravings if taken in reduced doses.

Copyright © Mometrix Media. You have been licensed one copy of this document for personal use only. Any other reproduction or redistribution is strictly prohibited. All rights reserved.
This content is provided for test preparation purposes only and does not imply an endorsement by Mometrix of any particular political, scientific, or religious point of view.

Nutrition

FAT-SOLUBLE VITAMINS

Fat-soluble vitamins that are integral in the body's growth, development, and immunity include the following:

- **Vitamin A (retinol)** aids growth, development, immune function, and maintains night vision. Sources include butter, egg yolks, cod liver oil, yellow and green leafy vegetables, and prunes. Deficiency causes night blindness, poor visual acuity, skin disorders, and bronchopulmonary dysplasia in low-birth-weight newborns.
- **Vitamin D (calciferol)** aids calcium and phosphorus absorption for bone and teeth formation and is necessary for normal growth and development. Sources include milk, cod liver oil, butter, and egg yolks. Sunlight activates Vitamin D. Deficiency causes rickets, osteomalacia (soft bones, bowed legs) and dental caries.
- **Vitamin E (tocopherols)** is an antioxidant found in sunflower seeds, wheat germ, egg yolks, vegetable oils, almonds, olives, and papaya. Deficiency causes hemolytic anemia of premature newborns.
- **Vitamin K (quinones)** is a necessary for normal clotting of the blood and is found in green leafy vegetables, meat, dairy products, alfalfa, fishmeal, oats, wheat, and rye. Deficiency causes hemorrhagic disease of the newborn. Caution must be taken if anticoagulants are being used as this may affect the clotting of the blood.

The small intestine absorbs fat-soluble vitamins, so patients who have had bowel resections, cystic fibrosis or malabsorption may have deficiencies. Excessive intake of fat-soluble vitamins may cause them to accumulate in fat and in the liver, which can be toxic.

WATER-SOLUBLE VITAMINS

Water-soluble vitamins that are integral in the body's growth, development, and immunity include the following:

- **Thiamin (B_1)** is found in whole grains, egg yolk, legumes, nuts, pork, and brewer's yeast. Deficiency causes beriberi, confusion, muscle weakness, and poor growth.
- **Riboflavin (B_2)** is in meat, whole grains, brewer's yeast, green vegetables, milk, and eggs. Deficiency causes growth retardation, cracked mouth, and light sensitivity.
- **Niacin (B_3)** is found in meat, fish and poultry, whole grains, dairy products, brewer's yeast, and legumes. Deficiency causes pellagra, dermatitis, and malabsorption.
- **Pantothenate (B_5)** is found in cheese and dairy products, eggs, peanuts, beef, fish, legumes, and soy. Deficiency causes dermatitis and depression.
- **Pyridoxine (B_6)** is in whole grains, nuts, legumes, eggs, meat, fish, bran, and yeast. Deficiency causes dermatitis, cracked mouth, insomnia, weakness, irritability, a strange gait, and seizures.
- **Biotin (B_7)** is in egg yolks, liver, brewer's yeast, and royal jelly. Deficiency is rare.
- **Folic acid (B_9)** is in green, leafy vegetables, organ meat, beef, whole grains and cereals, and legumes. Deficiency causes anemia, neural tube defects.
- **Cobalamin (B_{12})** is in liver, milk, and eggs. Deficiency causes pernicious anemia. Loss of balance and nerve damage.
- **Ascorbic acid (C)** is found in citrus fruits, strawberries, melons, and vegetables such as broccoli, peppers, tomatoes, potatoes, and green leafy vegetables. Deficiency causes scurvy, pyorrhea, bleeding gums, tooth and bone defects, and poor wound healing.

Copyright © Mometrix Media. You have been licensed one copy of this document for personal use only. Any other reproduction or redistribution is strictly prohibited. All rights reserved. This content is provided for test preparation purposes only and does not imply an endorsement by Mometrix of any particular political, scientific, or religious point of view.

MACROMINERALS AND TRACE MINERALS

The body requires seven macrominerals in large quantities, and some trace minerals are necessary for good health. The seven **macrominerals** are:

- **Calcium** for muscle contraction, conduction of nerve impulses, bone and tooth maintenance, and blood clotting
- **Phosphorous** for energy transfer, pH balance, and bone and tooth maintenance
- **Sodium** for fluid balance, function of nerves and muscles
- **Potassium** for fluid balance in the blood, acid-base balance, muscle building, and protein synthesis
- **Chloride** for pH balance and needed for digestive juices
- **Sulfur**, an essential component of protein that helps energy metabolism
- **Magnesium** for energy metabolism, muscle function, enzymes, and protein synthesis

Important **trace minerals** include:

- **Chromium** for metabolism of fats and carbohydrate
- **Cobalt** for red blood cell maintenance
- **Copper** for blood, nerves, bones, and immune function
- **Fluoride** to strengthen bones and teeth
- **Iodine** for thyroid function and metabolism
- **Iron** to make red blood cells and protein
- **Manganese** for formation of connective and skeletal tissue, reproduction, growth, and metabolism
- **Molybdenum** helps breakdown sulfites, nitrogen metabolism, enzyme function
- **Selenium** to protect against free radicals
- **Zinc** for immune response, tissue growth, and wound healing

CONDITION-SPECIFIC DIETARY GUIDELINES

Various diets exist to address the needs and deficiencies of specific conditions, including the following:

Weight loss	Diets vary: low carbohydrate, low fat, and/or low calorie. Most include more whole grains, vegetables, and fruit and less refined sugar and flour.
Diabetes mellitus	Patients eat 3 meals daily and sometimes two small snacks, but calories and portion size are usually limited. Patients avoid sugar and high carbohydrate foods and eat food high in fiber, lean meats/fish, vegetables, and limited amounts of fruit.
Hypertension	DASH diet (2,000 calories/day) is plant-focused and high in vegetables, fruits, and nuts and with limited fat, lean meats, and sweets/sugar.
Lactose intolerance	Diet is free of milk products (cheese, milk) because the patient lacks the enzyme necessary to metabolize milk. Some patients may take lactase tablets in order to tolerate milk products.
Gluten intolerance/ Celiac disease	Gluten is a protein found in wheat, rye, and barley, so patients must avoid all products containing these grains, including pastas, breads, and pastries. Gluten is commonly found in many prepared foods and seasonings (chicken broth, salad dressings, soy sauce, frozen foods), which must also be avoided.

Copyright © Mometrix Media. You have been licensed one copy of this document for personal use only. Any other reproduction or redistribution is strictly prohibited. All rights reserved. This content is provided for test preparation purposes only and does not imply an endorsement by Mometrix of any particular political, scientific, or religious point of view.

MEAL MODIFICATIONS

When the doctor admits a patient to a hospital, rehab, or hospice, check the chart for known allergies, religion, and other conditions that may affect eating. For example, patients with alcoholism and liver disease or who are nursing mothers may need extra calories and supplements, whereas patients with diabetes and PKU have dietary restrictions. Flag this information to alert the dietitian and nurse at the receiving facility by checking off the appropriate boxes on the meal card and admitting forms.

DYSPHAGIA

Esophageal **dysphagia** is difficulty swallowing. It is distinct from odynophagia, which is painful swallowing. Dysphagia can result from:

- Strictures, tumors, or foreign bodies
- Motility disorders, including achalasia
- Spasms of the esophagus

Patients present with difficulty swallowing, choking, or coughing during eating, chronic weight loss and aspiration pneumonia. The doctor diagnoses the cause of dysphagia with endoscopy, barium swallow, and manometric studies of the esophagus. Patients with stroke, Parkinson's disease, multiple sclerosis, Lou Gehrig's disease, myasthenia gravis, muscular dystrophy, and various palsies are prone to dysphagia in their end stages. The treatment approach depends on the underlying cause of the dysphagia, and may include physiotherapy to retrain swallowing muscles, acid blocking medications, surgery to remove obstructions, or placement of a gastrostomy tube.

EATING DISORDERS

Eating disorders are a health risk for young adult females (from puberty to age 40, most commonly) although males sometimes also have eating disorders, often presenting as excessive exercise. The most common eating disorders include:

- **Anorexia nervosa** is a profound fear of weight gain and severe restriction of food intake, often accompanied by abuse of diuretics and laxatives, which can cause electrolyte imbalances as well as kidney and bowel disorders and delay or cessation of menses. Anorexics may become emaciated and risk death. Self-image is severely impaired, and patients are often in denial.
- **Bulimia nervosa** includes binge eating followed by vomiting often along with use of diuretics, enemas, and laxatives. Gastric acids can damage the throat and teeth. While bulimics may maintain a normal weight, they are at risk for severe electrolyte imbalances that can be life threatening.

Treatment for both eating disorders may include psychotherapy, cognitive behavioral therapy, family therapy, nutritional counseling, and nutritional monitoring.

ANEMIA

Anemia is lack of blood or a deficiency in red blood cells. It occurs from increased red blood cell destruction from sickle-cell anemia, thalassemia, G6PD deficiency, autoimmune reaction, inherited disorders, hemolytic poison, or an enlarged spleen. Signs and symptoms of anemia are fatigue, thirst, rapid pulse, pallor, dizziness, sweating, shortness of breath, abdominal or chest pain, leg cramps, and syncope. Aplastic anemia results from suppressed bone marrow due to leukemia, radiation, or poisoning. Protein deficiency causes kwashiorkor anemia. Strict vegetarianism and

Copyright © Mometrix Media. You have been licensed one copy of this document for personal use only. Any other reproduction or redistribution is strictly prohibited. All rights reserved. This content is provided for test preparation purposes only and does not imply an endorsement by Mometrix of any particular political, scientific, or religious point of view.

chronic bleeding (e.g., heavy menstruation) deplete iron stores (ferritin), thereby causing iron deficiency anemia. Vitamin B_{12} deficiency causes pernicious anemia.

Humans need iron, folate, Vitamin B_6, Vitamin B_{12}, Vitamin C, Vitamin E, Vitamin K, riboflavin, copper, zinc, and protein to **manufacture blood in the bone marrow**. Even if these nutrients are adequate, the patient cannot produce sufficient blood without the hormone erythropoietin from the kidneys. Therefore, patients with end-stage renal failure who are on dialysis become anemic.

TPN

Many end-stage patients report anorexia (lack of appetite) and changes in the taste of food from medications, disease, or treatments. Anorexia means decreased food consumption, problems meeting the patient's nutritional needs, and distress for the patient's family. **Total parenteral nutrition (TPN)** replaces all or some of the patient's food with liquid nutrients delivered through a surgically implanted central line catheter in the subclavian vein under the collarbone, the jugular vein of the neck, the umbilical vein in the abdomen, or a PICC line in the arm. TPN can be given over the course of the day or overnight depending upon the patient's condition. A TPN bag will range in size from 500-3,000 mL and requires an infusion pump and IV pole to administer. TPN must be provided under the most sterile of conditions to reduce the risk for infection. There are many complications that can be associated with TPN including clotting issues, infection, and liver disease. Close monitoring by the healthcare team is essential. TPN can cause discord in the family and ethical issues for caregivers because it prolongs life artificially. TPN removes the patient's pleasure and sense of normalcy from eating.

Copyright © Mometrix Media. You have been licensed one copy of this document for personal use only. Any other reproduction or redistribution is strictly prohibited. All rights reserved.
This content is provided for test preparation purposes only and does not imply an endorsement by Mometrix of any particular political, scientific, or religious point of view.

Patient Education

PATIENT EDUCATION TECHNIQUES BY AGE

Age	Learning Issue	Teaching Solution
Infant	Non-verbal	Teach the parents or guardian.
Preschooler	Short attention span	Instruct with visuals (e.g., dolls) and role play. Tell parents to oversee treatment
5-8 yr	Longer attention span and eager for knowledge	Use short videos, visuals, and pictures.
9-12 yr	Good attention span, great curiosity, and some independence; rapid growth issues, such as mixed dentition; desire for group acceptance	Teach pairs or small groups, if confidentiality can be preserved. Use age-appropriate language to indicate respect.
13-15 yr	Peer pressure, interest in personal appearance, poor coordination, and bad eating habits	Give individualized instructions, motivation, and encouragement.
16-19 yr	Question authority, have busy schedules	Act as a friend and mentor. Explain disease process and anatomy.
20-60 yr	Individualized problems	Tailor instruction to the individual circumstances (e.g., pregnancy, depression, drug abuse).
60+ yr	Age-related problems (e.g., eyesight, memory, mobility, multiple prescriptions), fixed income, isolation, dependence on caregiver	Educate caregivers and patient. Emphasize avoiding triggers. Dispense free samples (promotions from suppliers). Register patient with wandering registry, if necessary.

ASSESSING READINESS TO LEARN

Reading body language is an important skill the medical assistant can use to assess a patient's stage of readiness. Assume that the patient is open to learning if his or her pupils are slightly dilated, signifying interest, and he or she leans forward and nods his or her head up and down in agreement. Look for direct eye contact, smiling, positive behavior, or a change in position from sitting back to leaning forward. Lowered eyes or looking away can mean fixation on something else or avoidance of the situation in an American-born patient, but in other cultures, direct eye contact is considered rude and challenging. Pursed lips may mean the patient is stressed, angry, or taking psychiatric drugs. Shaking the head from side to side may signal disagreement, while shrugging the shoulders can mean indifference or uncertainty. If the patient hangs his or her head down, this may indicate sadness, anxiety, or lordosis due to a deteriorating spine.

Copyright © Mometrix Media. You have been licensed one copy of this document for personal use only. Any other reproduction or redistribution is strictly prohibited. All rights reserved.
This content is provided for test preparation purposes only and does not imply an endorsement by Mometrix of any particular political, scientific, or religious point of view.

TEACHING POINTS FOR HEALTH TOPICS

The following are key teaching points for health topics:

- **Health and wellness**: Weight control, regular exercise, smoking cessation, intervention for substance use/abuse, support groups, resources
- **Nutrition**: Nutrients (fats, proteins, carbohydrates, vitamins, minerals), well-balanced meals, label-reading, and calories
- **Hygiene**: Hand-washing, dental care (brushing, flossing), bathing, and basic skin care
- **Treatment and medications**: Mode of administration, dosage, frequency, duration, and adverse effects
- **Preoperative care**: Any necessary preparation, such as showering, GI cleansing, fasting, and taking/withholding medications
- **Postoperative care**: Mobility, deep-breathing and coughing, wound care, medications, and restrictions on activities
- **Body mechanics**: Lifting, carrying, body alignment, avoidance of muscle strain
- **Personal/Physical safety**: Fall prevention, home safety measures, lighting, and medical ID bracelets

DIABETIC EDUCATION

Diabetic education should include the following:

- **Glucose monitoring**: Patients should understand how to use the monitor and read and understand the results. The patient should know how frequently to test glucose. The patient should be advised of unsafe lower and higher levels and when to contact the physician or 911.
- **Medications (oral hypoglycemics)**: Patients should know administration, dosage, schedule, and adverse effects.
- **Medications (insulin)**: Patients should know dosage, schedule, and adverse effects as well as sites for injection and site rotation. Patients should practice filling syringes or using prefilled syringes and giving injections under supervision.
- **Ketoacidosis/hypoglycemia**: Patients should be able to describe signs and symptoms of ketoacidosis and hypoglycemia and know what steps to take if these occur.
- **Foot care**: Patients should be advised to avoid going barefoot, to practice good hygiene, and to check feet daily for signs of irritation or infection.
- **Diet**: Patients should understand the prescribed diet and any limitations, such as avoiding sugar and refined carbohydrates. Patients must understand the importance of eating 3 meals daily and staying on the diet.

PATIENT EDUCATION FOR AT-HOME MONITORING
HOME ANTICOAGULATION MONITORING

Home **INR anticoagulation** monitoring is done with a small device that varies in size from 4.5 ounces to 28 ounces, depending on the manufacturer. The patient must prick a finger with a lancet to obtain a drop of blood, which is placed on a test strip or cuvette. This is inserted into the device for reading. The INR result is displayed in a digital screen. Medicare and most insurances cover the costs of the equipment if used at least one time weekly.

HOME CHOLESTEROL MONITORING

Various monitoring systems/devices exist for **at-home monitoring of cholesterol**. One type of device is similar to the anticoagulation monitor, and the procedure is similar: prick the finger with a

Copyright © Mometrix Media. You have been licensed one copy of this document for personal use only. Any other reproduction or redistribution is strictly prohibited. All rights reserved. This content is provided for test preparation purposes only and does not imply an endorsement by Mometrix of any particular political, scientific, or religious point of view.

lancet, place a drop of blood on a test strip, and place into an electronic monitor for results. Some monitoring systems require only a test strip, which changes color according to the cholesterol level. Some monitoring devices provide only total cholesterol while others provide total cholesterol, HDL, LDL, and triglyceride levels.

PATIENT INSTRUCTIONS FOR CRUTCHES, CANES, AND WALKERS

Crutches should be properly fitted before the client attempts ambulation. Correct height is one hand-width below axillae. The handgrips should be adjusted so the client supports the body weight comfortably with elbows slightly flexed rather than locked in place. The client should be cautioned not to bear weight under the axillae as this can cause nerve damage, but to hold the crutches tight against the side of the chest wall. The type of gait used depends on the type of injury.

A **cane** should be held in the opposite hand of the side of injury. When holding the cane in neutral position, the elbow should be bent at about a 15-degree angle and if holding the cane straight down to the side of the body, the top of the cane should be in line with the crease of the wrist.

The same is true of a **walker**, the elbow should be bent at 15 degrees when standing up straight and grasping the handles, and the handle grasps should be in line with to the crease of the wrists. The client should be able to move the walker forward without leaning over.

PATIENT INSTRUCTIONS FOR WHEELCHAIRS

Wheelchair instructions should include the following:

- Engage brakes before getting in or out of the wheelchair and ensure the footplates are folded up or swung to the side
- Secure feet on footplates before navigating, but never stand on them
- Check for obstacles before navigating
- Secure safety harness/lap straps as needed
- Use hand rims to navigate forward and backward
- Avoid steep inclines (greater than a one-foot rise per 12-foot distance) and avoid going up or down inclines diagonally
- Bend forward slightly when going up an incline and lean backward slightly when going down
- Avoid rocky, soft, or uneven surfaces and beware of slippery surfaces
- Engage brakes when stopped
- Avoid hanging anything from the chair handles as the weight may lead to imbalance and tipping backward
- Never attempt to navigate stairs or escalators
- Go backward into elevators
- Use a gripper to pick up items and avoid bending forward or reaching down or behind
- Transfer into a seat in a motor vehicle unless it is adapted for wheelchair use and contains a security system

PATIENT INSTRUCTIONS FOR SPLINTS AND SLINGS

With both splints and slings, the patient/caregiver should be advised to check circulation by noting the skin color below the injury. The pulse should be palpable. The affected limb below the injury should also be checked for sensation and any feeling of numbness or tingling, which may indicate

Copyright © Mometrix Media. You have been licensed one copy of this document for personal use only. Any other reproduction or redistribution is strictly prohibited. All rights reserved. This content is provided for test preparation purposes only and does not imply an endorsement by Mometrix of any particular political, scientific, or religious point of view.

impaired circulation. The patient should be able to freely move any digits below the injury (toes, fingers).

- **Splints**: Used to limit movement of a limb but are generally removable, so they may be worn during the day and removed at night or while bathing. Commercial splints are often applied and secured with Velcro straps, but some may be formed from casting material that is secured in place by compression bandages.
- **Slings**: Used to elevate the hand or wrist in order to prevent or reduce edema and prevent movement or to immobilize an arm to maintain bone alignment with a broken clavicle (collarbone). If a cast has been applied to an arm, the sling helps to redistribute pressure and reduce strain on the shoulder muscles. Slings are generally applied so that the arm lies bent at the elbow with the lower arm parallel to the floor.

EDUCATIONAL RESOURCES
OBTAINING READY-MADE PATIENT EDUCATION MATERIALS

Patients are entitled to **reliable information** about signs, symptoms, safety, and healthy behaviors. Print out information from the National Library of Medicine at http://www.nlm.nih.gov/. Obtain ready-made patient education materials from the drug or device manufacturer, which may include brochures, videos, demonstration models, self-evaluation quizzes, instruction manuals, and free samples. Contact a sales representative or call the supplier's order desk, and be prepared with the doctor's license number. For example:

- If the patient needs education on proper dental care, dispense a free brush, floss, and paste, which are available as a no-cost promotion from many suppliers.
- If the patient has allergies and needs to be taught to avoid triggers, send the patient home with a self-evaluation quiz and instructions to return with it to the next appointment.
- If the patient needs information about maintenance, spare parts, and operating procedures for medical devices, check the facility's computerized maintenance management system (CMMS).

RESOURCE MATERIALS FOR PARENTS, GUARDIANS, AND TEACHERS

Parents, guardians, and sometimes teachers and other caregivers are directly responsible for ensuring a patient receives his or her medication(s). Advise them to deal with only one pharmacy, if possible. If consistent compliance is desired, educate the parents about correct drug dosage, timing, administration technique, blood levels, adverse drug interactions, and prohibited foods and herbs. Inform the parents they must first discuss all changes in dose and medication type or drug withdrawal with the attending physician. If the attending physician is unavailable, advise the parents to ask for the doctor on call (locum tenens) and double-check with the pharmacist. Explain that abrupt withdrawal from some drugs can cause severe problems (e.g., neuroleptic malignant syndrome). Give the parents a written list of foods and herbs that could interact badly with the drugs. Parents' and guardians' attitude towards medication and therapeutic regimens highly influence their child. Utilize a translator, if necessary.

AVOIDING PREJUDICE IN PATIENT RESOURCE MATERIALS

The medical assistant often deals with patients who are not of his or her culture, race, religion, ethnicity, or socioeconomic status. **Multicultural skills** are, therefore, a job requirement for medical assistants in the United States. The *Ten Standards of Practice* require medical assistants to exercise compassion and place the welfare of the patient above all else. This means researching the specific cultures, learning their habits, traditions, and preferences. Remember that many immigrants in the United States continue their native practices from their country of origin. Utilize

Copyright © Mometrix Media. You have been licensed one copy of this document for personal use only. Any other reproduction or redistribution is strictly prohibited. All rights reserved. This content is provided for test preparation purposes only and does not imply an endorsement by Mometrix of any particular political, scientific, or religious point of view.

a translator to tailor existing English materials to the target population; do not merely translate material verbatim. Use street language if needed, and avoid medical jargon. To avoid prejudice in resource materials, review the *Patients' Bill of Rights* of 2010.

APPROPRIATE DOCUMENTATION OF PATIENT INSTRUCTION

Documentation of patient instruction should be done as soon as possible, including the date and time, a description of the instruction provided and the method used, the purpose, and the patient response. If a teaching plan is developed, this should be filed in the patient's record as well with a copy or record of any handouts or written instructions provided to the patient. In some cases of standardized instruction (such as wound care after a procedure), a checklist may be utilized to indicate the topics covered, but the checklist should also allow comments so that the medical assistant can indicate the effectiveness of the teaching. One method of assessing effectiveness is to have the person explain his or her understanding or do a return demonstration (such as for wound care). Follow-up should also be documented, such as when the patient returns to determine if the patient has demonstrated understanding or needs further instruction.

Copyright © Mometrix Media. You have been licensed one copy of this document for personal use only. Any other reproduction or redistribution is strictly prohibited. All rights reserved. This content is provided for test preparation purposes only and does not imply an endorsement by Mometrix of any particular political, scientific, or religious point of view.

Vital Signs

STABLE VITAL SIGNS

Stable vital signs (those maintained within the normal range for the individual's age) indicate good health (homeostasis). Ill or injured patients have vital signs outside the normal range. The severity of the illness or injury is often indicated by the variability of vital sign measurements. Wide variations mean the patient is unstable. Their vital signs should be checked every five minutes. For stable patients, vital signs can be checked less frequently, depending on the circumstance. The following parameters are considered vital signs:

- Pulse
- Respiration rate
- Blood pressure
- Oxygen saturation
- Temperature

PULSE

The pulse is a surge of blood through an artery that occurs when the heart contracts (during systole). The key **pulse points** are:

- **Apical**: Over the heart
- **Brachial**: In the elbow bend (most common site for palpation in children under 1 year)
- **Carotid**: In the neck (for pulse checks in unconscious patients; be sure to only palpate one side at a time to maintain perfusion to the brain)
- **Dorsalis pedis**: On top of the foot
- **Facial**: On the jaw under the mouth
- **Femoral**: In the groin (for pulse checks in unconscious patients)
- **Popliteal**: On the back of the knee
- **Posterior tibial**: On the back of the ankle
- **Radial**: On the anterior wrist below the thumb (most common site for palpation in patients older than 1 year)
- **Temporal**: On the temple
- **Ulnar**: On the anterior wrist below the little finger

Pulse **rate** varies by age:

Normal Resting Pulse Rate	Age
60-100 beats per minute	Adult
80-100 beats per minute	Child
100 beats per minute	Toddler
100-140 beats per minute	Infant under one year
up to 150 beats per minute	Newborn (neonate)

DISTAL PULSE AND PULSE DEFICIT

If a **distal pulse** cannot be felt in the patient's limbs, first utilize a doppler machine to find the pulse. If it still cannot be found, find the apical pulse in the chest. Count to the 5th rib space in the middle of the left side of the chest or midclavicular line. If the apical pulse is regular, count for 30 seconds and record the reading. If the apical pulse is irregular, count for a full minute and record the reading. Report an irregular pulse to the doctor to evaluate for possible pulse deficit. A **pulse deficit** occurs when the radial pulse in the wrist is slower than the apical pulse in the chest. A pulse

104

Copyright © Mometrix Media. You have been licensed one copy of this document for personal use only. Any other reproduction or redistribution is strictly prohibited. All rights reserved. This content is provided for test preparation purposes only and does not imply an endorsement by Mometrix of any particular political, scientific, or religious point of view.

deficit can indicate that the patient has weak heart contractions, which fail to transmit beats to the peripheral arterial system.

TACHYCARDIA AND BRADYCARDIA

Tachycardia is a pulse rate over 100 beats per minute, which may be caused by anxiety, fear, stress, pneumonia, anemia, low blood pressure, dehydration, fever, infection, hyperthyroidism, and heart conditions.

Bradycardia is a resting heart rate less than 60 beats per minute, which may be caused by a heart attack (MI), hypothermia, heat exhaustion, obstructive jaundice, skull fracture, malnutrition, hypothyroidism, and many adverse drug reactions. Olympic athletes may have bradycardia because their hearts are extremely efficient.

MEASURING RESPIRATIONS

Measuring respirations is done to assess the number of times per minute the patient breathes. Typically, when a person is made aware of his breathing, he does not breathe deeply or regularly. Do not tell the patient when measuring the respiration rate, as it may make them aware of their breathing and produce an inaccurate result. The ideal time to measure the patient's respiration rate is after checking the patient's pulse. Count the number of times the patient breathes, counting one rise and fall of the chest wall as one respiration. Count the number of breaths for one minute, noting the depth of the breath and any use of accessory muscles. Record the respiratory rate on the patient's chart.

INDICATIONS OF ABNORMAL RESPIRATIONS

The normal range for respiratory rate for adults is 12-20 breaths per minute. A number of factors may affect the rate of the patient's breathing. The patient may breathe more slowly if resting or if he is positioned on his back. Certain narcotics may also depress the respiratory drive, resulting in fewer breaths per minute. A rapid respiration rate may be caused by increased activity, pain, or stress. An elevated temperature or an infection may cause the patient's respiratory rate to be quicker. Other conditions, such as respiratory distress, fluid overload, or a heart attack, may also cause an elevated respiratory rate.

BLOOD PRESSURE

Increased blood pressure contributes to stroke and heart disease. Low blood pressure is associated with shock, trauma, bleeding, or severe infection. Blood pressure is defined by the following parameters:

- Normal adult blood pressure: Systole <120 mmHg, diastole <80 mmHg
- Prehypertension: Systole 120-129, diastole <80
- Hypertension stage 1: Systole 130-139, diastole 80-89
- Hypertension stage 2: Systole ≥140, diastole ≥90
- Hypotension (low blood pressure): 90/50 or less

Copyright © Mometrix Media. You have been licensed one copy of this document for personal use only. Any other reproduction or redistribution is strictly prohibited. All rights reserved. This content is provided for test preparation purposes only and does not imply an endorsement by Mometrix of any particular political, scientific, or religious point of view.

False BP reading can occur from the following:

- **Incorrect cuff size**: If the patient is obese, use a thigh cuff on the upper arm. Bariatric blood pressure cuffs also exist. If the patient is a child, use a pediatric cuff.
- **Deflating the cuff more rapidly** than 2–3 mmHg per second can inhibit the ability to accurately record both systole and diastole.
- **Venous congestion** makes it difficult to hear the blood pressure sounds. Elevating the patient's arm after positioning the cuff but before inflating it can decrease venous congestion.
- Loud **environmental noises**
- **Operator error**

ANEROID SPHYGMOMANOMETER

Blood pressure is measured as systolic and diastolic pressure by means of a stethoscope and an **aneroid sphygmomanometer** (portable blood pressure cuff). For example, if the reading is 120/80 mmHg, 120 is the systole, and 80 is the diastole. The first Korotkoff sound the medical assistant hears is the systole; the last Korotkoff sound is the diastole. Position the blood pressure cuff so it is 1-2 cm from the antecubital fossa and two fingers can slide between the cuff and the arm. The width of the cuff bladder should exceed the diameter of the patient's arm by 20% or more. Place the stethoscope's diaphragm over the patient's brachial artery of the same arm, and insert the earpieces into one's ears. Inflate the cuff quickly, in 7 seconds or less. Deflate the blood pressure cuff slowly, at a rate of 2-3 mmHg per second. Listen for the "lub" and "dub," while mentally noting the mmHg when each sound was made. Remove the cuff and stethoscope. Record the measurement in the patient's chart immediately.

OXYGEN SATURATION

Pulse oximetry non-invasively measures a patient's oxyhemoglobin (oxygen saturation) level using a small clip-like device with a light that measures the oxygen saturation of the site it is attached to. This is a painless method of monitoring an individual's respiratory status and perfusion over a period of time when attached continuously, or in a single moment as part of a physical assessment. Attach the oximeter sensor to one of the patient's first three fingers (index, middle or ring). If the patient's hands are damaged, use a toe or earlobe. Consider using the forehead, nose, or other parts of the foot only as a last resort. Normal range should fall between 95% and 100%, although patients with certain conditions, such as COPD, may have a chronically lower saturation. If a patient's oxygen saturation falls below normal range persistently, the medical assistant must inform the doctor that the patient is hypoxic. Many pulse oximeters also measure the patient's heart rate at the same time. A pulse oximeter is not accurate if the patient is very anemic, has poor circulation (due to being cold or having vascular abnormalities), is edematous, moves a lot, or wears artificial nails or very dark nail polish. Adjust the room temperature, lighting, and move electronic equipment to get a good reading.

Copyright © Mometrix Media. You have been licensed one copy of this document for personal use only. Any other reproduction or redistribution is strictly prohibited. All rights reserved.
This content is provided for test preparation purposes only and does not imply an endorsement by Mometrix of any particular political, scientific, or religious point of view.

BODY TEMPERATURE

A live patient's body temperature is measured to determine if he or she is storing and releasing heat properly, to detect abnormally high or low body temperatures, and to assess the effectiveness of some types of medications. The coroner measures temperature to determine time of death. Adult normal temperature ranges are as follows:

- Normal range: 97-99 °F (36.1-37.2 °C)
- Hypothermia (too cold): <95°F (<35 °C)
- Pyrexia (fever): >100.4 °F (>38 °C)
- Hyperpyrexia (lethal fever): >106.7 °F (>41.5 °C)

Temperature is at its lowest around 4:00 a.m. and highest around 6:00 p.m. Temperature spikes often occur after meals. Ovulation in women creates a temperature rise of 0.5-1.0 °F when measured before arising from bed in the morning (basal body temperature). Individual temperature differences in healthy people are due to the rate of metabolism. Patients with hypothyroidism tend to be cold. Body temperature differs at different sites. Normal oral temperature is 98.6 °F, while rectal temperature is 0.5-1.0 °F higher than oral temperature, and axillary temperature is usually 0.5-1.0 °F lower than oral temperature. Do not take the patient's oral temperature for 30 minutes after eating or drinking, as it will be raised with hot food, and lowered with cold drinks.

Copyright © Mometrix Media. You have been licensed one copy of this document for personal use only. Any other reproduction or redistribution is strictly prohibited. All rights reserved. This content is provided for test preparation purposes only and does not imply an endorsement by Mometrix of any particular political, scientific, or religious point of view.

Physical Examination

PHYSICAL EXAMINATION/HEALTH ASSESSMENT

Collect subjective data: Subjective data is the personal information that is given by the client, such as symptoms, feelings, perceptions, preferences, beliefs, values, and ideas. Subjective data includes biographical information, physical symptoms related to each body system, past health history, family health history, and personal health and lifestyle practices.

Collect objective data: Objective data is directly observed by the examiner, such as physical characteristics, measurements (blood pressure, heart rate, respiratory rate, temperature, height, weight), range of motion of joints, appearance, behavior, and results of laboratory testing. Objective data is obtained by general observation and by using the four physical examination techniques.

The **four physical examination techniques** include the following:

- **Inspection**: Involves looking at the patient and patient's body and determining color, shape, size, and abnormalities (such as scars, birthmarks, bruises, swellings, and other injuries)
- **Palpation**: Using the hands and fingers to touch and feel body parts, such as palpating the abdomen to feel for the liver margins
- **Percussion**: Tapping a part of the body with fingers or an instrument to test reflexes or to assess hollow organs (such as the lungs)
- **Auscultation**: Using a stethoscope to listen to the heart, the lungs, and the abdomen in order to assess for abnormalities

EXAMINATION POSITIONS

The following are positions for examination:

- **Supine**: A lateral/horizontal lying position, where the patient is lying on the back, face up. This position is utilized when examining the patient's abdomen.
- **Fowler's/Semi-Fowler's**: A sitting position where the patient is sitting upright at 90° (Fowler's) or leaning back slightly (Semi-Fowler's). This position is used when examining the patient's ears, nose, and throat, in addition to during dental procedures and the auscultation of the posterior lung lobes.
- **Trendelenburg**: Also known as shock position, where the patient is supine (face up) with the feet elevated and the head down. If the patient faints when his or her blood is drawn, then place him or her in a left side-lying Trendelenburg position to increase blood flow to the brain and reverse syncope. Place a patient with an air embolism from an IV in the Trendelenburg position to decrease the chance that the embolism will push further into the pulmonary circulation.
- **Sims**: A left side-lying position that often benefits the patient suffering with abdominal distension or ascites from liver disease.
- **Orthopneic**: Also known as the tripod position, the patient is seated upright and leaning forward to allow easy respiration. Avoid placing a patient with breathing difficulty (dyspnea) in the supine position (reclining on the back). The orthopneic position is good for EKG patients with labored breathing to minimize artifacts on the tracing.

Copyright © Mometrix Media. You have been licensed one copy of this document for personal use only. Any other reproduction or redistribution is strictly prohibited. All rights reserved.
This content is provided for test preparation purposes only and does not imply an endorsement by Mometrix of any particular political, scientific, or religious point of view.

SEATED POSITION

HIGH FOWLER'S POSITION

SEMI FOWLER'S POSITION

SUPINE POSITION

PRONE POSITION

SIMS POSITION

TRENDELENBURG POSITION

KNEE-CHEST POSITION

Copyright © Mometrix Media. You have been licensed one copy of this document for personal use only. Any other reproduction or redistribution is strictly prohibited. All rights reserved.
This content is provided for test preparation purposes only and does not imply an endorsement by Mometrix of any particular political, scientific, or religious point of view.

BODY POSITIONS AND DRAPING FOR TREATMENTS/SURGERY

Body positions utilized for treatments/surgical procedures may include:

- **Knee-chest**: The patient kneels on the exam table, placing the head and shoulders on the bed, with the head turned to one side. The trunk is elevated with a 90-degree angle between the body and the hips. The weight of the body is supported by the knees and chest.
- **Prone**: The patient lies face down with the abdomen touching the bed and the head turned to one side.
- **Lithotomy**: Patient lies flat on back (supine) with feet and legs elevated in stirrups, exposing the genital area for examination or treatment of the urogenital organs and anus. The arms are extended alongside the trunk.
- **Dorsal recumbent**: The patient lies flat on the back with the knees bent and the feet resting flat on the bed so that the knees are elevated.

Draping depends on the position and type of procedure but should completely cover the patient until the procedure begins. Sterile draping should follow established protocol, exposing only the area that requires access.

PEDIATRIC EXAM

Components of a pediatric exam may vary somewhat according to the patient's age and size:

- **Height and weight**: The infant's height will be measured according to length with the infant lying in supine position.
- **Head circumference**: This is measured on infants and children until about 3 years of age to assess growth of the skull and indications of hydrocephalus (increased fluid in the brain).
- **Chest circumference**: This is also measured until about age 3. Under one year, the head circumference is usually 2-3 inches greater than chest circumference, but they equalize between ages 1 and 2.
- **Vital signs**: Apical pulse is used for children under 5; blood pressure is usually omitted on infants and small children. Oral temperatures are only taken on children ages 5 and older; tympanic or axillary temperature on infants, toddlers, and preschoolers; and rectal temperature on infants when necessary.
- **Eye examination**: A special Snellen Eye Chart with pictures or the letter E is used for small children.
- **Scoliosis exam**: Conducted between ages 8 and 10.
- **Immunizations**: The immunization record should be checked and appropriate immunizations administered.

Copyright © Mometrix Media. You have been licensed one copy of this document for personal use only. Any other reproduction or redistribution is strictly prohibited. All rights reserved. This content is provided for test preparation purposes only and does not imply an endorsement by Mometrix of any particular political, scientific, or religious point of view.

CHILD'S HEIGHT, WEIGHT, AND HEAD CIRCUMFERENCE

The child's height, weight, and head circumference are compared to a standard growth chart to obtain the child's percentile. For example, if the child's measurements fall within the 60th percentile for height, then he or she is taller than 60% of American children of the same age and he or she is shorter than 40% of American children of the same age. To collect the data, use the following techniques:

- If the child struggles, the medical assistant should hold him or her and step on the scale. The medical assistant can then subtract his or her weight from the total to obtain the child's weight in pounds or kilograms. One kilogram equals 2.2 pounds.
- For an infant or child unable to stand, lay the child face up on a measuring mat with his or her head gently touching the headpiece. Gently straighten the infant's leg and place the sliding foot positioner on the sole of the foot. If no adjustable measuring device is available, gently place the child's head against the wall, straighten the legs, and then place a tape measure against the wall and measure to the child's heels to obtain the height in inches or centimeters. One centimeter equals 0.39 inches.
- Always record occipital-frontal circumference (OFC) in centimeters. Place a non-stretchy tape measure above the eyebrows, extend it above the ears, and note the place where the ends meet at the back of the child's head.

OB-GYN EXAM

PELVIC EXAM/PAP SMEAR

The supplies needed for pelvic exam and Pap smear include the following:

- Gloves
- Vaginal speculum
- Lubricant
- Cervical brush, spatula, and/or combination cytobrush
- ThinPrep solution or slide with fixative.

The **procedure** is as follows:

1. Explain the procedure and verify that the patient is not menstruating and has not had a douche or sexual intercourse for at least 24 hours, as these activities may interfere with test results.
2. Ask the patient to empty bladder and undress below the waist or completely (if breast exam included) and put on a gown. Instruct the patient into lithotomy position with feet in stirrups and to cover with draping.
3. Warm the speculum and provide supplies to the physician/nurse practitioner, who will insert the vaginal speculum and scrape some cells from the cervix and place them in the ThinPrep solution or on a slide for examination.

The patient may experience slight discomfort and should be advised she may have slight bleeding after the procedure. The Pap smear will be normal (negative) or abnormal (positive), meaning that abnormal cells were found. The Pap smear may also be used to test for human papillomavirus but cannot be used to detect other sexually transmitted diseases.

Copyright © Mometrix Media. You have been licensed one copy of this document for personal use only. Any other reproduction or redistribution is strictly prohibited. All rights reserved. This content is provided for test preparation purposes only and does not imply an endorsement by Mometrix of any particular political, scientific, or religious point of view.

PRENATAL EXAMS

Supplies needed for prenatal exams (initial and subsequent) are same as for Pap smear and also include:

- Venipuncture supplies: tourniquet, collection tubes, syringe, gloves
- Pregnancy test, urine specimen container

The **procedure** is as follows:

1. Obtain height, weight, and vital signs.
2. Obtain a clean-catch urine specimen and carry out dipstick urinalysis for glucose and protein.
3. Collect blood samples (if done in-house) for complete blood count; blood typing/Rh factor; syphilis; rubella titer; HIV, hepatitis B, and possibly hepatitis C titers; and blood chemistry. Complete pregnancy test.
4. Prepare, position, and drape patient and assist with pelvic exam, Pap smear, pelvimetry, vaginal cultures for STDs, and assessment of fetal heart rate and gestational age.

The physician/nurse practitioner should discuss fetal screening (triple or quad screen), timing of subsequent examinations, and procedures. At **subsequent visits** (usually every 4 weeks until month seven and then every 2-3 weeks), the fundal height, fetal heart rate, and fetal development will be assessed along with the mother's weight and urine for protein and glucose.

- Elevate head of examining table 15-25° to prevent hypotension.
- Assist with vaginal exam if discharge or spotting has occurred.
- Set up ultrasound if used to assess fetus.

POSTNATAL EXAM

Supplies needed for postnatal exam (usually at 6 weeks postpartum) include:

- Gloves
- Venipuncture supplies
- Vaginal speculum
- Lubricant
- Contraceptive supplies (if indicated)

The **procedure** is as follows:

1. Obtain height, weight, and vital signs.
2. Ask patient about lochia and cramping or other discomfort.
3. Collect blood sample (if done in-house) for hemoglobin and hematocrit.
4. Ask the patient to undress from the waist down or completely (if doing a breast exam), put on a gown, and position on examining table with drape.
5. Assist physician/nurse practitioner with pelvic exam.
6. Assist physician/nurse with insertion of contraceptive device if the patient wishes either procedure:
   a. **Contraceptive implant device**: Expose upper arm, and set up sterile field with antiseptic, syringe with needle, local anesthetic, contraceptive implant trocar kit, gauze pads, and tape.
   b. **IUD**: As for pelvic exam but with sterile field and antiseptic, uterine tenaculum, uterine sound, sterile scissors, and IUD kit.

Copyright © Mometrix Media. You have been licensed one copy of this document for personal use only. Any other reproduction or redistribution is strictly prohibited. All rights reserved. This content is provided for test preparation purposes only and does not imply an endorsement by Mometrix of any particular political, scientific, or religious point of view.

PROCTOLOGY EXAM

Examination of the anus, rectum, sigmoid, and colon is generally carried out after a GI prep that typically includes laxatives and sometimes enemas to cleanse the bowel of fecal residue. Patients are typically positioned in the left Sims position. Elements of **proctology** include:

- **Proctoscopy**: A 10- to 12-inch instrument 1 inch in diameter is used to examine the anus and rectum. It is commonly used to examine for the cause of rectal bleeding, presence of hemorrhoids and indications of rectal cancer. It may also be used to obtain a biopsy and identify or remove polyps or other abnormalities.
- **Sigmoidoscopy**: Longer (extends about 20"), thinner (1/2") and more flexible than the proctoscope, the sigmoidoscope is used to examine the rectum and the sigmoid colon. The sigmoidoscope includes a distal light and camera. Use is similar to proctoscope.
- **Colonoscopy**: Similar to the sigmoidoscopy but longer (50-64 in) so that examination of the entire colon is possible. Used for diagnostic purposes and for removal of polyps.

CYSTOSCOPY

Cystoscopy assesses the urethra, bladder, and associated structures using an endoscope. It is used to diagnose urinary problems, such as cancer, retention, infections, obstruction, strictures, and bleeding. Tissue biopsy as well as irrigations or instillations may be done through the endoscope. The patient may be asked to fast or have a special diet before the test, and may also need to stop taking anticoagulants or aspirin for a period of time. The procedure may be done under a local anesthesia or with conscious sedation.

The **procedure** is as follows:

1. An intravenous line is inserted.
2. Patient is positioned in supine position with feet in stirrups.
3. A topical anesthetic gel is placed in urethral meatus with a catheter.
4. The cystoscope is inserted through the urethra into the bladder.
5. Sterile water or saline may be instilled in the bladder to allow better visualization.
6. A biopsy or urine specimen may be obtained.
7. Cystoscope is removed.

VISUAL ACUITY TESTING

To test an individual's visual acuity, both distance and near vision must be assessed. Start with the assessment of **distance vision**. Tape a line on the floor exactly 20 feet from a well-lit eye chart. Place the Snellen chart at the patient's eye level. Perform the test first with the patient's glasses or contact lenses in place. Position the patient at the floor line. Give the patient an eye pad or paper cup. Tell the patient to keep both eyes open, but to cover the right eye with the pad or cup. Stand beside the eye chart and point to the letters. Ask the patient to read the letters aloud, line by line, from the top down. The line on which a patient makes an error is his or her visual acuity for distance. Record the reading beside the line in the patient's chart (e.g., 20/50). The top number is the distance the patient stands from the chart, 20 feet. The bottom number indicates the distance from which a person with normal vision could read the same line. For example, a patient with 20/40 vision can read the line 20 feet away that a person with normal sight can see clearly from 40 feet away. Repeat with the left eye. Tell the patient to remove his/her glasses or contact lenses. Provide a sink, soap, towel, lens case and saline, if the patient with contacts requires them. Repeat the test without glasses or contact lenses.

To test **near vision**, repeat the test with a Jaeger card held 14 inches from the patient's face.

Copyright © Mometrix Media. You have been licensed one copy of this document for personal use only. Any other reproduction or redistribution is strictly prohibited. All rights reserved. This content is provided for test preparation purposes only and does not imply an endorsement by Mometrix of any particular political, scientific, or religious point of view.

REFRACTIVE ERRORS OF VISION

Normal visual acuity (VA) is 20/20, meaning the patient can read the eighth line down on a Snellen eye chart from a distance of 20 feet away. The **refractive errors of vision** that may obstruct this vision include the following:

- **Myopia**: The patient sees nearby objects clearly but objects in the distance are blurry because the eye is too long. The patient can read the Jaeger card but not the Snellen wall chart and requires glasses for driving and distance vision.
- **Presbyopia**: Around age 45, the aging patient's lenses become inelastic and his or her eyes do not focus well on nearby objects. The patient can see the Snellen wall chart well, but not the Jaeger card, and requires reading glasses.
- **Hyperopia**: The eye may be too small or the focusing power too weak, so the patient is unable to see objects nearby (far-sighted). The patient can read the Snellen chart, but not the Jaeger card, and requires glasses.
- **Astigmatism**: The patient's cornea and/or lens are not smooth; they have irregular curvatures, with flat and steep sections that blur sections of the visual field.

COLOR BLINDNESS AND ISHIHARA TEST

Color blindness is an inherited condition affecting 12% of men of European descent and 0.5% of women. There is no treatment, but the patient can wear glasses with red-orange filters to see cooked meat and ripe fruit. An **Ishihara test** measures Color Vision Deficiency (CVD) in a patient's sight. Color blindness is an inaccurate term because there are degrees of color loss. Many people with excellent visual acuity can see some colors but cannot distinguish differences in complementary colors, such as red and green or blue and yellow. Some people see colors well in one eye but not in the other. Seeing totally in shades of gray is a very rare condition. The U.S. Army uses colorblind people to detect camouflage. At night, colorblind people tend to see better than people with normal vision. To test for color blindness, the medical assistant seats the patient in a well-lit room and holds 10 Ishihara plates 75 centimeters (almost 30 inches) from the patient's eyes. The plates look like dotted discs from a distance. A number is hidden in the dots that colorblind people cannot see. The individual is asked to read the number on each plate in order to determine which colors, if any, the individual is unable to see.

AUDIOLOGY TESTING

Audiology testing measures the ability of the patient's inner ear to hear sounds through varying degrees of loudness (intensity) and vibration speed (tone). The audiometer measures **intensity** in decibels (dB) and **tone** in hertz (Hz or cycles per second).

A whisper is 20 Hz and 20 dB. Prolonged sounds louder than 85 dB cause hearing loss. A loud concert is 100 dB. The bass plays at 50 Hz, and the high violin plays at 10,000 Hz. Normal hearing range is 20-20,000 Hz. Speech ranges from 500-3,000 Hz.

If an adult cannot hear a ticking watch or a whisper, he or she needs an audiology test, which takes about 10 minutes. The doctor taps a tuning fork and holds it on the sides of the patient's head to find if the sound conducted through air is heard. The tuning fork is also held behind the patient's ear on the mastoid bone and tapped to find if the sound conducted by vibration through bone is heard. The medical assistant conducts the portion of the hearing test with the audiometer by placing earphones on the patient, connecting them to the audiometer, and attaching a bone oscillator to the patient's mastoid bones. Pure tones are emitted through one earpiece at a time, and the intensity is controlled by the medical assistant. The patient either raises one hand or presses a button when he or she hears a tone. The minimum intensity the patient needs to hear each tone is

Copyright © Mometrix Media. You have been licensed one copy of this document for personal use only. Any other reproduction or redistribution is strictly prohibited. All rights reserved. This content is provided for test preparation purposes only and does not imply an endorsement by Mometrix of any particular political, scientific, or religious point of view.

recorded on a graph. The patient should be able to hear 250-8,000 Hz at 25 dB or lower. If he or she cannot hear below 25 dB, then hearing loss is present.

PULMONARY FUNCTION TESTS

Pulmonary function tests (PFTs) measure how much air the patient's lungs can hold, how fast air can be moved in and out of the patient's lungs, and how well the lungs retain oxygen and discard carbon dioxide. Use an interpretation table, because PFT varies by age, body mass, gender, and race. Seat the patient. Place a clip over his or her nose. The patient inhales to full capacity and exhales completely into a spirometer for 6 seconds. Repeat twice and take the best reading out of three, measured in liters.

- **Tidal volume** (TV) is the volume of one normal inhalation and exhalation.
- **Inspiratory reserve volume** (IRV) is the most volume the patient can inhale after a complete breath.
- **Expiratory reserve volume** (ERV) is the most volume a patient can exhale forcefully after one normal exhalation.
- **Residual volume** (RV) is the amount of air remaining in the lungs after the patient exhales forcefully.
- **Minute volume** (MV) is the air inhaled and exhaled in one minute of normal breathing.
- **Vital capacity** = TV + IRV + ERV
- **Total lung capacity** = TV + IRV + ERV + RV

INTRADERMAL SKIN TESTING

Intradermal skin testing is often done to test for TB and allergies. Injections are given with the needle bevel facing upward and inserted slowly at a 10-15° angle under the skin without aspiration. When the fluid is injected, a wheal should form and then the needle slowly withdrawn, leaving the wheal intact. The skin may be gently patted with a swab but pressure should not be applied to the wheal.

ALLERGY TESTING

When preparing to do an allergy skin test on a patient, wait until the patient's serology results come back from the lab because skin pricking could cause an antibody reaction that would result in a false positive outcome. Check the patient's existing allergy alerts recorded in the chart, particularly for latex and contrast dye, before proceeding. Keep an Epi-pen handy, in case the patient has an anaphylactic reaction. Ask the patient if he or she is taking antihistamines (e.g., Benadryl), which invalidate the results. Use a drop of normal saline on the skin as a negative control and histamine as a positive control. Follow a template for applying allergens to the skin (pollen, dander, mold, etc.) so they are recognizable after application. Scratch each application site gently with a separate needle. Wait 15 minutes. If the skin reddens at a scratch site, there is an IgE antibody on mast cells and the patient is allergic to the substance.

ALLERGY INJECTIONS

Allergy injections are administered to build tolerance to the substance causing an allergic response. Dosages of allergens are calculated individually and administered in slowly increasing dosages. Injections are subcutaneous with a 28-gauge, 1/2-inch allergy syringe because IM injection increases the risk of severe reaction. Patients must be observed for 20-30 minutes after injections so that emergency treatment can be administered if an allergic reaction occurs (rash, edema, itching, shortness of breath). Injections are usually administered 2 times weekly for about 15 weeks and then monthly for about 5 years.

Copyright © Mometrix Media. You have been licensed one copy of this document for personal use only. Any other reproduction or redistribution is strictly prohibited. All rights reserved. This content is provided for test preparation purposes only and does not imply an endorsement by Mometrix of any particular political, scientific, or religious point of view.

Procedures

EYE IRRIGATION

The **supplies** required for eye irrigation include the following:

- Gloves
- Sterile irrigant solution
- Irrigating syringe or water pick
- Basin
- Disposable underpad
- Sterile gauze
- Towel

The following is the **procedure** for performing eye irrigation:

1. Wash hands.
2. Ask the patient to remove glasses or contact lenses.
3. Position the patient lying down and turned to the side of the eye to be irrigated or, if sitting, with the head turned to the affected side. Place a disposable underpad and towel under the patient's head or on the patient's shoulder if sitting.
4. Place a curved basin beside or beneath the affected eye (ask patient to help hold in place if sitting).
5. Wash hands again and apply gloves.
6. Cleanse eye from inner canthus to outer with damp gauze.
7. Prepare irrigating syringe or water pick and hold eye open with thumb and index finger.
8. Ask the patient to look upward or stare at fixed point and begin the irrigation from the inner to the outer canthus, allowing the solution to flow over the eye and into the basin, usually using about 500 mL solution.
9. Wipe eyelids with dry gauze from inner to outer canthus.
10. Discard supplies.

EAR IRRIGATION

The **supplies** required for ear irrigation include the following:

- Gloves
- Irrigating syringe or Elephant ear wash
- Curved basin
- Irrigating solution
- Disposable underpad
- Towel
- Cotton balls
- Otoscope

The following is the **procedure** for performing ear irrigation:

1. Wash hands and apply gloves.
2. Warm the prescribed solution to body temperature.
3. Check ear with otoscope if indicated to check location of earwax.
4. Position the patient in sitting position with their head tilted to affected side.
5. Place a disposable underpad and towel on the patient's shoulder.

Copyright © Mometrix Media. You have been licensed one copy of this document for personal use only. Any other reproduction or redistribution is strictly prohibited. All rights reserved. This content is provided for test preparation purposes only and does not imply an endorsement by Mometrix of any particular political, scientific, or religious point of view.

6. Prepare the syringe or elephant ear wash and check that the solution is as prescribed (may contain hydrogen peroxide and alcohol with water).
7. Hold a curved basin under the ear.
8. Insert the irrigating tip and begin irrigation, aiming solution toward the roof of the ear canal and catching the solution as it returns in basin.
9. Continue for the duration prescribed or until the earwax is removed.
10. Dry the outer ear with cotton balls.
11. Use the otoscope to check ear for irrigation effectiveness.
12. Assess the patient for dizziness or nausea.
13. Properly dispose of supplies and gloves.

NEBULIZER TREATMENTS

A nebulizer is a therapeutic device that allows the patient to inhale medication in mist form. The purpose of **nebulizer treatments** is to alleviate difficulty breathing (dyspnea) associated with lung diseases such as asthma, emphysema, lung cancer, and Chronic Obstructive Pulmonary Disease (COPD). Examples of nebulizer medication are Pulmicort Repsules (budesonide) and Atrovent (ipratropium). The medical assistant must check the regulations in the state in which they practice, as some states do not permit medical assistants to administer medication. Assist the RN in nebulizer administration by preparing the patient for treatment. Position the patient, clean and assemble the nebulizer apparatus, and encourage the patient in deep breathing and coughing exercises before and after treatment. Recognize side-effects of nebulizer therapy, including a rapid heart rate, dry mouth, and headache.

DRESSING CHANGE

The **supplies** required for a dressing change include the following:

*   Gloves (non-sterile)
*   Gloves (sterile)
*   Sterile dressings
*   Tape
*   Bandage scissors

The following is the **procedure** for performing a dressing change:

1. Wash hands and apply non-sterile gloves.
2. Place disposable underpad under the area of the wound if on an extremity or under the body if the wound is located on the chest, abdomen, or back.
3. Inspect the dressing for soiling, discharge, and loosened edges.
4. Cut the outer dressing with bandage scissors if necessary, loosen tape, and remove the dressing by pulling toward the center of the wound and lifting. Note any drainage on the inner dressing.
5. Examine the wound.
6. Remove gloves and wash hands.
7. Set up sterile field with all required dressing supplies.
8. Wash hands or use alcohol rub, and apply sterile gloves.
9. Cleanse the wound if prescribed.
10. Place the sterile dressing over the wound and utilize bandaging as appropriate for the site, securing the dressing with tape or other wrapping.
11. Dispose of all supplies, removed dressings, and gloves in a biohazard container.

Copyright © Mometrix Media. You have been licensed one copy of this document for personal use only. Any other reproduction or redistribution is strictly prohibited. All rights reserved. This content is provided for test preparation purposes only and does not imply an endorsement by Mometrix of any particular political, scientific, or religious point of view.

SUTURE/STAPLE REMOVAL

The **supplies** required for a suture/staple removal include the following:

- Gloves
- Suture removal kit or staple removal device
- Antiseptic as prescribed or NS
- Steri-strips, if necessary

The following is the **procedure** for performing a suture/staple removal:

1. Verify the type and number of sutures or staples in the patient's record.
2. Wash hands and apply non-sterile gloves.
3. Set up suture/staple removal kit and dressings if needed on sterile field.
4. Position the patient so that the wound is easily accessible.
5. Remove the dressing, if present.
6. Remove gloves, wash hands or use alcohol rub and apply sterile gloves.
7. Cleanse the incision with the prescribed solution or NS by wiping with dampened gauze or premoistened swabs.
8. Using forceps, lift the suture knots upward and hold them with one hand while slipping scissors underneath and clipping sutures with other hand.
9. Pull the sutures out using straight forceps and lay the removed sutures on gauze for counting.
10. If removing staples, slip the staple remover under the staples and press handle to compress and remove. Lay the staples on gauze for counting.
11. Cleanse the incision as prescribed and apply Steri-strips if indicated.
12. Apply a dressing if necessary, to protect the area; otherwise, leave open to air.
13. Verify the suture/staple count and dispose of all supplies, removed dressings, and gloves in a biohazard container.

SURGICAL PROCEDURES

SURGICAL TRAY PREPARATION

The **supplies** required for a surgical tray preparation include the following:

- Mayo stand
- Sterile surgical pack
- Sterile gloves or sterile transfer forceps

The following is the **procedure** for performing a surgical tray preparation:

1. Wash hands.
2. Adjust the height of Mayo stand.
3. Place the surgical pack on the Mayo stand and check its sterilization tape for color change and date.
4. Remove tape and pull the first flap away from body (the outer inch of wrap is considered unsterile). Pull the side flaps, grasping the corners only, and then pull the last flap toward the body. Do not allow the corners to fall back over the sterile field as they are now contaminated and any flap that has been below the sterile field is considered unsterile.

Copyright © Mometrix Media. You have been licensed one copy of this document for personal use only. Any other reproduction or redistribution is strictly prohibited. All rights reserved. This content is provided for test preparation purposes only and does not imply an endorsement by Mometrix of any particular political, scientific, or religious point of view.

5. If adding liquid to a container in the sterile field, open the bottle before donning sterile gloves. Grasp the bottle by the label side, remove the lid and place it open side up on counter. If the bottle was opened previously, pour a small amount of liquid into a waste container, such as an emesis basin.
6. Apply sterile glove to non-dominant hand and pick up sterile container into which liquid is to be poured and step back from the sterile field.
7. Pour liquid into container holding the bottle 2-6 inches above container, being careful not to touch the container or splash. Replace the sterile container onto the sterile field.
8. Recap the bottle with non-gloved hand.
9. Apply other sterile glove or open sterile pack of transfer forceps to move supplies about the sterile field.
10. Cover sterile field with sterile drape if not using immediately.

ANTISEPTIC SKIN PREP

Infection control prior to surgical procedures is critical in preventing dangerous postoperative complications. The procedure for **antiseptic skin preparation** includes the following:

1. Wash hands and ensure surgical attire covers arms. Open a sterile basin and pour solution or open package of pre-moistened antiseptic swabs.
2. Wash hands (again) or use alcohol rub and apply sterile gloves.
3. Prep the skin with the solution in circular motions from incision site outward or from the least contaminated area to most (such as toward anus) in a large enough area to accommodate any extension of incision.
4. Prep all surfaces of surgical site.
5. Allow the prepped surfaces to dry completely.
6. Remove the prep solution from the skin with sterile water and gauze sponge unless it is to be left on the tissue and dry with gauze sponge.
7. Apply draping, framing the surgical site on all four sides and placing a fenestrated (windowed) drape over the incision site.

SURGICAL ASSISTING IN NON-STERILE PROCEDURES

Responsibilities of the medical assistant when assisting in **non-sterile procedures** include the following:

- Reassure the patient
- Assist others in fastening gowns
- Obtain supplies and place them on the sterile field (using appropriate technique)
- Adjust lighting, facemasks, glasses for others
- Hold specimen containers

SURGICAL ASSISTING IN STERILE PROCEDURES

When assisting with sterile procedures, first the medical assistant must be familiar with sterile field boundaries. Areas with sterile drapes are sterile fields and anything within that field is sterile. The individual's sterile field, including hand position, is limited to above the waist and below the neck. Anything below the level of the operating table or sterile field is unsterile.

Copyright © Mometrix Media. You have been licensed one copy of this document for personal use only. Any other reproduction or redistribution is strictly prohibited. All rights reserved. This content is provided for test preparation purposes only and does not imply an endorsement by Mometrix of any particular political, scientific, or religious point of view.

Responsibilities of the medical assistant when **assisting in sterile procedures** include the following (the assistant may be gloved and gowned or just gloved, depending on the procedure):

- Ensure sterile field is not contaminated
- Pass instruments to physician and receive instruments
- Hold retractors
- Pass sponges to physician
- Take used sponges from physician and lay out for later counting
- Suction or sponge blood or drainage from surgical field
- Prepare suture/staple materials
- Apply dressing

COMMON SURGICAL INSTRUMENTS

Common surgical instruments that the medical assistant should be familiar with include the following:

Forceps	Tools used to hold, grasp, or pull tissue, supplies, or other instruments (such as a needle). The jaws may be blunt, sharp, or toothed. Hemostats are forceps with narrow jaws used to grasp blood vessels and control bleeding. Needle holders grasp needles during suturing. Foerster and Bozeman forceps grasp gauze sponges. Tissue and dressing forceps (like giant tweezers) grasp tissue or sponges. Splinter forceps with very sharp tips remove foreign bodies from tissue; ear forceps remove foreign bodies from ears. Tenaculum forceps have sharp curved points to grasp tissue. Biopsy forceps have a long rod that can pass through an endoscope and a cutting instrument at the end to take a tissue sample.
Scissors	Tools used to cut tissue and supplies. Metzenbaum and Mayo scissors have sharp straight blades. Spencer suture scissors have one straight blade and one curved at the end to hook sutures for removal. Lister bandage scissors are angled to slide under bandages with a blunt tip on the bottom blade.
Scalpels/Blades	Surgical knives used to cut tissue. A straight scalpel/blade is used to make an incision and a curved scalpel/blade to excise tissue. Scalpels may be disposable or have reusable handles with disposable blades.
Retractors	Tools used to hold wounds open with smooth, toothed, or rake-like tips. Retractors come in various sizes and shapes and some are self-retaining.
Probes/Sounds	Long thin tools used to probe a wound to show depth and identify foreign objects.
Curettes	Instruments with a metal loop at the end to scrape tissue, such as to remove fetal tissue or to remove earwax.
Endoscopes	Instruments used to examine the interior of a body cavity or hollow organ. There are many different types, but they generally have a long flexible tube with a light source and camera at the end. A laryngoscope examines the throat; a cystoscope, the bladder; and a colonoscope, the colon.

Copyright © Mometrix Media. You have been licensed one copy of this document for personal use only. Any other reproduction or redistribution is strictly prohibited. All rights reserved.
This content is provided for test preparation purposes only and does not imply an endorsement by Mometrix of any particular political, scientific, or religious point of view.

COMMON MEDICAL INSTRUMENTS

The medical assistant must have knowledge of the use of the following **medical instruments**:

Catheter	Used to insert into a body part for drainage, most often into the bladder to drain urine or to obtain a urine specimen
Endoscope	Inserted into body openings (mouth, nose, urethra, rectum) to examine and to obtain a biopsy or carry out a minor operative procedure
IV start kits	Used to prepare the skin and insert an intravenous line
Kidney dish/basin	Used to collect fluids used in irrigations (such as of ear or eye) and for emesis
Nasogastric tube	Inserted through the nose and to the stomach for decompression and drainage; may also be used for gastric lavage
Otoscope	Used to examine the ear canal, the tympanic membrane, and the nares
Nebulizer	Nebulizers convert liquid medication into an aerosol that can be inhaled, such as for treatment of asthma and COPD
Sphygmo-manometer	Used to monitor patients' blood pressure, usually applied to the upper arm
Stethoscope	Used to listen to the heart, the lungs, the bowel sounds, and the carotid arteries

PREPARING PATIENT FOR SAFE MEDICAL IMAGING

Medical imaging includes x-rays (radiographs), CAT scan (computerized axial tomography), MRI (magnetic resonance imaging), ultrasound, and contrast and barium studies. **Preparing the patient for safe medical imaging** includes the following considerations:

- Check the patient's allergy alerts recorded in the chart, particularly for latex and contrast dye, and alert the radiology technologist (RT) if necessary.
- If the patient may be pregnant, perform a pregnancy test before imaging and inform the patient and RT if it is positive.
- Tell the patient to wear loose, comfortable clothing. Explain that he or she may need to don a gown because metal snaps, zippers, buttons, and fasteners interfere with imaging.
- Dentures, hearing aids, eyeglasses, hairpins, credit cards, watches, jewelry, and keys must be placed in the locker provided or left with an attendant because they interfere with imaging.
- Metal jewelry worn in body piercings and new tattoos are dangerous because they heat up during MRI scans. The patient must remove the jewelry and may need to wait until the dye of a new tattoo becomes safe before imaging.
- Contact the RT for specific directions that vary by test and relay them to the patient (e.g., fast 8 hours, drink a liter of water, take a laxative and enema the night before).

Copyright © Mometrix Media. You have been licensed one copy of this document for personal use only. Any other reproduction or redistribution is strictly prohibited. All rights reserved. This content is provided for test preparation purposes only and does not imply an endorsement by Mometrix of any particular political, scientific, or religious point of view.

Wound Care and Dressing Changes

CLASSIFICATION OF WOUNDS BY CAUSE

Wounds can be classified in various ways. The most common classification of wounds is that according to cause:

- **Vascular wounds:** Vascular changes can result in wounds that occur most commonly in the lower extremities, such as those that result from arterial insufficiency and ischemia, those that relate to changes in the lymphatic system, and those related to venous insufficiency.
- **Neuropathic wounds:** Neuropathic changes that occur with chronic diseases, such as diabetes, and chronic alcoholism can decrease sensation and circulation, resulting in ulcerations.
- **Pressure ulcers:** Shear friction and pressure, especially over bony prominences such as the sacral area and heels, causes erosion of the tissue.
- **Traumatic wounds:** Trauma often results in contaminated wounds.
- **Surgical wounds:** Surgery can result in wounds that are originally contaminated or originally clean, depending upon the type of surgery and the reason.
- **Infected wounds:** Inflammation and infection may result in deteriorating wounds or fistulas.
- **Self-inflicted wounds:** Vary widely, from minor cuts to traumatic gunshot wounds.
- **Dysfunctional healing wounds:** Hypergranulation/keloid formation can change the character of a wound and prevent adequate healing.

STAGING SYSTEM FOR PRESSURE ULCERS

The National Pressure Injury Advisory Panel developed a staging system to ensure that definitions for pressure ulcers were standardized.

- **Stage I: Non-blanchable erythema**: Intact, reddened area that does not blanch.
- **Stage II: Partial thickness**: Destruction of the epidermis and/or dermis. This type of injury may be an intact blister, ruptured blister, or an open ulcer if it has a pinkish or a reddish wound bed.
- **Stage III: Full thickness skin loss**: Epidermis and dermis have experienced loss and the injury now extends through to the subcutaneous fat tissue.
- **Stage IV: Full thickness tissue loss**: Damage has progressed to the bone, muscle, or tendons.
- **Unstageable/Unclassified**: Injury is present and involves full thickness, but cannot be staged until slough is removed.
- **Suspected Deep Tissue Injury**: Discolored skin that is still intact but has been damaged. The injury is likely deeper than a stage one injury, but the epidermis is still intact, and therefore the depth cannot be visualized.

Copyright © Mometrix Media. You have been licensed one copy of this document for personal use only. Any other reproduction or redistribution is strictly prohibited. All rights reserved. This content is provided for test preparation purposes only and does not imply an endorsement by Mometrix of any particular political, scientific, or religious point of view.

STAGE I   STAGE II   STAGE III

STAGE IV   SUSPECTED DEEP TISSUE INJURY   UNSTAGEABLE/ UNCLASSIFIED

FACTORS THAT AFFECT SKIN'S ABILITY TO HEAL

AGE

Age is an important consideration when evaluating the skin because the characteristics of the skin change as people age. An infant 's skin is thinner than an adult's because, while the epidermis is developed, the dermis layer is only about 60% of that of an adult and continues to develop after birth. The skin of premature infants is especially friable, allowing for transepidermal water loss and evaporative heat loss. During adolescence, the hair follicles activate and the thickness of the dermis decreases about 20% and epidermal turnover time increases, so healing slows. As people continue to age, Langerhans' cells decrease in number, making the skin more prone to cancer, and the inflammatory reactions decrease. The sweat glands, vascularity, and subcutaneous fat all decrease, interfering with thermoregulation and contributing to dryness and irritation of the skin. The epidermal-dermal junction flattens, resulting in skin prone to tearing. The elastin in the skin degrades with age and solar exposure. The thinning of the hypodermis can lead to pressure ulcers.

LOTIONS, OILS, AND SOAPS

Lotions, oils, and soaps all have an effect on the skin. Many oils and lotions are used to increase hydration of the skin. These can include oil baths, which have a minimal effect on hydration but do increase the skin-surface lipids. Lipids are the fatty substances that surround skin cells, and those in the outer layer of skin, the stratum corneum, with fatty acids form the water barrier to retain skin hydration and soften skin. Sebum, produced by the sebaceous glands, is also a lipid. Applying lotion increases the hydration of the epidermis, giving the skin a smoother appearance, and moisturizing lotions also increase the lipids, providing some protection. Alkaline soaps, on the other hand, removes the lipid coating of the skin for about 45 minutes after a normal washing and may increase dryness and susceptibility to bacterial infection. Alcohol and acetone also remove the lipid coating and can increase dehydration of the skin. Acidic cleaners are less irritating than either neutral or alkaline cleaners.

Copyright © Mometrix Media. You have been licensed one copy of this document for personal use only. Any other reproduction or redistribution is strictly prohibited. All rights reserved. This content is provided for test preparation purposes only and does not imply an endorsement by Mometrix of any particular political, scientific, or religious point of view.

SUN EXPOSURE

Sun exposure is one of the primary factors in aging of the skin, referred to as photoaging or dermatoheliosis. Tanning occurs when ultraviolet radiation (UVR) damages the epidermis and stimulates the production of melanin as a protective mechanism to prevent damage to deeper layers of skin. When the melanin is overpowered, sunburn results, damaging the outer layers of the skin and sometimes the DNA of the skin cells, which can lead to cancer. There are several effects of photoaging that should be noted in assessment:

- Decrease in elasticity and strength
- Dry, rough, wrinkled skin
- Fine veins on face and ears
- Freckles and large brown macules (solar lentigines, liver spots) on face, and exposed areas, such as hands and arms and white macules on exposed areas of upper and lower extremities
- Benign lesions, such as actinic and seborrheic keratoses
- Malignant lesions, such as basal cell and squamous cell carcinoma

MEDICATIONS

Medications are a frequent cause of dermatologic effects that can impair the integrity of the skin:

- **Photosensitivity** can be either photoallergic with exposure to ultraviolet radiation causing an allergic reaction, usually with rash, erythema, edema, and pruritis or phototoxic with the drug being converted into a toxin that causes edema, pain, and pronounced erythema. Thiazide diuretics and conjugated estrogens often cause photosensitive reactions.
- **Allergic reactions** may involve rash, urticaria or more complex reactions, such as serum sickness. Amoxicillin alone or with clavulanate causes a high rate of these reactions.
- **Erythema multiforme** has been caused by nifedipine, verapamil, and diltiazem (calcium channel blockers).
- **Toxic epidermal necrolysis** with full-thickness loss of epidermis can be caused by ciprofloxacin.
- **Thinning or atrophy of the skin** because of a loss of collagen and telangiectasia (spider veins) are associated with oral, topical, and inhaled corticosteroids.

LOCAL FACTORS

Local factors that may impact the healing process include:

- **Local infection**: Invasion of the wound by microorganisms, such as *Staphylococcus aureus, MRSA, Pseudomonas,* and *Escherichia coli,* not only slows healing but may cause the wound to erode and increase in size, increasing the risk of systemic infection. Inflammation is a normal part of the healing process, but prolonged inflammation delays healing.
- **Repeat trauma**: If a wound is not adequately protected or if the patient is not positioned correctly, further erosion of the wound may occur.
- **Impaired tissue oxygenation**: Conditions that result in vasoconstriction or low blood flow to the area (such as PAD, blood clot, and hypotension) of the wound can impair healing or worsen the wound. Wounds are typically hypoxic initially because of disruption of blood flow and increased need for oxygen, but this triggers angiogenesis and release of growth factors, which should increase oxygenation unless other factors are present.

Copyright © Mometrix Media. You have been licensed one copy of this document for personal use only. Any other reproduction or redistribution is strictly prohibited. All rights reserved. This content is provided for test preparation purposes only and does not imply an endorsement by Mometrix of any particular political, scientific, or religious point of view.

SYSTEMIC FACTORS

Systemic factors that may impact the healing process include:

- **Inadequate nutrition:** A diet with adequate nutrition and protein is necessary for healing, so inadequate diet may slow the healing process.
- **Obesity**: Patients who are overweight are at increased risk of pressure sores because of compression of tissues, and have slower rates of healing as well as increased risk of infection.
- **Chronic disease**: Some diseases, such as diabetes mellitus and hypertension may impair healing.
- **Systemic infection**: Whether originating from the wound or elsewhere, a systemic infection impairs healing
- **Decrease in sex hormones** (usually associated with age): Low levels of androgens and estrogen slow healing of wounds.
- **Stress**: Emotional stress increases glucocorticoids and reduces cytokines at the wound, impairing healing.

CLOSURE OF DEAD SPACE

Dead space is the defect of soft tissue left behind after debridement or excision of a space-occupying lesion. Dead space may also occur if portions of the wound separate beneath the skin after primary closure, leaving an open pocket if air/fluid becomes trapped between tissue layers. Closure of the dead space is essential because it promotes healing and decreases the risk of infection. Treatment options vary depending on the location, extent of the dead space, and the cause, but may include application of a compression bandage (using care not to apply excessive pressure that may impair oxygenation), insertion of a drain (open or closed, active or passive), and/or aspiration of fluid contents (seroma) of the dead space. Negative pressure wound therapy may be utilized for large wounds. Dead spaces open to the surface should be completely filled with suitable wound packing material (depending on the extent of drainage) but should be lightly packed so as to avoid pressure on healthy tissue. Patients may need to restrict activity during treatment for dead space.

WOUND EDGE OPTIMIZATION

Chronic wounds may take weeks or months to heal, so wound edge optimization is essential to healing. If the wound edges are not advancing or there are indications of undermining or deterioration, this may indicate that the wound cells are nonresponsive and that there are abnormalities of protease activities. Wound optimization methods include careful wound assessment and adequate debridement of the wound to remove necrotic tissue through sharp excision or enzymatic debridement, such as with collagenase, which debrides and promotes epithelialization. Maintaining appropriate moisture balance is also important as excessive moisture may cause maceration and deterioration of the wound while inadequate moisture may result in desiccation of the wound and slowed epithelialization. The choice of dressing, therefore, may affect the healing process. If infection occurs appropriate antimicrobials (systemic or topical) may be necessary. In some cases, bioengineered skin or skin grafts may be appropriate. Additionally, edema slows healing and increases the risk of bacterial colonization and must be controlled, such as through compression therapy. Wound exudate should be controlled because exudate, especially with chronic wounds, depresses cell proliferation (fibroblasts, keratinocytes).

Copyright © Mometrix Media. You have been licensed one copy of this document for personal use only. Any other reproduction or redistribution is strictly prohibited. All rights reserved. This content is provided for test preparation purposes only and does not imply an endorsement by Mometrix of any particular political, scientific, or religious point of view.

MAINTAINING A WARM AND MOIST WOUND ENVIRONMENT

One of the basic principles of current wound care is the use of occlusive dressings that keep the wound warm and moist. There are a number of reasons for keeping a healing wound warm and moist:

- **Reduction in dehydration** allows cells such as neutrophils and fibroblasts to carry out their functions in wound repair, as they require a moist environment. This also results in less cell death.
- **Angiogenesis** requires a moist environment and low oxygen tension, which is found in occlusive dressings.
- **Autolytic debridement** with proteolytic enzymes is enhanced in a moist environment.
- **Re-epithelization** of tissue occurs because the epidermal cells are able to spread across the surface of the wound.
- **Reduction in microorganisms** because of the seal provided by occlusive dressings decreases infection.
- **Pain reduction** results from the protection of the nerve endings and the need for fewer dressing changes.

PERIWOUND SKIN PROTECTION

The area extending about 4 cm from the wound edges is the periwound tissue and it is especially vulnerable to irritation from drainage and adhesive. The periwound tissue should be evaluated for increased warmth and erythema as well as signs of maceration from exposure to exudate. Moisture-associated and adhesive associated skin damage can be prevented and treated by gentle cleansing of the periwound tissue with NS or water and application of a skin barrier. Moisture-retentive dressings help to keep the wound surface moist but avoid excessive wetness and can wick fluid away from the periwound tissue. Dressing changes should be minimized to prevent stripping of periwound skin. Barriers may include:

- **Alcohol-based skin sealants**: Provide a sticky surface to help adhesives adhere and provide some skin protection. Available in wipes and spray.
- **Creams/Ointments**: May contain petrolatum, zinc oxide or dimethicone and are applied in a thin layer to the skin and covered with absorptive dressings or applied in the perineal area to prevent skin irritation from incontinence.
- **Topical corticosteroids**: Used for allergic reactions, such as to adhesives.

WOUND CLEANSING WITH EACH DRESSING CHANGE

Microorganisms, contaminants, and cellular debris in a wound can significantly delay healing and increase inflammation. Antiseptics such as hydrogen peroxide, acetic acid, povidone-iodine, or sodium hypochlorite (Dakin solution) are toxic to developing fibroblasts and interfere with healing over time. They are sometimes used and rinsed with saline for a short period of time to control heavily infected wounds. The current standard is to use irrigation to deliver normal saline in a manner forceful enough to break the adhesion of debris to the wound bed yet gentle enough to prevent injury to developing cells. Pressures of at least 5-15 psi delivered by mechanical irrigators (such as pulsatile lavage) are needed for effective cleansing. Higher pressures can cause penetration of the fluid into tissues. When utilizing a needle and syringe for manual irrigation, the irrigation pressure is based on the size of both the needle and the syringe:

- Irrigation using a 12 mL syringe and a 22-gauge needle will deliver a force of 13 psi.
- The use of a 35 mL syringe and a 19-gauge needle will deliver 8 psi and is more effective than using a bulb syringe when mechanical irrigation is not available.

126

Copyright © Mometrix Media. You have been licensed one copy of this document for personal use only. Any other reproduction or redistribution is strictly prohibited. All rights reserved. This content is provided for test preparation purposes only and does not imply an endorsement by Mometrix of any particular political, scientific, or religious point of view.

CLEANSING A WOUND BY SOAKING

Soaking is a beneficial way to cleanse a wound that has a large amount of necrotic debris or contamination. Contamination must be removed from new wounds to avoid excess inflammation that will delay wound healing. Soaking softens any necrotic tissue and helps to ease it away from the healthy tissue at the bottom of the wound bed. It also helps to loosen contaminants that are embedded in the wound. Antiseptic agents should not be used in the soaking solution. Soaking may be accomplished using any container that will hold the wound area, or by whirlpool. The container must be disinfected well prior to and after the soaking. It may take several soaks to remove tough, dry eschar and once the necrotic material has been removed soaking should be discontinued, as it will then delay healing.

BASIC DRESSING REQUIREMENTS

The basic dressing requirements, regardless of the type, are the following:

- Maintain a moist environment in order to promote healing.
- Absorb wound drainage and preventing leakage.
- Increase wound temperature to promote healing.
- Provide a protective barrier to prevent mechanical injury to the wound.
- Provide a protective barrier to prevent colonization and infection with microorganisms.
- Allow exchange of gases and fluids.
- Retain and absorb odor of wound or drainage.
- Remove easily without causing additional trauma to the wound or disrupting the healing process.
- Debride wound of dead tissue and exudate.
- Provide protection without toxicity or causing sensitivity reactions.
- Provide a sterile protective covering for the wound.

The dressing that directly covers the wound may be inadequate to absorb large amounts of drainage, so sometimes additional secondary dressings are needed.

WOUND DRESSING SELECTION

The proper dressing for a wound may change over time depending on wound characteristics:

- The wound environment's moisture content may call for a dressing that either wicks away too much moisture or provides moisture to a dry wound to enhance epithelialization.
- Slough and dry eschar calls for a dressing that will enhance debriding.
- The presence of tunneling or undermining will require a packing material.
- Some wounds need dressings that are absorbent and deodorizing to control exudate.
- Control and prevention of infection is important in some wounds.
- Dressings must allow oxygen, water, and carbon dioxide to be exchanged between the environment and the wound.
- Dressings need to provide warmth as well.
- Dressings must not adhere to or harm the wound tissues but must be kept in place reliably without harming skin around the wound.

Copyright © Mometrix Media. You have been licensed one copy of this document for personal use only. Any other reproduction or redistribution is strictly prohibited. All rights reserved. This content is provided for test preparation purposes only and does not imply an endorsement by Mometrix of any particular political, scientific, or religious point of view.

CATEGORIES OF DRESSINGS AND METHODS OF SECURING DRESSINGS

Dressings are considered primary if they are next to the wound surface and secondary if they are used to cover the primary or to secure the dressing. There are three main types of dressings to consider when determining which will be the most effective for a particular type of wound:

- **Traditional topical dressings** that are used primarily to cover the wound, such as gauze and tulle.
- **Interactive dressings**, such as polymeric films, are generally transparent so that the wound can be observed and are permeable to water vapor and oxygen but provide an effective barrier for microorganisms, such as hyaluronic acid, hydrogel, and foam dressings.
- **Bioactive dressings** provide substances that directly promote wound healing, such as hydrocolloids, alginates, collagens, and chitosan.

Securing a dressing depends on the health of the surrounding skin and the type of dressing. Skin protection and tape may be appropriate. Some are self-adherent. Tubular dressings or wraps can help to secure dressings with fragile skin.

GAUZE DRESSINGS

Gauze dressings are made from cotton, rayon, or polyester, and are frequently used with primary closure where there is little or no exudate and the purpose is to provide protection of the partial or full-thickness wounds or those with cavities or tracts. They may be sterile or non-sterile. In the past they were used for wet to dry dressings, but wet to dry dressings have little use in current wound care unless the wound is very small because the gauze adheres to the wound and can disrupt granulation or epithelization. Wet to moist saline gauze dressings are sometimes used to treat wounds but are less effective than hydrocolloid dressings. Gauze dressings may be used as secondary dressings with another type of dressing in direct contact with the wound or as packing to fill dead space in combination with amorphous hydrogel or other dressings. When used to fill space, the gauze should be fluffed to avoid causing excess pressure.

TULLE OR IMPREGNATED GAUZE DRESSINGS

Tulle dressings, also known as paraffin gauze, (Jelonet®, Paranet®) are open weave gauze that are coated with paraffin so they do not adhere to the wound, but are suitable only for flat or shallow wounds. They may be useful for people with sensitive skin. When these are placed in contact with the wound, secondary dressings may be used to absorb exudate.

Impregnated gauze may contain antimicrobials, medications, nutrients, and moisture (such as normal saline). Commonly used gauzes are impregnated with petrolatum, zinc oxide, and iodoform. They are used for partial or full-thickness wounds or those infected or with cavities or tracts. The choice of gauze depends upon the needs of the wound. They should be loosely packed into cavities and avoid contact with intact skin as they may cause maceration because of the moisture content of the dressing. Exudate should be carefully monitored so dressings can be changed as needed.

Copyright © Mometrix Media. You have been licensed one copy of this document for personal use only. Any other reproduction or redistribution is strictly prohibited. All rights reserved. This content is provided for test preparation purposes only and does not imply an endorsement by Mometrix of any particular political, scientific, or religious point of view.

FOAM DRESSINGS

Foam dressings are made of semi-permeable hydrophilic foam and sheet forms may have an impermeable barrier. They come in a wide variety of sizes and shapes (wafers, rolls, pillows, films) depending upon the manufacturer. Some types have a charcoal layer to control odor. Foam dressings provide a warm, moist environment and provide cushioning. Foam dressings may be used for partial and full-thickness wounds. Non-sheet forms are used as packing and are appropriate for minimal to heavy exudate. When used as packing, a secondary non-occlusive dressing is secured over the foam. They are used for leg ulcers as well as pressure sores. Because they are intended for wounds with exudate in order to provide the appropriate environment for healing, they are not suitable for dry epithelializing wounds or those with eschar. Sheet forms can be used as secondary dressings with alginates, pastes, or powders. Some have adhesive borders. Foam dressings are changed every 2-7 days, depending on the dressing type and the wound.

SEMI-PERMEABLE FILM DRESSINGS

Semi-permeable film (OpSite®, Tegaderm®, Polyskin II®) dressings are composed of polyurethane with a coating of acrylic adhesive so the dressing will adhere to the skin. These types of dressings are frequently used over intravenous sites to allow observation of tissue. They are suitable only for shallow partial-thickness wounds that have little or no exudate because they are not able to absorb; therefore, they are not suitable for infected wounds. They are permeable to air and water vapor but provide a barrier to pathogenic agents and liquid. The tissue under the dressing is maintained in a warm moist environment, encouraging autolysis. The dressings are comfortable and may be left in place for up to 1 week although some people may develop local irritation from the adhesive. Semi-permeable film may be used as a protective dressing and is often used for stage I and II pressure ulcers.

ALGINATES OR OTHER FIBER GELLING DRESSINGS

Alginates (AlgiSite M®, Sorbsan®, Aquacel®, Hydrofiber®) are very absorbent dressings made from brown seaweed. Through ion exchange, they absorb drainage and form a hydrophilic gel that conforms to the size and shape of the wound, so they are useful for full-thickness wounds with moderate to heavy exudate or slough, such as pressure ulcers and cavity wounds, especially if there is undermining or tunneling. They are effective for infected and foul-smelling wounds. Alginates are sold in sheet form or fibers for packing. Alginate dressings or packing fibers are loosely packed into the wound to allow for swelling and then secured with a secondary dressing. They are usually changed once daily. Alginates serve to cushion and protect the wound as well as contain exudate. They are easier to remove than gauze dressings used for packing and cause less discomfort. Alginates need differing times to gel with some requiring 24 hours, so they are not interchangeable.

HYDROCOLLOID DRESSINGS

Hydrocolloids (DuoDerm®, Restore®, Tegasorb®) are sheets or wafers of absorbent adherent material with an occlusive coating so that they provide a barrier to moisture. They are used for clean granulating wounds that are partial and full thickness with minimal to moderate amounts of drainage. They may be used with pastes or alginates. Hydrocolloids come in various sizes and shapes and can be cut to fit, overlapping the wound by 2-3 cm. They are usually changed about every 2-5 days. Hydrocolloid material may be stiff and should be warmed between the hands to soften before application. Some hydrocolloids emit an unpleasant odor when active. Because the dressings are occlusive, infected wounds should be observed carefully for signs of infection with anaerobic bacteria. They may be used with compression for venous ulcers but are not recommended for third degree burns. Hydrocolloids may cause hypergranulation tissue to form.

Copyright © Mometrix Media. You have been licensed one copy of this document for personal use only. Any other reproduction or redistribution is strictly prohibited. All rights reserved. This content is provided for test preparation purposes only and does not imply an endorsement by Mometrix of any particular political, scientific, or religious point of view.

HYDROGEL DRESSINGS

Hydrogel dressings (AquaForm®, Curasol®, Hypergel®, Elastogel®, Vigilon®, Intrasite® gel) are produced in amorphous form, supplied in tubes, or impregnated in packing strip materials. They are also produced in sheet form, with or without adhesive border. The have a high moisture content with water or glycerin with hydrophilic sites allowing them to absorb exudate and provide a warm, moist wound environment. Hydrogels are used for partial and full-thickness wounds, dry to small amounts of exudate, necrotic and infected wounds. They are applied directly to the wound and provide rehydration and autolysis, effectively and quickly debriding the wound. They are usually used with a secondary dressing, such as gauze or films. Dressings may be changed every 1-3 days, depending upon the type of product used. Hydrogels are contraindicated for wounds with heavy exudate as the leakage may cause maceration of periwound tissue or candidiasis.

CONTACT LAYER DRESSINGS

Contact layers (Dermanet®, Mepitel®, Tegapore®) are composed of woven polyamide net and may be coated with silicone (Mepitel®). They adhere lightly to the wound but have pores that allow exudate to pass through to absorbent secondary dressings. They are particularly useful in wounds in which adherence of dressings to the tissue may pose problems, such as with abrasions, second degree burns, grafts, full-thickness granular wounds, and skin damaged by radiotherapy or steroids. They may be used with negative pressure wound therapy. They protect the wound base but are not recommended for shallow or dry wounds. Usually, the contact layer stays in place for up to a week while the secondary absorbent dressings are changed more often. If exudate is extremely viscous, it may not penetrate the net and can build up beneath the contact layer. Some types of contact layers may need to be kept moistened with normal saline so they don't adhere to the wound base.

COMPOSITE DRESSINGS

Composites are combination dressings that are frequently used to secure primary dressings or with other dressings, such as alginates. The material in composites varies from one dressing to another, but usually consists of some type of impermeable exterior barrier to prevent leakage of exudate, an absorptive layer (*not* alginate, foam, hydrocolloid, or hydrogel), a semi-adherent or non-adherent surface for covering the wound, and an adhesive rim to secure the dressing to the periwound tissue. Used alone, they are most suitable for partial or shallow full-thickness wounds but used with other dressings they are suitable for larger wounds with minimal to large amounts of exudate. A paper backing must be removed prior to application. They are usually changed about 3 times a week or more often if needed for wounds with larger amount of exudate.

ABSORPTIVE DRESSINGS AND WOUND FILLERS

Absorptive dressings (Surgipad®, Tendersorb®, ABD® pad, Exu-dry®) are composed of cellulose, cotton, or rayon fibers. Some have adhesive borders. They are highly absorptive and are intended for wounds that have moderate to heavy drainage. They are changed every 1-2 days.

Wound fillers (Biafine WDE®, DuoDerm® Sterile Hydroactive Paste, Multidex® Maltodextrin Wound Dressing) are composed of starch copolymers in numerous different forms, such as pastes, granules, beads, gels, and powders. They fill dead space in shallow wounds, hydrate, providing a warm moist environment, and absorb exudate. They soften necrotic tissue and aid debridement. Wound fillers are indicated for partial and shallow full-thickness wounds with minimal to moderate exudate and can be used for both infected wounds and uninfected wounds. They are used with secondary dressings, such as films and hydrocolloids. Wound fillers are not recommended for use in dry, eschar-covered, or tunneled wounds. Dressings are usually changed daily.

Copyright © Mometrix Media. You have been licensed one copy of this document for personal use only. Any other reproduction or redistribution is strictly prohibited. All rights reserved. This content is provided for test preparation purposes only and does not imply an endorsement by Mometrix of any particular political, scientific, or religious point of view.

WOUND POUCHES

Wound pouches (Convatec® Wound Manager, Hollister® Wound Manager) are adapted from ostomy appliances and work in a similar way to contain heavy exudate from fistulas, wounds, drains, and tubes. The pouches provide a skin barrier to protect the skin and a drainage spout so that the pouch can be attached to straight drainage and a bedside bag. The pouch provides odor control as well. The opening in the pouch is cut to fit around the wound and paste, such as Stomahesive®, is applied about the cut opening to ensure seal. The skin is usually wiped with a skin barrier prior to application, and any skin crevices are filled with paste. Forceps are used to feed drains or tubes through the opening of the pouch. Pouches are usually changed about every 4-7 days or when there is leakage or drainage under appliance.

Copyright © Mometrix Media. You have been licensed one copy of this document for personal use only. Any other reproduction or redistribution is strictly prohibited. All rights reserved.
This content is provided for test preparation purposes only and does not imply an endorsement by Mometrix of any particular political, scientific, or religious point of view.

Therapeutic Modalities

COMPLEMENTARY AND ALTERNATIVE MEDICINE

Complementary medicine is a group of diagnostic and therapeutic disciplines that is used in conjunction with conventional Western medicine. Examples of **complementary medicine** include acupuncture, aromatherapy, biofeedback, chiropractic, hypnosis, massage, naturopathy, nutrition therapy, osteopathic manipulation, qi gong, reflexology, Reiki, traditional Chinese medicine, and yoga. Complementary medicine is often useful to relieve pain after surgery when conventional Western methods are not sufficient. The complementary method acts to complement conventional medicine.

Alternative medicine is used instead of conventional Western medicine. Examples of alternative medicine include dietary supplements, herbs, magnet therapy, vitamin megadoses, and spiritual healing.

Complementary and alternative medicine (CAM) often lacks the support of scientific research studies, instead relying on anecdotal evidence. Patients should be encouraged to discuss their use of complementary and alternative treatments during the collection of their history due to the possible interactions that alternative methods (specifically herbal and dietary supplements) have with standard medications.

HEAT TREATMENTS

Externally applied **heat sources** penetrate only the superficial layers of the skin (1-2 cm after about 30 minutes) but are believed to relax deeper muscles by reflex, decrease pain, and increase metabolism (there has been evidence suggesting a 10% increase in oxygen consumption for every 1 °C increase in skin temperature). Therapeutic temperature range for heat therapy is 40-45 °C (104-113 °F). Various methods of heat therapy exist:

- **Hot packs** utilize dry heat (hot water bottles, microwaved heat packs, and heating pads). Hot packs are applied for 15-20 minutes at a time.
- **Moist heat packs**, such as cloth moistened with warm water, are placed on the skin and secured by several layers of towels to provide insulation, applied for 15-30 minutes at a time.
- **Paraffin (wax) baths** (at temperatures of 52-54 °C or 126-130 °F) involve the hand, foot, or elbow being dipped 7 times, cooling between dippings, and then wrapped with plastic and towels for 20 minutes.
- **Whirlpool baths** are used to increase circulation and promote healing. Water temperature is 35-40 °C (95-104 °F, adjusted for the individual) and should be deep enough to completely submerge the affected part. The body part should be cleaned with soap and water before immersion for about 20 minutes.
- **Heat lamps** provide deep heat that differs from superficial heat in that the heat penetrates 3-5 cm deep and is generated internally using ultrasound, short wave, and microwave diathermy rather than applied to the surface of the skin.

Copyright © Mometrix Media. You have been licensed one copy of this document for personal use only. Any other reproduction or redistribution is strictly prohibited. All rights reserved.
This content is provided for test preparation purposes only and does not imply an endorsement by Mometrix of any particular political, scientific, or religious point of view.

COLD TREATMENTS

Therapeutic cold treatment is used to cool the surface of the skin and underlying subcutaneous tissues in order to decrease blood flow, pain, swelling and metabolism. Initial response to cold therapy causes vasoconstriction to occur within the first 15 minutes, but if the tissues are cooled to -10 °C (14 °F), then the body responds with vasodilation. Cryotherapy affects sensory response so the person will at first feel cold, which progresses to burning, aching, and finally to numbness and tingling. Treatment is usually given for 15-30 minutes. Treatment options include:

- **Ice packs** such as refrigerated gel packs (-5 °C or 23 °F) or plastic bags filled with water and ice chips are applied directly to the skin for 10-15 minutes for superficial cooling and 15-20 minutes for greater penetration.
- **Cold compress**: A towel or heavy gauze compress is dipped in an ice and water slurry and then applied to the affected area to provide cold therapy, but this is best used only for emergency situations when ice packs are unavailable, as the compress must be changed frequently as the skin warms the towel rapidly.

RANGE-OF-MOTION EXERCISES

Range-of motion exercises are active or passive exercises intended to maintain mobility of joint, muscles, and tendons by moving the joints through all of their normal ranges:

- **Neck (pivot joint)**: Flexion, extension, lateral flexion, and rotation
- **Shoulder (ball and socket joint)**: Flexion, extension, abduction, adduction, circumduction, and external and internal rotation
- **Elbow (hinge joint)**: Flexion, extension, supination, and pronation
- **Wrist (condyloid joint)**: Flexion, extension, abduction, and adduction
- **Hands and fingers (condyloid and hinge joints)**: Flexion, extension, abduction, and adduction
- **Thumb (saddle joint)**: Flexion, extension, abduction, adduction, and opposition (touching finger tips)
- **Hip (ball and socket joint)**: Flexion, extension, abduction, adduction, circumduction, and internal and external rotation
- **Knee (hinge joint)**: Flexion and extension
- **Ankle (hinge joint)**: Flexion and extension
- **Foot (gliding joint)**: Eversion and inversion
- **Toes (hinge, gliding)**: Flexion and extension
- **Trunk (gliding)**: Extension, lateral flexion, and rotation

Copyright © Mometrix Media. You have been licensed one copy of this document for personal use only. Any other reproduction or redistribution is strictly prohibited. All rights reserved. This content is provided for test preparation purposes only and does not imply an endorsement by Mometrix of any particular political, scientific, or religious point of view.

First Aid, BLS, and Rapid Response Procedures

STANDARD CRASH CART EQUIPMENT

A standard crash cart contains a green oxygen tank, masks, airway options, a defibrillator, and resuscitation drugs. One crash cart should be available per floor. The location of each floor's crash cart should be known by all staff members. In an emergency, the medical assistant's duties are to:

- Tell the receptionist to call an ambulance (911) and notify the doctor, or if there is no receptionist, the medical assistant should handle these tasks directly.
- Place the patient in recovery position (side-lying) while retrieving the crash cart, or staying with the patient in recovery position while directing another staff member to retrieve the crash cart.
- Reposition the patient in the Trendelenburg position, lying on the back with feet raised above chest level if they are dizzy or briefly loss consciousness but are otherwise arousable.
- Apply direct pressure to a wound to stop bleeding, if necessary.
- Position the nasal cannula over the patient's ears, or into the nares, with tubing to the side. If utilizing a mask, it should fully cover the nose and mouth. Fasten the mask firmly. Administer oxygen immediately, from 2-4 L/min. If the patient is still conscious, encourage slow deep breaths, inhaling and exhaling fully.
- Try to calm and comfort the patient. Cover the patient with a blanket to help prevent shock. Screen the patient from public view.
- Palpate the radial pulse if the patient is not responsive. If no pulse is present and the patient is not breathing, initiate CPR, starting with 30 compressions, followed by 2 rescue breaths.
- The doctor or registered nurse will intubate the unconscious patient and administer resuscitation drugs. Assist as required.
- If there is no receptionist, wait at the door to guide the ambulance attendants to the patient.

AED

An **automated external defibrillator (AED)** can revive an individual that is in specific types of cardiac arrest, providing it is applied within four minutes and damage is not extensive. Continue CPR until the unit is charged. The patient must be on a flat, dry surface. Connect the pads of the AED to the patient, as illustrated on the unit. Press the "analyze" button first for a readout, to ensure the unit is ready and electroshock is appropriate. Announce, "stay clear of the patient" while the AED is analyzing the patient's rhythm. Restart chest compressions if defibrillation is contraindicated (in the case of asystole or ventricular tachycardia with a palpable pulse). The unit indicates by tone or light that it is ready to shock the patient. The AED display shows when defibrillation occurs. Check the pulse after the third shock. If there is a pulse, check the airway, breathing, and circulation and move the patient into recovery position. If there is no pulse, continue CPR. The defibrillator will continue to provide instructions through this process. When the defibrillator announces that it is analyzing, the patient must not be touched. Continue CPR as directed by the AED. The unit indicates when to stop defibrillation.

CHOKING VICTIM AND HEIMLICH MANEUVER

If a patient is reclined, anesthetized, or eating, a **foreign body airway obstruction** (FBAO) may occur. The universal distress signal for FBAO is clutching of the throat with both hands. If the patient does this, suspend treatment immediately. A choking patient cannot speak. Breathing is difficult or absent. The mouth may be blue (cyanotic). Ask the patient to sit up and cough. If he or she cannot force out the foreign body independently, call for help. Perform the **Heimlich maneuver** to open the blocked airway. If the patient is conscious, stand behind him or her. Wrap

Copyright © Mometrix Media. You have been licensed one copy of this document for personal use only. Any other reproduction or redistribution is strictly prohibited. All rights reserved. This content is provided for test preparation purposes only and does not imply an endorsement by Mometrix of any particular political, scientific, or religious point of view.

the arms around the patient's abdomen. Make one hand into a fist and grasp the other hand firmly over it. Deliver a series of swift subdiaphragmatic thrusts, until the airway is clear or the patient falls unconscious. The patient requires follow-up medical treatment in case the airway was damaged.

ABDOMINAL THRUSTS IN UNCONSCIOUS PATIENT WITH AIRWAY OBSTRUCTION

If a patient with foreign body airway obstruction (FBAO) becomes **unconscious** during the standing Heimlich maneuver, phone Emergency Medical Services (EMS) immediately. Brain death occurs in 4-6 minutes. Place the patient on his or her back. Don gloves. Lift the tongue and jaw and if the object is visible, sweep the mouth with the fingers to remove the foreign body. If the object is not visible, it is no longer advised to do a blind sweep due to the risk of pushing the object further into the airway. Next, initiate CPR starting with 2 rescue breaths, and followed by 30 chest compressions, repeating this process until Emergency Medical Services arrive.

SINGLE-RESCUER CPR FOR ADULT VICTIM

Call Emergency Medical Services (911) before beginning **cardiopulmonary resuscitation (CPR).** Only perform CPR on a patient with cardiac arrest, who is unresponsive, with no pulse or breathing. Don gloves, if possible. Place the patient supine on the floor. Look, listen, and feel for the patient's breathing and pulse. If there is no pulse, immediately start chest compressions at a 30:2 compression-breath ratio. If there is a pulse, but no breathing, open the patient's airway by inclining the head back and raising the chin. Place a resuscitation mouthpiece into the patient's mouth. Pinch the nose closed. Inflate the lungs with two breaths. Observe the chest's rise and fall. Check the carotid pulse after administering the rescue breaths. If the pulse has been lost, kneel beside the patient. Landmark the xiphoid process at the end of the sternum (breastbone), where the ribs meet. Place palms over the breastbone. Compress 30 times, followed by two breaths. After four cycles, check the carotid pulse again. Pulse checks should never be longer than 10 seconds. Continue until the patient regains a pulse/breathing or until a rescuer with higher training arrives to provide relief. Discard the mouthpiece. Document CPR in the patient's chart.

BLEEDING

When direct pressure on an injury does not stop **bleeding**, exert indirect pressure with the flats of the fingers or thumb on the nearest pulse (pressure point). Compressing the artery against a bone where they are both close to the skin surface usually stops bleeding. If the fingers are insufficient, use the heel of the hand. Indirect pressure results in inadequate blood flow to an area and can cause tissue damage from ischemia. Use indirect pressure cautiously. Applying pressure to the carotid artery can cause cardiac arrest or stroke. The brachial artery is the pressure point to control bleeding in the forearm. The femoral artery is the pressure point to control bleeding from the leg. The subclavian artery controls upper chest and neck bleeding. The temporal artery and facial artery control bleeding in the face and neck.

Only use a tourniquet to control bleeding when all other methods have failed, and only on the extremities, not the trunk or head. Write the letters TK and the time the tourniquet was applied on the patient's forehead. Release the tourniquet every 5 minutes to allow circulation. The patient may lose the limb due to ischemia.

Copyright © Mometrix Media. You have been licensed one copy of this document for personal use only. Any other reproduction or redistribution is strictly prohibited. All rights reserved. This content is provided for test preparation purposes only and does not imply an endorsement by Mometrix of any particular political, scientific, or religious point of view.

BURNS

The types of burns include thermal, chemical, electrical, radiation, and mechanical. There are also various degrees (representing severity) of burns:

- A **first-degree** (superficial) burn is damage to the epidermis with reddening and moderate pain.
- A **second-degree** (partial-thickness) burn involves the epidermis and dermis with reddening, blistering, and severe pain.
- A **third-degree** (full-thickness) burn extends through the epidermis, dermis, and deep tissues, such as muscle and bone. It may be leathery and white or charred, and is not painful where nerves are destroyed.

Take care to assess for signs of a respiratory tract burn (inhalation injury), which produces sooty nasal hairs, nostrils, or lips and a hoarse voice or stridor. Respiratory arrest may be impending and the patient should be treated accordingly.

To begin treatment for a first- or second-degree burn, remove the patient from the burning agent. Gently remove clothing and jewelry from the affected area, provided they are not sticking, because burns swell. If there is chemical powder, brush it from the patient with cardboard so it does not react with water. Flush the burn with cool water for 20 minutes. If skin is sloughing, immerse the burn in cold water. Do not use ice. If the burn cannot be flushed or immersed, wrap it in clean cloth soaked in cool water. After the burn has cooled, the wound should be loosely covered with sterile gauze. An over-the-counter pain reliever such as ibuprofen or acetaminophen should be given. For major burns, call 911 immediately. The patient needs an antibacterial silver bandage, an analgesic, and possibly IV fluid replacement therapy.

RULE OF NINES

The Rule of Nines is often used when transcribing burns:

- In an **adult**, each part of the body contributes the following percentage to the entire body surface area: Perineum, 1%; each leg, 18%; each arm, 9%; chest and abdomen, 18%; back and buttocks, 18%; and head, 9%.
- In a **child**, each part of the body contributes the following percentage to the entire body surface area: Each leg, 14%; each arm, 9%; chest, abdomen, and groin, 18%; back and buttocks, 18%; and head, 18%.
- In an **infant**, each part of the body contributes the following percentage to the entire body surface area: Each leg, 14%; each arm, 9%; chest and abdomen, 18%, back and buttocks, 18%, and head, 18%. The palm of the hand and groin are *each* 1% of the entire body surface.

The doctor uses the Rule of Nines to determine when to give fluid resuscitation (20-25%) and when to transfer the patient to the burn unit. Burns to the face and palms are usually critical.

> **Review Video: <u>Rule of Nines</u>**
> Visit mometrix.com/academy and enter code: 846800

Copyright © Mometrix Media. You have been licensed one copy of this document for personal use only. Any other reproduction or redistribution is strictly prohibited. All rights reserved.
This content is provided for test preparation purposes only and does not imply an endorsement by Mometrix of any particular political, scientific, or religious point of view.

DIABETIC COMA AND DIABETIC SHOCK

Diabetic coma results from prolonged high blood sugar (hyperglycemia) caused by excessive sugar or carbohydrates and not enough insulin in patients with diabetes mellitus. Initially, the patient's mental status alters. He or she is confused, thirsty, and exhibits drunken behavior. The patient urinates frequently and may vomit. He or she complains of nausea and abdominal pain. The skin is flushed and dry. The patient snores when he or she eventually sinks into coma. Ketones will be present in the urine, the blood sugar level will be elevated, and the patient's breath may have a fruity odor. This patient requires immediate attention and insulin. Fluid replacement is required. The doctor should be informed immediately.

Diabetic shock is also known as insulin shock and results from sudden low blood sugar (hypoglycemia, glucose less than 70 mg/dL) through fasting, overexertion, alcohol ingestion, stress, or drug reactions. The patient displays nervousness, irritability, shaking, cold sweats, and complains of hunger. Loss of consciousness often follows. In this case, stop the procedure. The rule of 15 should be followed, where 15 grams of carbohydrate are administered (orally if the patient can tolerate it), then the blood glucose can be rechecked in 15 minutes. Give 4 ounces of orange juice, or a glucose drink, 3-4 glucose tablets, or 6-8 Lifesavers candies immediately. A delay may cause the patient to become unresponsive and require glucagon injections or hospital treatment for acidosis. If the blood glucose is still low after 15 minutes, this process should be repeated.

FRACTURES

A fracture is a break or disruption in the integrity of a bone that occurs when force or weight are applied to the bone that exceed the bone's ability to remain structurally intact. Fractures occur from direct or indirect trauma, or due to diseases (e.g., cancer and osteoporosis) and congenital states such as contractures. Fractures are frequently associated with adjacent soft tissue injuries. Fractures are classified as either **open** or **closed**.

Older fracture classifications still used in transcriptions include:

Transverse (right angled to the axis)	Comminuted (splintered)	Greenstick (twisted immature bones)	Spiral (twisted, as in a skiing accident)	Displaced (complete separation; ends no longer align)
TRANSVERSE	COMMINUTED	GREENSTICK	SPIRAL	DISPLACED

Copyright © Mometrix Media. You have been licensed one copy of this document for personal use only. Any other reproduction or redistribution is strictly prohibited. All rights reserved. This content is provided for test preparation purposes only and does not imply an endorsement by Mometrix of any particular political, scientific, or religious point of view.

Additional terms used to describe fractures include:

- Simple (skin intact, no bone contact with air)
- Compound (bone protrudes through skin)
- Compacted (bone ends are jammed together)
- Compression (where the patient loses height because the spine fuses)
- Oblique (diagonal to the axis)
- Linear (parallel to the axis)
- Incomplete (bone is still joined at some points)
- Complete (bone fragments are completely separated)

LOCATING AND TREATING A FRACTURE

Observe the patient for:

- **Angulation**: bones shifted out of their normal position
- **Deformity** or swelling
- **Guarding**: holding the injured body part or favoring it
- **Inability** to use the part
- **Paradoxical breathing movements**
- **Rotation**: a bone fragment turned around its central axis

The goals of the medical assistant are to:

- **Immobilize** the area with bandages or splints to prevent further injury and pain
- **Identify** the mechanism of injury
- **Call EMS** for transportation to the nearest Emergency Room for x-ray

Look for associated injuries, such as flail chest and pneumothorax. If it is an open fracture, apply a dressing to control bleeding, prevent further contamination, and minimize psychogenic shock, because the patient does not have to look at the injury. Burns that cause fractures are critical. Fractures or dislocations involving the vertebral column can cause spinal cord injuries and paralysis so do not move the patient. Clear yellow cerebrospinal fluid or blood leaking from the ear, nose, or eyes indicates a skull fracture.

Copyright © Mometrix Media. You have been licensed one copy of this document for personal use only. Any other reproduction or redistribution is strictly prohibited. All rights reserved. This content is provided for test preparation purposes only and does not imply an endorsement by Mometrix of any particular political, scientific, or religious point of view.

POISONING

Rapid treatment of poisoning most commonly involves activated charcoal. Syrup of ipecac, a medication that used to be recommended by pediatricians to treat poisoning, induces vomiting. More recent studies have not been able to provide evidence that ipecac prevents impending poisoning, and have found frequent misuse in the home environment. For that reason, it is no longer recommended. Activated charcoal pills or slurry absorb poison and are more often recommended to treat poisoning.

- If it **burned** the esophagus on the way down (e.g., petroleum distillates or lye), then it will burn on the way up. Therefore, dilute the corrosive poison with 2 cups of water or milk. Do not induce vomiting.
- If the patient ingested **cyanide, a medication, or a non-corrosive substance** AND is completely **conscious**, then activated charcoal is administered to absorb and clear it from the body. The medical assistant may give water and multiple doses of charcoal (charcoal slurry) to dilute and absorb the residue.
- When the doctor arrives, assist him or her with gastric lavage and neutralizing the ingested substance, if required. Depending on the pH, the doctor may neutralize a base with vinegar or lemon juice, or neutralize an acid with baking soda.

SEIZURES

Epilepsy is an electric storm in the brain from uncontrolled, synchronized firing of neurons. Epilepsy can be acquired from head injury or innate, from neural membranes abnormally permeable to sodium and potassium. Anticonvulsants such as carbamazepine (Tegretol), phenobarbital (Luminal) and phenytoin (Dilantin) are used to control epilepsy.

An **absence seizure** is a generalized seizure, formerly called petit mal, with no specific focus in the brain. The patient stares, lip smacks, and blinks for a few seconds. Absences begin and end without warning and are difficult to discern because there is no after-effect. However, a 3 Hz spike and wave discharges result on an EEG. Absence seizures interfere with learning. The patient is unaware of what occurred during the seizure. Youths ages 7-19 are prone to seizures from flashing strobe lights at discos and flickering TV patterns. A famous case is the December 1997 Pokémon episode that sent 700 children to hospital; 500 had confirmed seizures.

Tonic-clonic seizure (formerly grand mal) is a convulsion involving the entire brain. An aura may precede the seizure (smell, lights, or other warning symptom). In the tonic phase, muscles contract, breathing is irregular, and skin is blue tinged from lack of oxygen (cyanosis). The patient loses bladder control. In the clonic phase, limbs jerk from quick muscle contraction and relaxation. After the seizure, the patient is limp, extremely drowsy, regains consciousness gradually, and is confused (referred to as the postictal phase). Recovery takes hours.

STROKE

Signs and symptoms of stroke (cerebrovascular accident or CVA) include the following:

- Disruptions in vision
- Trouble speaking or expressing thoughts
- Headache
- Weakness affecting one side of the body
- Difficulty walking
- Numbness or tingling on one side of the body

Copyright © Mometrix Media. You have been licensed one copy of this document for personal use only. Any other reproduction or redistribution is strictly prohibited. All rights reserved. This content is provided for test preparation purposes only and does not imply an endorsement by Mometrix of any particular political, scientific, or religious point of view.

Loss of consciousness is rare. The patient may be having a transient ischemic attack (TIA or mini-stroke), which is a warning of an impending stroke. Call the EMS (911) immediately if a stroke is suspected. Do not administer anything orally, as this patient is at risk for aspiration. Place the patient in recovery position with the affected side down, the head slightly elevated, and cover him or her with a blanket. Retrieve the crash cart. Paramedics will ask the patient to smile, to extend the arms for 10 seconds with the eyes closed, and to repeat a phrase to assess the progression of the stroke. Approximately 33% of patients who experience a transient ischemic attack will have recurrent attacks.

Complete stroke (CVA) is diagnosed if neurological signs and symptoms last more than 24 hours. It is imperative to obtain medical care as soon as possible to improve outcome. Tissue Plasminogen Activator (tPA) should be started immediately if appropriate. It can only be given within 3-4 hours of symptoms starting (depending on specific exclusion criteria) to reduce the chance for long term disability, hence receiving medical attention as soon as possible. Approximately 5% of patients who have a transient ischemic attack will have a cerebrovascular accident within one month, and 30% will have a cerebrovascular accident within one year.

> **Review Video: Overview of Strokes**
> Visit mometrix.com/academy and enter code: 310572

SYNCOPE

Syncope is characterized by fainting due to a temporary loss of consciousness caused by a disruption in the blood flow to the brain. The insufficiency of blood results in a lack of oxygen in the brain. When the patient falls into horizontal position, blood flow to the brain is restored and the problem corrects itself. After a patient regains consciousness, place the patient in recovery position. Alert the doctor and phone EMS (911) if necessary. Syncope may result from the following:

- Emotional stress/fear
- Physical pain
- Standing in one position for too long
- Overheating
- Dehydration
- Exhaustion
- Rapid changes in blood pressure
- Heart disease
- Neurological disorders
- Lung disease
- Adverse reaction to medication

If syncope occurs with exercise or is associated with irregularities in heart rhythm, it can indicate a serious health problem. Sharp muscle contractions called myoclonic jerks may occur with syncope. This is not true seizure activity. Bradycardia and increased vagal tone are often seen in cases of syncope.

Copyright © Mometrix Media. You have been licensed one copy of this document for personal use only. Any other reproduction or redistribution is strictly prohibited. All rights reserved. This content is provided for test preparation purposes only and does not imply an endorsement by Mometrix of any particular political, scientific, or religious point of view.

WOUNDS

The following are different types of wounds and their proper treatment:

- **Contusion**: A raised bruise (hematoma). Treat contusions during the first 48 hours by applying cold packs for 15 minutes on and 15 minutes off, taking acetaminophen or ibuprofen, and elevating the area. Warm washcloths help after the second day.
- **Laceration**: A long break in the surface of the skin. The edges of a laceration may be linear (smooth) or stellate (irregular). A laceration is caused by a knife blow, glass, or a surgeon's scalpel and usually requires sutures.
- **Abrasion**: A scrape or scratch of the outer layer of the skin. Friction burns and rug burns are types of abrasions. Wash the wound and remove gravel with forceps.
- **Avulsion**: A flap of tissue that is torn away from the main body of tissue, which often requires sutures.
- **Puncture**: A small, deep perforation of the skin caused by teeth, needles, icepicks, small caliber bullets, and other narrow, sharp objects. The doctor irrigates and probes the puncture.
- **Amputation**: The body part is completely detached. Wrap the amputated part in a sterile dressing and place in a labeled plastic bag on ice. A surgeon may be able to reattach it.

ADDITIONAL MISCELLANEOUS MEDICAL EMERGENCIES

Condition	Response
Cold exposure	Remove from cold environment, remove any wet clothing, wrap in warm blankets, begin CPR if no pulse obtained after 30-45 seconds of assessment, and utilize AED if it indicates need to defibrillate. In the case of frostbite, remove jewelry and manually stabilize the affected area; do NOT break blisters, rub or massage the area, apply heat, rewarm the area if it may refreeze, allow the individual to walk, or give anything to the individual by mouth.
Heat exposure	Remove from heat; use evaporative cooling techniques or ice packs to axilla, groin, and neck; rehydrate (half glass of water every 15-20 minutes). Administer oxygen if needed.
Joint dislocations	Splint and immobilize area, apply cold compress, place in position of comfort. Do NOT force into correct position.
Asthmatic attack	Elevate head, monitor respiratory status, assist with inhaled bronchodilator (albuterol).
Hyper-ventilation	Reassure patient, encourage patient to slow their breathing and try to relax. If a paper bag is available, have the patient inhale and exhale into a paper bag to prevent alkalosis.
Animal bite	Control bleeding, flush with NS (100-200 mL of irrigant per inch of wound).
Concussion	Elevate head, monitor vital signs and level of consciousness.

Copyright © Mometrix Media. You have been licensed one copy of this document for personal use only. Any other reproduction or redistribution is strictly prohibited. All rights reserved. This content is provided for test preparation purposes only and does not imply an endorsement by Mometrix of any particular political, scientific, or religious point of view.

Phlebotomy

Laboratory Procedures and Specimen Collection

VENIPUNCTURE
EQUIPMENT
Routine adult venipuncture equipment includes the following:

- Completed requisition with a physician's signature and billing information
- Soap, water, and towels for hand washing
- Sufficient evacuated blood tubes with the right color stopper
- One 21- or 22-gauge cannula, 1.5" length
- Plastic vacutainer holder with a Luer lock hub
- Isopropyl alcohol or povidone-iodine swab
- Clean, dry cotton balls
- Band-aid or Micropore tape, if the patient is allergic to adhesive
- Tourniquet (rubber Penrose catheter or blood pressure cuff)
- Kidney basin or tray to hold the specimen during collection
- Latex or vinyl gloves
- Pen with indelible ink
- Plastic biohazard bag with outer pouch for the requisition
- Well-buttoned lab coat to protect clothing
- Reclining chair or bed to support the patient
- Certain tests require chemical additives, ice, or a hot water bath
- Sharps disposal container
- Garbage can

PATIENT IDENTIFICATION AND CONSENT PROCEDURES
Patient identification and consent procedures include the following:

1. If the patient requires an interpreter, provide one.
2. Identify oneself to the patient.
3. Tell the patient which doctor requested the blood sample.
4. Explain in general terms of what is going to be done.
5. Check the patient's armband or health card to confirm identity.
6. Verify the correct spelling of the patient's name and date of birth.
7. If there is any discrepancy between the patient's written identification and the requisition, STOP. Get a doctor or nurse who knows the patient to confirm the identity, and note this on the requisition.
8. A conscious, adult patient has the right to refuse treatment. If the medical assistant proceeds with collection after the patient has refused it, they can be charged with battery. Mark "PATIENT REFUSED" with initials, the date and time on the requisition, return it to the patient's chart, and inform the charge nurse at once. If the patient is unconscious, the law considers the medical assistant to have been given implied consent.

Copyright © Mometrix Media. You have been licensed one copy of this document for personal use only. Any other reproduction or redistribution is strictly prohibited. All rights reserved. This content is provided for test preparation purposes only and does not imply an endorsement by Mometrix of any particular political, scientific, or religious point of view.

PREPARATION

Preparation for a venipuncture is as follows:

1. Check the expiration dates on all tubes, cannulae and swabs. Get fresh products if any have expired.
2. Wash, dry, and glove the hands.
3. Place the equipment in the kidney basin on an easily accessible table, not on the bed where they can break if the patient rolls over.
4. Select the patient's arm that has no intravenous fluid drip or injury.
5. Tie the tourniquet around the patient's bicep, or inflate a blood pressure cuff to 20 mmHg.
6. Ask the patient to clench a fist. Palpate the veins in the ante cubital fossa.
7. If the arm turns blue, or if the patient complains the tourniquet is too tight, loosen it immediately. Wait until the arm returns to a normal color before reapplying. Prolonged or repeated use of the tourniquet or blood pressure cuff can result in artificially high calcium levels in the specimen.

DRAWING BLOOD

Procedures for drawing blood include the following:

1. Position the patient's arm on a pillow so blood flows downwards. Tell the patient to remain still.
2. Apply tourniquet and cleanse the planned needle insertion site with an alcohol pad, allowing the alcohol to air dry.
3. Retract the skin from the site by anchoring the vein using the non-dominant hand below the insertion site.
4. Uncap the 21- or 22-gauge cannula. Rest the first tube inside the holder. Do not push it onto the hub.
5. Insert the cannula, bevel up, into the vein at a 30° angle until flash of blood is visualized.
6. Grasp the holder with one hand. Push the tube onto the hub with the other. Blood flows automatically into the evacuated tube when the stopper is pierced and stops when its vacuum is depleted.
7. Detach the filled tube from the hub and invert the tube several times to mix the anticoagulant and blood.
8. Place the filled tube in the kidney basin.
9. Release the tourniquet. The tourniquet should not be applied for longer than one minute to prevent hemoconcentration.
10. Rest cotton over the puncture site.
11. Remove the cannula while still on the end of its holder, without unscrewing it. Apply steady pressure to the wound for 4-6 minutes to stop bleeding—longer if the patient is taking anticoagulant drugs like aspirin or coumadin.
12. Ask the alert patient to continue applying pressure after the first minute and dispose of the used equipment in appropriate containers. Elevate the puncture slightly to help slow bleeding, but do not bend the arm. Apply a band-aid.

Copyright © Mometrix Media. You have been licensed one copy of this document for personal use only. Any other reproduction or redistribution is strictly prohibited. All rights reserved.
This content is provided for test preparation purposes only and does not imply an endorsement by Mometrix of any particular political, scientific, or religious point of view.

Mometrix

BLOOD COLLECTION BY CAPILLARY PUNCTURE

Capillary puncture is suitable when a very small quantity of blood is required and the patient has difficult veins. Examples of when capillary puncture is appropriate include:

- Newborn PKU
- Diabetic glucose via glucometer
- Anemic hemoglobin via hemoglobinometer
- Bleeding time before surgery

Capillary puncture is inappropriate for blood cultures or large quantities because the site clots quickly.

Perform newborn capillary puncture with a short point lancet on the lateral or medial plantar heel surface to avoid nicking the calcaneus (heel bone) and causing osteomyelitis. The infant may require a foot amputation if the site becomes gangrenous. Older infants can have the plantar surface of their big toes pricked with a short point lancet. Children and adults have the distal phalanx palmar surface pricked with a long point lancet.

PROCEDURE

Wash the puncture site with warm water to dilate capillaries. If the site remains cold, apply a chemical warming pack. Wrap the pack in a cloth so it does not directly contact the infant's thin skin. Swab the site with alcohol. Puncture the skin quickly with a lancet. Draw blood into the Microtainer tube by capillary action and GENTLE squeezing in the following order:

Color	Additive	Order of Draw	# of Inversions
Lavender	EDTA	First	Mix 20 times
Dark Green	Lithium Heparin	Second	Mix 10 times
Mint Green	PST	Third	Mix 10 times
Gold and Amber	SST	Fourth	Do not mix
Red	None	Last	Do not mix

The order of draw is different than that used for venipuncture because capillary blood is more likely to clot or hemolyze during collection.

Wiping the puncture with alcohol to encourage bleeding when the wound has already clotted will dilute the specimen. Vigorous squeezing can cause interstitial fluid to leak into the specimen and dilute it, or hemolysis of red blood cells, giving a false result.

CULTURE AND SUSCEPTIBILITY TESTING

Sensitivity testing is also called **culture and susceptibility testing (C&S)**. Wash hands. Don gloves and a lab coat. Sterilize a loop. Streak body fluid (stool, urine, blood, sputum, or wound drainage) across an agar plate with the loop. Rotate the loop and streak again so the bacteria are evenly distributed across the agar. Tissue may also be placed directly on media by the RMA. Incubate at body temperature (37 °C) for 24-48 hours.

If growth occurs, the lab distinguishes normal flora from pathogens by chemical and enzyme tests. A lab tech inoculates pathogens with antimicrobials to see if they can be killed (susceptible), or cannot be killed (resistant). If the antimicrobial that works best requires high doses (intermediate), it is likely to be toxic to the patient. The doctor initially prescribes the antimicrobial to which the pathogen is susceptible, except if the patient is allergic to it. The doctor consults with a pharmacist and microbiologist to choose the least toxic alternative, but the intermediate dose may need to be

Copyright © Mometrix Media. You have been licensed one copy of this document for personal use only. Any other reproduction or redistribution is strictly prohibited. All rights reserved.
This content is provided for test preparation purposes only and does not imply an endorsement by Mometrix of any particular political, scientific, or religious point of view.

given over a long time and the patient may suffer side-effects. If the pathogen is resistant to many antimicrobials, then expensive intravenous combination therapy may be the only effective treatment.

LIPID PROFILE

A lipid profile tests for hyperlipidemia, elevated fats and oils in the blood which clog blood vessels and result in heart attack, stroke, and ischemia. Routinely screen men over 35, women over 45, and younger patients with risk factors or a significant family history of cardiovascular disease.

Lipid	Normal Value
LDL cholesterol (bad cholesterol)	High: >160 mg/dL Borderline high: 130-159 mg/dL Near optimal: 100-129 mg/dL Optimal: <100 mg/dL
HDL cholesterol (good cholesterol)	Male: >40 mg/dL Female: >50 mg/dL
Total cholesterol	Desirable: <200 mg/dL Borderline high risk: 200-239 mg/dL High risk: ≥240 mg/dL
LDL/HDL ratio	<4
Triglycerides	Normal: <150 mg/dL Borderline high: 150-200 mg/dL High: >200 mg/dL

Instruct the patient to fast for 12-14 hours before testing. Random lipids are inaccurate because fatty meals spike them. Treatment is diet modification, exercise, weight loss, niacin supplements, statins for cholesterol (Lipitor, Mevacor), and fibrates for triglyceride (Lopid, Tricor).

SPECIMEN LABELING AND COMMON PRESERVATION METHODS

Appropriate specimen labeling and preservation is critical in obtaining accurate results and readings:

- **Specimen labeling**: Before collecting a specimen, the patient's identity should be confirmed with two identifiers (name and birthdate). Every specimen container must have a label directly attached at the time and point of collection. The following information must be on each specimen: Patient's first and last name, medical record number, date of birth, date and time of collection, and initials of person collecting the sample. Infant samples also require the mother's first name, infant's gender, and infant's ID band number. Some labels may contain a barcode and/or the physician's name as well.
- **Preservation**: Some specimens may be stored in the refrigerator, including urine and stool specimens, after being properly labeled. Fresh tissue specimens should be inserted into a container holding the fixative already with volume 20:1 in comparison with specimen. The container should be gently agitated for a few minutes after the specimen is inserted to ensure penetration.

Copyright © Mometrix Media. You have been licensed one copy of this document for personal use only. Any other reproduction or redistribution is strictly prohibited. All rights reserved. This content is provided for test preparation purposes only and does not imply an endorsement by Mometrix of any particular political, scientific, or religious point of view.

TOOLS AND METHODS OF SPECIMEN PREPARATION AND EXAMINATION

Tools and methods of specimen preparation and examination include the following:

Incubator	Equipment used to store cell and tissue cultures in a temperature-controlled environment for optimal growth. Shaking incubators provide a shaking platform and agitation to promote cell growth.
Centrifuge	Equipment used to spin and separate components of a specimen, such as blood, placed inside in a vial.
Microscope	Used to examine slides of tissue to note microscopic elements, such as abnormal cells, and wet mounts to identify microscopic organisms.
Culture inoculation	Procedure by which a specimen is applied to an agar plate or injected into a liquid medium for a bacterial culture.
Microbiologic slides (wet mount)	A sample, such as vaginal discharge, is placed on a slide and a drop of water or NS placed on top of the specimen before the top slide is carefully put in place. This method is especially useful for viewing and identifying motile (moving) microscopic organisms.

GRAM-POSITIVE AND GRAM-NEGATIVE BACTERIA

Bacteria are either gram-negative or gram-positive. Identifying this quality is important in planning treatment:

- **Gram-negative**: Thin-walled bacteria that turns **RED** when Gram stained from absorbing crystal violet, pink safranin, and fuchsin. Lipopolysaccharide in their walls repels blue stain. Lipid-A is the endotoxin found outside the cell wall. Parts include: flagellum (motility), pilus (adherence, conjugation), capsule (protection), peptidoglycan wall (support, shape), cytoplasmic membrane, and periplasmic space (holds enzymes and proteins). Examples: *Escherichia coli, Klebsiella pneumoniae, Pseudomonas aeruginosa, Haemophilus influenzae, Enterobacter aerogenes.*
- **Gram-positive**: Thick-walled bacteria that turns **VIOLET-BLUE** when Gram stained. Walls contain teichoic acid and a membrane that increase virulence. Examples: group B streptococcus, *Staphylococcus aureus* and *epidermidis,* and *Listeria monocytogenes.* Most bone infections (osteomyelitis) are caused by Gram-positive bacteria.

Copyright © Mometrix Media. You have been licensed one copy of this document for personal use only. Any other reproduction or redistribution is strictly prohibited. All rights reserved. This content is provided for test preparation purposes only and does not imply an endorsement by Mometrix of any particular political, scientific, or religious point of view.

Laboratory Standards and Regulations

OCCUPATIONAL SAFETY AND HEALTH ADMINISTRATION (OSHA)

OSHA stands for Occupational Safety and Health Administration. It is an organization designed to assure the safety and health of workers by setting and enforcing standards; providing training, outreach, and education; establishing partnerships; and encouraging continual improvement in workplace safety and health.

SDS (formerly MSDS) stands for **Safety Data Sheets**. These sheets are the result of the "Right to Know" Law also known as the OSHA's HazCom Standard. This law requires chemical manufacturers to supply SDS sheets on any products that have a hazardous warning label. These sheets contain information on precautionary as well as emergency information about the product.

OSHA REGULATIONS REGARDING LABORATORY SERVICES

The Occupational Safety and Health Administration (OSHA) requires that facilities provide safe medical equipment and devices. OSHA also regulates workplace safety, including disposal methods for sharps, such as needles, and blood disposition. OSHA requires that standard precautions be used at all times and that staff be trained to use precautions. OSHA requires procedures for post-exposure evaluation and treatment and availability of hepatitis B vaccine for healthcare workers. OSHA defines occupational exposure to infections, establishes standards to prevent the spread of bloodborne pathogens, and regulates the fitting and use of respirators. OSHA requires the use of needleless blood transfer devices as a means of decreasing the risk of needlestick injuries and infection as part of OSHA's Bloodborne Pathogen Standard. Sharps used for blood draw should have sharps injury protection devices whenever possible. Needles without this protection should never be recapped as this increases risk of needlestick. States may have their own OSHA-approved programs but must meet the minimum standards developed by OSHA.

LABORATORY STANDARDS AND INTEGRITY ASSESSMENT

Laboratory standards are established by a number of agencies, including OSHA, which establishes safety standards; the EPA, which established good laboratory practices; CLSI, which provides global laboratory standards; and ISO-9000, which establishes standards for quality management. Laboratory standards are norms or requirements stablished for the profession. **Integrity assessment** is carried out to determine if a laboratory is meeting standards or has engaged in fraud or misconduct (as opposed to accidents or errors), such as through:

- Failure to properly carry out procedures
- Falsification of records or measurements, incomplete documentation, manipulation of data
- Violation of standards or rules of conduct, violations of codes of ethics
- Misrepresentation of quality assurance results
- Failure to adequately calibrate equipment
- Failure to retain samples for required time
- Improper storage of reagents, samples, and supplies
- Failure to follow standard operating procedures
- Alterations of log book
- Employment of personnel without appropriate license or certification

Integrity assessment may include reviewing data, comparing manual logs with computer logs, conducting an audit trail, carrying out unannounced audits, encouraging and supporting whistleblowers.

Copyright © Mometrix Media. You have been licensed one copy of this document for personal use only. Any other reproduction or redistribution is strictly prohibited. All rights reserved.
This content is provided for test preparation purposes only and does not imply an endorsement by Mometrix of any particular political, scientific, or religious point of view.

CLSI, CLIA AND CDC

The **Clinical and Laboratory Standards Institute (CLSI)** provides standards for a wide range of performance and testing and covers all types of laboratory functions and microbiology. These standards are used as a basis for quality control procedures. Standards include: Labeling, security/information technology, toxicology/drug testing, statistical quality control, and performance standards for various types of antimicrobial susceptibility testing.

In the United States, all laboratory testing, except for research, is regulated by the CMS (Centers for Medicare and Medicaid) through **Clinical Laboratory Improvement Amendments (CLIA).** CLIA is implemented through the Division of Laboratory Services and serves approximately 244,000 laboratories. Laboratories receiving reimbursement from CMS must meet CLIA standards, which ensure that laboratory testing will be accurate and procedures followed properly.

The Centers for Disease Control and Prevention (CDC) is a federal agency that supports health promotion, prevention, and health preparedness. The CDC partners with CMS and the FDA in supporting CLIA programs.

ADDITIONAL AGENCIES AND THEIR RESPONSIBILITIES

National Accrediting Agency for Clinical Laboratory Sciences: The agency responsible for approving and accrediting clinical laboratory science and similar healthcare professional education programs.

College of American Pathologists: The primary organization for board-certified pathologists serving to represent the interests of the public, as well as pathologists and their patients by fostering excellence in the pathology and laboratory medicine practice.

The Joint Commission: A large organization that aims to improve the quality of care provided to patients through implementing healthcare accreditation standards and other supportive services aimed at improving the performance of healthcare organizations

SOP FOR LABORATORIES

Each laboratory should draw up a **standard operating procedure document (SOP)** that outlines all the processes and procedures associated with reception of a sample and processing, including:

- **Specimen collection processes**: PPE, patient identification, collection tubes, collecting procedures, need for special handling, labeling, transporting specimens, criteria for rejecting inadequate sample, protocols for adverse reactions.
- **Chain of custody**: Labeling, storing, packing, and transporting.
- **Sample reception**: Specimen identification, logging, specimen condition, specimen accountability, retention times.
- **Rejection criteria**: Incorrect collection tube, leaking tube, incorrect labeling, incorrect sample for test, volume inadequate, order unverified, mismatch between order and labeling.
- **Delivery** (from reception to processing); Process for delivery to correct department, specimen retention policies.
- **Processing**: Procedures for testing, accountability standards, storage, and retention policies.
- **Reporting**: Methods of reporting and timeframes.

Copyright © Mometrix Media. You have been licensed one copy of this document for personal use only. Any other reproduction or redistribution is strictly prohibited. All rights reserved.
This content is provided for test preparation purposes only and does not imply an endorsement by Mometrix of any particular political, scientific, or religious point of view.

ECG and Other Diagnostic Tests

Electrocardiography

ELECTROCARDIOGRAPH

An electrocardiograph machine records the heart's electrical activity on an **electrocardiogram** (EKG or ECG). The EKG monitors heart rate, patterns of heartbeats, the size and location of the chambers of the heart, and helps to diagnose heart conditions. The EKG is a non-invasive, painless, inexpensive way to determine if there is any damage to the heart muscle (myocardium) or electrical conduction system. The cardiologist uses the EKG to determine if drug therapy or pacemaker implants are having the desired effect. The P wave on an EKG corresponds to the atria contracting. The QRS complex corresponds to the ventricles contracting. The T wave is repolarization.

For a resting EKG, position the patient lying down, face up. If the patient has difficulty breathing (dyspnea), prop the patient's head up with pillows. For a stress test, 12-15 leads are attached to the patient, who runs on a treadmill. For a Holter monitor, 3-5 leads are used, and the results of the EKG are recorded on a telemetry device worn around the patient's neck for 24-48 hours.

Review Video: EKG Rhythms – Reading the Graph
Visit mometrix.com/academy and enter code: 872282

Copyright © Mometrix Media. You have been licensed one copy of this document for personal use only. Any other reproduction or redistribution is strictly prohibited. All rights reserved.
This content is provided for test preparation purposes only and does not imply an endorsement by Mometrix of any particular political, scientific, or religious point of view.

SECTION OF HEART MONITORED IN EACH EKG LEAD

An EKG lead is the wire and electrode that connects the patient to the electrocardiograph machine (also abbreviated ECG). A standard 12-lead EKG actually has only 10 wires and electrodes, which record 12 electrical vectors:

- **Unipolar Leads:**
  - Augmented Vector Right (AVR) [right atrial view]
  - Augmented Vector Left (AVL) [lateral view]
  - Augmented Vector Foot (AVF) [inferior view]
  - Precordial chest lead V1 [anterior view]
  - Precordial chest lead V2 [anterior view]
  - Precordial chest lead V3 [septal view]
  - Precordial chest lead V4 [septal view]
  - Precordial chest lead V5 [lateral view]
  - Precordial chest lead V6 [lateral view]

- **Bipolar Leads:**
  - Limb lead I [lateral view]
  - Limb lead II [inferior view]
  - Limb lead III [inferior view]

Copyright © Mometrix Media. You have been licensed one copy of this document for personal use only. Any other reproduction or redistribution is strictly prohibited. All rights reserved.
This content is provided for test preparation purposes only and does not imply an endorsement by Mometrix of any particular political, scientific, or religious point of view.

TECHNIQUES FOR PATIENTS WITH SPECIAL CONDITIONS

Capturing an EKG on a patient with special conditions requires the following considerations:

- **Amputee**: If the patient has an amputated limb, or a limb is not accessible for an electrode due to a dressing or wound, the priority is that the EKG leads are placed symmetrically on the body. For instance, if the right wrist of a patient is amputated, place the RA and LA electrodes on the soft tissue below the shoulder joint.
- **Pacemaker**: If a patient has a pacemaker, be sure not to place the electrode directly atop the pacemaker to avoid interference with the EKG reading. Place the electrode 3-5 inches from the pacemaker and place the RA electrode symmetrically on the other side of the body.
- **Piercings**: It should be advised that patient's remove all jewelry possible. Body piercings present a particular risk during EKG's and may be ripped out unintentionally after being snagged on the lead wires.

ARTIFACTS ON THE EKG TRACING

The two most common **causes of artifact** on the EKG tracing are easily preventable:

- **Loose Leads**: Electrodes may not have sufficient adhesion to the body, due to body hair, perspiration or oil on the skin, or lead location. To avoid this problem, quickly shave heavy body hair and wipe the skin of any perspiration or dampness. Use alcohol pads to effectively remove oil from the skin and allow the alcohol to dry. Select flat locations for electrode placement to prevent bending and folding of the electrode.
- **Patient Movement**: Patient movement, such as shivering, coughing, or speaking, can cause a wandering baseline on the EKG reading. To avoid this, communicate with the patient prior to initiating the EKG reading, asking them to keep still. Also notify any of the health care members that may be working on the patient, so that they can step back and refrain from moving the patient during EKG capture. Make sure the patient is warm to prevent shivering.

CAPTURING AN EKG

Steps for capturing an EKG include the following:

1. Introduce oneself and confirm the identity of the patient using two patient identifiers.
2. Explain the procedure, clarifying in layman's terms that the EKG will be capturing a picture of the heart rhythm that will involve no pain. Talk through the steps that will be taken, including describing the "stickers" (electrodes) that will be placed on the patient.
3. Turn on the EKG machine and fill in the required patient data, including name, age, sex, and indication for the EKG.
4. Attach the electrodes to the patient in the appropriate locations, ensuring to avoid bony prominences and dense fatty tissue/muscle. Shave the patient if necessary. Pat the patient's skin dry if perspiration is evident and use an alcohol pad if the patient's skin is oily. Attach the leads to the electrodes, paying attention to their labels: LA, LL, RA, RL and V1-V6.
5. Review the EKG preview screen to ensure all leads are properly placed and without artifact. Some EKG machines will alert for artifact. Remind the patient (and providers who are interacting with the patient) not to move or speak while the image is acquired.
6. Initiate capture. Wait patiently while the EKG machine acquires and prints the EKG. Tear the EKG report from the printer.
7. Review the EKG for artifact or malfunctioning leads.
8. Clean the EKG machine with the proper disinfectant based on the precautions required by the patient's condition. Remove the EKG and the EKG machine from the patient's room, and return to proper location.

Copyright © Mometrix Media. You have been licensed one copy of this document for personal use only. Any other reproduction or redistribution is strictly prohibited. All rights reserved.
This content is provided for test preparation purposes only and does not imply an endorsement by Mometrix of any particular political, scientific, or religious point of view.

CLEANING AND STORAGE OF THE EKG MACHINE

Following the EKG, the medical assistant must disinfect the EKG machine. The EKG machine is used across patient rooms; therefore, all bacteria must be removed prior to removing the EKG machine and using it on another patient. While wearing gloves, disinfect the machine using the proper disinfectant identified for this patient based on their level of isolation. Wipe down the entire machine, being sure to wipe each wire and lead. Remove gloves, wash hands, and exit the patient room with the EKG machine. Every unit should have a docking station for their EKG machine. It is the responsibility of the medical assistant to know where this docking station is located. Return the EKG machine to the docking station and plug it in to the power source to ensure power is available for the next EKG ordered. Apply a "clean" tag to the EKG machine to confirm that it has been properly disinfected after patient use.

PERMANENT RECORD OF EKG FOR PATIENT'S CHART

While **recording the EKG**, mark the leads on the top while changing the dial to different lead settings. To make a permanent record of a strip EKG, cut it to fit an 8.5" x 11" mounting card that fits in the chart. Examine the recording, and find one accurate representative example of each lead for the permanent record (I, II, III, AVR, AVL, AVF, V1, V2, V3, V4, V5, and V6). The example must not wander from the baseline, should contain any ectopic beats, and must contain a 1-milivolt standard deflection for comparison to the wave height. If there is a run of irregular beats, include it as a fold-over. Cut the example to fit the appropriate section of the mounting card. Peel back the cover over the adhesive, and press the cutting onto the card. Include a long rhythm strip from Lead II. Note if the patient is taking cardiac drugs, such as digoxin, or if he or she had difficulty breathing (dyspnea) or complained of chest pain during the recording.

Copyright © Mometrix Media. You have been licensed one copy of this document for personal use only. Any other reproduction or redistribution is strictly prohibited. All rights reserved.
This content is provided for test preparation purposes only and does not imply an endorsement by Mometrix of any particular political, scientific, or religious point of view.

Other Diagnostic Tests

URINE COLLECTION PROCEDURES

ROUTINE URINALYSIS

Below are the common urine dipstick tests in routine urinalysis. Normal values are bracketed:

1. **Blood** (negative): Intact or hemolyzed red blood cells indicate bleeding due to infection, menstruation, paroxysmal hemoglobinuria, or trauma.
2. **Glucose** (negative): Uncontrolled diabetes and women with gestational diabetes spill sugar into their urine when their renal threshold is exceeded.
3. **Ketones** (negative): Uncontrolled diabetes, extreme dieters, and starving people produce ketones in urine when their bodies burn fat instead of sugar.
4. **Leukocytes** (negative): White blood cells indicate infection.
5. **pH** (5-9): Acidic urine helps the bladder resist infection. Alkaline urine encourages bacterial growth.
6. **Protein** (up to 8 mg/dL): Albumin is shed from the kidneys if the nephrons are damaged. Trace protein can be from genitals or feces.
7. **Nitrites** (negative): Some bacteria, like E-coli, produce nitrites after eating nitrates, so this is an indicator of infection.

If kidney stones, infection, or damage is suspected, then a microscopic urinalysis is performed with the routine urinalysis for casts, crystals, and cells.

MICROSCOPIC URINE EXAMINATION

On microscopic urinalysis, assess for:

1. **Red blood cells (RBC)**: Up to two RBC at low-power field are normal. Five or more indicate tumor, infection, glomerulonephritis, or trauma; this is recorded as microscopic hematuria.
2. **White blood cells (WBC)**: Up to four WBC at low-power field are normal. Five or more indicate a urinary tract infection.
3. **Casts**: Negative or occasional hyaline casts are normal. Record many hyaline casts as proteinuria. The cast types and diseases they indicate are WBC, pyelonephritis; RBC, glomerulonephritis; waxy and granular, non-specific; broad casts, chronic renal failure; and fat casts, nephritic syndrome.
4. **Crystals**: None are normal. Urate crystals indicate gout. Phosphate and calcium oxalate crystals appear in hyperparathyroidism and malabsorption conditions. "Coffin lid" struvite casts occur with urea-splitting bacteria. Tyrosine or cystine indicates metabolic disease or poisoning.
5. **Bacteria**: Normal urine is sterile, with no bacteria. Many indicate a urinary tract infection (UTI).
6. **Artifacts**: Squamous cells from the vagina, cotton fibers from clothes, and starch granules from baby powder are all examples of extraneous artifacts

RANDOM AND MIDSTREAM URINE COLLECTIONS

Random urine is used at any time of day for a routine checkup, in any clean container. It does not require a sterile container nor does it require a lid if it will be tested immediately, only if it will be transported or stored. Urine is generally tested in the chemistry department. Routine checkup tests include blood, protein, glucose, ketones, and pH. Hands should be clean and free of contaminants that could affect the results.

Copyright © Mometrix Media. You have been licensed one copy of this document for personal use only. Any other reproduction or redistribution is strictly prohibited. All rights reserved. This content is provided for test preparation purposes only and does not imply an endorsement by Mometrix of any particular political, scientific, or religious point of view.

Midstream urine can also be collected at any time of day but requires a sterile, lidded container. It is used for bacteriology studies to diagnose bladder and kidney infections. The patient cleans the urinary opening (meatus), voids a little urine, collects the midstream of urine, and voids the remainder in the toilet. If hands touch the inside of the container, the specimen may be contaminated and produce a false positive.

PLATING A MIDSTREAM URINE SAMPLE

The procedure for plating a midstream urine sample for culture and sensitivity testing (MSU for C&S) is described below:

1. Touch the outside of the MSU container only.
2. Open an agar plate; do not touch the inner surface or lid.
3. Dip a sterile swab or loop in the urine.
4. Press the swab or loop lightly across the surface of the agar to plant the possible bacterial infection for culture.
5. Close the plate tightly. Label it with the patient's name, date and time, physician's name, and test ("urine for C&S").
6. If the specimen will be sent to an outside lab, refrigerate it until pickup. If testing it onsite, place it in an incubator for 24-48 hours so the microbiologist can make a determination about the infection.
7. If growth occurs, a microbiologist places several small circles of paper impregnated with different antibiotics on the plate.
8. If the bacteria are sensitive to the medication, a small area surrounding the paper circle will have no apparent growth.
9. If bacteria are resistant, growth is uninhibited.

MANUAL HEMOGLOBIN TEST FOR HEMODIALYSIS PATIENT

When performing a manual hemoglobin test for a hemodialysis patient, test the hemoglobinometer with known controls first. Polish a clean hemocytometer slide with lens paper. Fill a blue-ringed, unheparinized capillary tube with blood. Place one drop of blood on the hemocytometer slide. Roll the heparinized, wooden hemolysis stick over the blood drop until the blood is hemolyzed and transparent (about 30 seconds). Place the cover slip over the slide. Slide them together into the hemoglobinometer. Look through the viewer. Adjust the light until the two fields are exactly the same color. (Most hemoglobinometers use green and black.) Read the scale (usually on the side of the meter) and record the hemoglobin level. Normal values are 12-16 g/dL for women, and 14-16 g/dL: for men. Disassemble the slide and cover slip. Sanitize, disinfect, polish, and case them. Wipe the test area and outside of the hemoglobinometer with disinfectant. Hemoglobinometer readings with capillary blood show about 10% false-positives for anemia, as compared to venous Coulter Counter readings. Hemoglobinometers are for point-of-care testing for "ballpark" estimates.

HEMATOCRIT TEST

A hematocrit (Hct) test separates the blood cells from the plasma in a centrifuge as part of a complete blood count (CBC). Hct indirectly measures red blood cell (RBC) mass, so if the RBCs are of normal size, then the Hct should confirm the RBC count. Patients with macrocytic, microcytic, or iron deficiency anemia with small RBCs will not have parallel Hct and RBC counts. Report results as Packed Cell Volume (PCV), meaning the percentage by volume of packed red blood cells in whole blood. Normal values for venous blood are: Males 42-52%; females 36-48%. Microhematocrit readings from capillary tubes are a little higher. Infants have higher hematocrits than adults because they have more macrocytic RBC's. An abnormal hematocrit suggests follow-up tests must be done for a firm diagnosis. Low hematocrit readings (less than 30%) may indicate many diseases,

Copyright © Mometrix Media. You have been licensed one copy of this document for personal use only. Any other reproduction or redistribution is strictly prohibited. All rights reserved. This content is provided for test preparation purposes only and does not imply an endorsement by Mometrix of any particular political, scientific, or religious point of view.

including adrenal insufficiency, anemia, burns, Hodgkin's disease, leukemia, or poisoning. High hematocrit can be from erythrocytosis, polycythemia vera, or shock.

MONITORING RBC, WBC, AND PLATELETS

The medical assistant performs a quality control test on the Coulter counter every 8 hours by manually comparing RBC, WBC, and platelet counts on a smear against the machine's reading for the same patient. The patient's blood may be normal, but the machine could report an incorrect result if the quality of the stain used was poor (too acidic or alkaline), the specimen was diluted incorrectly, or the machine's calculation was inaccurate.

Test	Normal Values
RBC count	Infants: 3-5 million cells per microliter of blood (cells/mcL)—varies greatly from newborn to toddler Adult males: 4.35-5.65 million cells/mcL Adult females: 3.92-5.13 million cells/mcL, but lower in pregnancy
WBC count	3,400-10,000 WBC's per microliter (cells/mcL) Differential: 1% basophils, 1-3% eosinophils, 50-70% neutrophils, 15-40% lymphocytes, and 2-8% monocytes
Platelets	Infants: 200,000-475,000 per mcL Adults: 150,000-450,000 per mcL

MONITORING PATIENTS ON ANTICOAGULATION

The three tests used to monitor patients who take the blood thinner (anticoagulant) coumadin are **INR**, **PT**, and **PTT**. Note that PT and PTT are being phased out in favor of INR.

INR (international normalized ratio) checks clotting Factor VII to I. It standardizes different tissue factors (thromboplastin) used worldwide for testing. Normal INR is 0.9-1.2. If a patient has an INR under 0.8, there is little bleeding (due to rapid clotting). If a patient has an INR of 3.0-4.5, there is heavy bleeding (hemorrhage). Most patients on anticoagulant therapy (coumadin, heparin, and warfarin) are kept with an INR of 2.0-3.0, depending on their condition. If the patient is very likely to develop blood clots, the doctor may push the INR to 3.5. Therapeutic INR is checked every 4-6 weeks. Prolonged INR may be due to bile deficiency, cirrhosis of the liver, lack of Vitamin K, or small intestine disease.

Normal PT (prothrombin time) is 10-12 seconds. Therapeutic value for patients on coumadin is 13-18 seconds. PT checks Factor VII to I.

Normal PTT (partial thromboplastin time) is 25-38 seconds. Therapeutic value for patients on coumadin is 38-76 seconds. PTT checks Factor XII to I.

Copyright © Mometrix Media. You have been licensed one copy of this document for personal use only. Any other reproduction or redistribution is strictly prohibited. All rights reserved. This content is provided for test preparation purposes only and does not imply an endorsement by Mometrix of any particular political, scientific, or religious point of view.

ESR

An erythrocyte sedimentation rate (**ESR** or **sed rate**) measures how far blood cells with anticoagulant (EDTA or sodium citrate) will fall in a clump (aggregate) in a Westergren or Wintrobe tube in one hour, due to changes in plasma proteins (Rouleaux formation). Normal RBC's do not form Rouleaux, and they settle slowly. Normal values are as follows:

- Males <50 years of age: 0-15 mm/hr
- Males >50 years of age: 0-20 mm/hr
- Females <50 years of age: 0-20 mm/hr
- Females >50 years of age: 0-30mm/hr
- Children: 0-10 mm/hr

If RBC's settle quickly, the Rouleaux indicates some type of inflammation, necrosis, or parasites are present and further tests are required, but a sed rate does not definitively diagnose a disease. A high ESR can indicate many diseases: Anemia, arthritis, cancer, heart attack, lupus, pelvic inflammatory disease, kidney disease, pneumonia, poisoning with heavy metals, syphilis, thyroid disease, toxemia, and tuberculosis. A low sed rate can result from heavy blood loss.

C-REACTIVE PROTEIN

C-reactive protein (CRP) is a globulin required to resist bacterial infections and inflammation. CRP binds to dying cells to activate the complement system, triggering it to fight infection and disease. Young people normally have a CRP less than 10 mg/L. Pregnant women, the elderly, and patients with mild viral infections or inflammation have a slightly elevated CRP of 10-40 mg/L. However, CRP rises in 6 hours after a severe infection or inflammation occurs, up to 200 mg/L, and peaks in 48 hours. People with massive burns or overwhelming bacterial infections have CRP levels over 200 mg/L. CRP is elevated in patients with rheumatic fever, heart disease, colon cancer, pneumonia, tuberculosis, lupus, diabetes, vasculitis, rheumatoid arthritis, septic arthritis, and osteomyelitis. Athletes who train excessively decrease their CRP and become more susceptible to infections as a result. To perform a CRP test, draw 10 mL of blood in a red stoppered tube. The immunohistochemistry lab performs an ELISA latex agglutination test to measure the C-reactive protein level. A positive result indicates only inflammation somewhere in the body.

BLOOD SUGAR MONITORING

The following tests monitor blood sugar for suspected or confirmed diabetes:

- **Fasting blood sugar**: Instruct the patient to fast for 8 hours before collection. Do not drink excessive water, as it dilutes the blood (and therefore the sugar level). Normal fasting blood sugar is less than 100 mg/dL. Use a grey stoppered tube because the oxalate preservative stops the blood cells from eating sugar.
- **2 hr. p.c.**: Two hours post cibum (after eating). After the fasting blood collection, the patient takes a normal meal and returns for a second collection exactly 2 hours after it was finished. Blood sugar should peak two hours after eating (postprandial), and then drop precipitously.
- **HbA1c**: A test for glucose bound to hemoglobin in red blood cells over their 120-day lifespan. It is a snapshot of blood glucose control for the past three months and can help to evaluate the effectiveness of strategies being used to control diabetes such as medication or diet.
- **GTT**: A 3- or 5-hour glucose tolerance test diagnoses hyperglycemia (high blood sugar) that is a precursor to diabetes. Collect blood and urine fasting, 30 minutes after a glucose drink was finished, and at 1 hour, 2 hours, and 3 hours. Occasionally it is ordered at 4 and 5 hours.

Copyright © Mometrix Media. You have been licensed one copy of this document for personal use only. Any other reproduction or redistribution is strictly prohibited. All rights reserved.
This content is provided for test preparation purposes only and does not imply an endorsement by Mometrix of any particular political, scientific, or religious point of view.

PREGNANCY TESTING

Beta Human Chorionic Gonadotropin (beta-hCG) is the substance the lab tests urine or blood for to confirm female pregnancy or gestational tumors, or testicular tumors in males. It is performed preoperatively as a precaution for women of childbearing age.

Qualitative hCG just confirms the pregnancy, as it is detectable one week after conception. Tell the patient to collect the first morning urine sample, if possible, because it is the most concentrated at that time. Avoid taking diuretics or the antihistamine promethazine, because it could create a false-negative result. The patient should tell the doctor if they take drugs to control epilepsy or Parkinson's disease, or tranquilizers or hypnotics to induce sleep, because they can cause false-positive results. At least 50 mL is required in a clean jar. The specimen must not be contaminated with stool, menstrual blood, semen, or prostate extractions.

Quantitative hCG helps diagnose ectopic or failing pregnancy, ovarian or testicular tumors, or monitors a woman after a miscarriage. Draw a red stoppered tube of blood for the lab. High levels of beta-hCG in blood indicate tumor progression. Low levels indicate effective cancer treatment.

VAGINAL SWAB FOR MATERNAL STREP B

The procedure to collect a vaginal swab for maternal strep B is described below:

1. Wash and glove hands.
2. The patient should be informed that two swabs will be collected to ensure there is no danger to her newborn.
3. Tell the patient to remove her trousers and panties, but she may retain a skirt.
4. Cover the patient with a clean drape for modesty.
5. Position her face up on the exam table and move her buttocks to the bottom edge.
6. The patient must spread her legs widely, so if she has difficulty, place her feet in the stirrups.
7. Do not use lubricant.
8. Gently open her labia with one hand.
9. Clean mucous away from the mother's cervix with a clean, dry vaginal swab. Discard the swab.
10. Apply a Strep B swab to her cervix for 10 seconds to collect a sample.
11. Place it in the media container.
12. Snap off the end of the stick so the lid fits tightly.
13. Label the vial with the patient's name and date.
14. Give the patient a disposable wipe to clean herself before departing.

STOOL COLLECTION PROCEDURES
O&P AND PINWORM

Stool for ova and parasites (O&P) is a test that assesses for worms (helminths) and protozoa that can cause anemia in feces samples, such as tapeworm and round worms. Give the patient a clean jar containing an ounce of formalin. Tell the patient to use a popsicle stick to mix a teaspoon of stool with the preservative and return it, tightly capped and labeled, to the lab.

Pinworms are white, thread-like parasites usually contracted by children from sand boxes in which infected cats and dogs have defecated. The child often scratches his/her itchy bottom and grinds the teeth while sleeping. Give the parent a stool container containing a pinworm paddle, or tell the parent to use a jar with clear tape. When the child sleeps, use a flashlight to visualize the anus. Female tapeworms leave the bowel to lay eggs around the anus at night. Gently touch the paddle or

157

Copyright © Mometrix Media. You have been licensed one copy of this document for personal use only. Any other reproduction or redistribution is strictly prohibited. All rights reserved. This content is provided for test preparation purposes only and does not imply an endorsement by Mometrix of any particular political, scientific, or religious point of view.

tape to the anus and place it in the jar. Cap tightly. Wash hands well. Return the labeled jar to the lab.

OCCULT BLOOD AND GUAIAC

Patients who use aspirin regularly or have ulcers may lose microscopic amounts of blood in their feces. The lab examines stool smears on a mail-in card for **occult blood**. Provide the patient with an occult blood kit. Instruct the patient to follow the enclosed diet for three days before collection, as foods that cause bleeding must be avoided (e.g., cantaloupe, turnip, broccoli and horseradish). Tell the patient to place plastic wrap under the toilet seat and defecate. Use the enclosed popsicle sticks to smear thin samples of stool from three consecutive bowel movements on the three windows in the card. The patient mails the card back to the lab in the envelope provided.

Guaiac also detects occult blood, but is collected by the doctor in the office during a rectal examination with a gloved finger. The doctor wipes the soiled glove across a window that contains guaiac resin on a card and adds two drops of peroxide. If the sample oxidizes (turns blue) in 2 seconds or less, the patient is losing blood.

These two tests are not reliable tests for bowel cancer.

SPUTUM CULTURE

Sputum is phlegm (mucous) and other matter expelled from the lungs and trachea. It should contain as little saliva from the mouth as possible. Sputum can be cultured (C&S) to identify an infection, such as pneumonia. Sputum can be examined microscopically to identify cancer or a disease-causing agent, such as asbestos fibers. If the doctor orders sputum for AFB (acid fast bacilli stain), then the lab searches for bacteria that cause tuberculosis. Drink fluids the night before specimen collection, to encourage secretions. Collect the specimen upon arising, because sputum collects in the air passageways during sleep. Tap on the chest. Cough deeply. If unable to produce any sputum, try inhaling steaming salt water. If any sputum arises, spit it into a sterile cup. Cap it tightly and label it. Bring the sputum to the lab immediately for testing. If unable to transport it immediately, refrigerate it up to 3 days. The doctor may order specimen collection on 3 consecutive days.

KIDNEY (RENAL) FUNCTION TESTS

The following are kidney (renal) function tests and their normal values:

- **BUN**: Blood urea nitrogen (BUN) is a nitrogenous waste byproduct of amino acid metabolism. Urea is the end product. BUN is normally excreted by the kidneys at 7-20 mg/dL. Patients with end-stage renal disease (ESRD) have BUN levels between 60-100 mg/dL and are monitored monthly.
- **Creatinine**: Creatinine is the end-product of muscle metabolism and is normally removed by the kidneys at 0.7-1.5 mg/dL. High creatinine (over 1.5 mg/dL) and BUN (over 20 mg/dL) means the patient has a kidney disease (e.g., glomerulonephritis, pyelonephritis, stones, tubular necrosis, or tumors).
- **Protein**: A normal serum protein test includes total protein 6-8 g/dL, albumin 3.5-5.0 g/dL, and globulin 2.5-3.0 g/dL. Albumin deficiency causes swelling (edema) and can be from protein malnutrition, kidney or liver, and disease. Low globulin indicates severe burns, malnutrition, or kidney or liver disease.
- **Urea**: Carbamide, a nitrogenous waste product of protein metabolism made by the liver from ammonia and aspartic acid (an amino acid). Healthy kidneys eliminate about 10 g of urea daily. Purified urea is used as a diuretic, pressure reducer, and antiseptic.

Copyright © Mometrix Media. You have been licensed one copy of this document for personal use only. Any other reproduction or redistribution is strictly prohibited. All rights reserved. This content is provided for test preparation purposes only and does not imply an endorsement by Mometrix of any particular political, scientific, or religious point of view.

24-HOUR CREATININE CLEARANCE TEST

The 24-hour creatinine clearance test determines if kidneys are damaged by measuring their output of creatinine against the blood level. If the kidneys do not filter properly, creatinine output in the urine decreases and blood levels increase. In a normal male, creatinine clearance results fall between 110 and 150 mL/min; in normal females, they are between 95 and 125 mL/min. A BUN-to-creatinine ratio between 15:1 and 20:1 is a normal finding.

Patients should be instructed to prepare for the test in the following way: Two days before and during the test, do NOT eat more than 8 ounces of red meat, take Vitamin C, drink caffeine, or exercise strenuously. Discard the first morning urine in the toilet. Note the start time. Collect all urine in the jug up to and including the same time the next morning. Keep the jug on a bucket of ice or in the refrigerator. Note the time of the last collection. Return to the lab the next morning to have a blood creatinine level drawn for comparison.

Drugs that affect the test include diuretics, vitamin C, levodopa, Tagamet, Mefoxin, Dilantin, Garamycin, quinine, procainamide, amphotericin B, and tetracycline.

LIVER FUNCTION TESTS

ALP (Alkaline Phosphatase) normally ranges from 40-129 IU/L in adults and up to 300 in children with growing bones. Doctors use ALP to differentiate between bone and liver diseases. ALP increases in bone fractures and Paget's disease, liver cancer, hyperparathyroidism, hyperphosphatasia, infarcted bowel, and rheumatoid arthritis. ALP decreases in pernicious anemia, celiac disease, hypothyroidism, low serum phosphorous (hypophosphatemia), and malnutrition.

ALT (Serum Alanine Aminotransferase) normally ranges from 7-55 IU/L. ALT increases in liver disease. AST:ALT ratio should be 1:1. If it is greater than 1:1, this can indicate cirrhosis, congestion, or tumors of the liver. If the ratio is less than 1:1, suspect hepatitis or mononucleosis.

AST (Serum Aspartate Aminotransferase) normally ranges from 8-48 IU/L. AST increases in conditions that affect the heart such as congestive heart failure, liver such as chronic alcohol or drug abuse or cirrhosis, muscles such as muscular dystrophy, or pancreatitis.

Bilirubin normally ranges from 0.1-1.2 mg/dL (0.3-1.0 mg/dL for individuals under 18 years of age). It is a reddish-yellow bile pigment created when the liver breaks down old red blood cells, and is stored in the gall bladder. Excess bilirubin causes jaundice. The medical assistant can artificially lower bilirubin by leaving a specimen tube exposed to light at room temperature for one hour, shaking the specimen, or allowing air bubbles in it.

TESTS FOR MONONUCLEOSIS

Epstein-Barr virus (EBV) causes mononucleosis. The **Monospot** heterophile antibodies test confirms the patient is in the early stage of mononucleosis (2-9 weeks). To perform a Monospot, drop capillary or venous blood on a glass slide. Mix with guinea pig kidney antigen to absorb Forssmann antibodies. Mix with beef red blood stroma to absorb non-Forssman antibodies. Mix with horse blood. Guinea pig agglutination means the patient has early mononucleosis. Beef should not agglutinate. Monospot can be false-negative on children under 10, or before two weeks of infection. False-positives are caused by adenovirus, Burkitt's and Hodgkin's lymphomas, cytomegalovirus, hepatitis, HIV, leukemia, lupus, pregnancy, rheumatoid arthritis, rubella, and toxoplasmosis. Monospot may not detect an infection that is older than six months.

Copyright © Mometrix Media. You have been licensed one copy of this document for personal use only. Any other reproduction or redistribution is strictly prohibited. All rights reserved. This content is provided for test preparation purposes only and does not imply an endorsement by Mometrix of any particular political, scientific, or religious point of view.

If the patient has late-stage mono, the doctor orders EBV antibody titer, CBC, and throat swab. To perform a titer, serially dilute blood serum or other body fluids with saline. Negative is less than 1:40 EBV and no IgM antibodies are present. Positive is greater than 1:40 and antibodies are present. IgM indicates the active phase of mono. IgG antibodies mean the patient is recovering from mononucleosis.

TEST FOR STREP THROAT

Often, acute pharyngitis results from group A streptococci. **Strep throat** especially affects children 5-15 years old in the winter and spring. Strep throat can develop into rheumatic fever when it travels through the bloodstream to destroy the heart, joints, and kidneys. "Super Strep" strains are resistant to antibiotics. To perform a Quidel QuickVue rapid strep test:

- Swab the patient's tonsils and pharynx for no more than five seconds with the swab in the kit. Use a tongue depressor to avoid swabbing the cheeks and tongue. The patient will gag briefly.
- Place the swab in the test cassette chamber.
- Crush the extraction reagent delivery device.
- Mix the extraction solutions until they turn green.
- Add the solution to the top rim of the swab chamber.
- Stand the swab upright in the chamber so capillary action draws the solution up to the rabbit reagent pad.
- Read the window at five minutes. A red stripe on the reagent strip indicates strep infection. The control is the blue line next to the letter C, and it should always appear. The absence of a red line indicates no strep infection. A positive result means the patient requires antibiotic treatment to avoid rheumatic fever.

TEST FOR TUBERCULOSIS

The tests that identify tuberculosis (TB) are a positive **Mantoux skin test** or **QFT-G blood test**. Both must be confirmed by chest x-ray and sputum culture to determine whether the TB is active or latent. 10% of exposed persons with positive Mantoux tests develop active TB infection. Employers offer prophylaxis with Isoniazid (INH) if a medical assistant is exposed to an active TB case.

To perform the two-step Mantoux skin test:

- Week 1: The medical assistant injects 0.1 mL of 5 units of tuberculin intradermally in the patient's forearm.
- 2-3 days later: The patient returns to have the test read. A negative test has no redness or swelling.
- Week 2 or 3: The medical assistant repeats the test again to prevent identification of a booster reaction as a positive TB result.

Patients with AIDS, lupus, renal failure, or kidney transplant have false-negative reactions to Mantoux. The patient who received BCG vaccine against TB will have a false-positive reaction. Ask the registered nurse to perform the QFT-G blood test for these patients, instead of Mantoux.

Copyright © Mometrix Media. You have been licensed one copy of this document for personal use only. Any other reproduction or redistribution is strictly prohibited. All rights reserved. This content is provided for test preparation purposes only and does not imply an endorsement by Mometrix of any particular political, scientific, or religious point of view.

COLLECTING A WOUND CULTURE

To obtain a wound culture, first gather a biohazard waste bag, a microbiology requisition, a cleansing pack, and a sterile dressing. Use a red-stoppered swab for MRSA testing and a charcoal swab for all other tests.

1. Wash and glove hands and don personal protective equipment (PPE).
2. Create a sterile field with drapes; examine the wound.
3. Note in the patient's chart the presence of pus; foul odor; discharge; cellulitis; discoloration; delayed healing; friable, granulated tissue; increased pain to touch; pocketing; or wound enlargement.
4. Wet the swab with sterile saline and rotate it 360° across the wound in a zigzag.
5. Place the swab in the media and cap tightly.
6. Clean the wound with disinfectant (e.g., Betadine) and dress it.
7. Discard soiled articles and doff PPE.
8. If the patient is taking antibiotics, note it on the requisition.
9. Do not refrigerate the swab; transport it to the lab immediately.

Copyright © Mometrix Media. You have been licensed one copy of this document for personal use only. Any other reproduction or redistribution is strictly prohibited. All rights reserved.
This content is provided for test preparation purposes only and does not imply an endorsement by Mometrix of any particular political, scientific, or religious point of view.

General Office Procedures

Office Communication

CORRECT COMMA USE

Commas separate parts of a sentence that need to be emphasized or isolated so that the sentence will make sense. Commas set apart afterthoughts ("You look marvelous, my dear"), interrupting elements ("It makes sense, I think, to go ahead with the plan"), transitional phrases ("Roger, on the other hand, was prepared for action"), or descriptive expressions ("My new book, *Feeling Young Again*, is available in paperback"). Commas set the year apart in a representation of the date, and set apart all of the abbreviations and titles that follow a person's name.

Do not use a comma to set a verb apart from its object or complement. Do not use a comma to separate adjectives from their succeeding nouns or to separate a noun from the prepositional phrase that follows it. Commas can be used to divide two independent clauses in a sentence when the clauses are connected by *and*, *but*, *or*, or *nor*. Commas can divide three or more items in a series or more than one adjective that is being used to modify the same noun.

CORRECT SEMICOLON USE

Semicolons are meant to be used between independent clauses in a sentence whenever there is not conjunction such as *and* or *but*. Use a semicolon between clauses whenever one of the clauses has several commas, and the addition of another comma separating the two clauses has the potential to make the sentence unclear. Semicolons should be used to separate the independent clauses in a sentence any time the conjunction between the two sentences is *besides*, *consequently*, *nevertheless*, *however*, or *therefore*. It is also appropriate to use semicolons to separate the items in a list when the items in that list contain commas; for instance, a list of dates that includes the years should be separated by semicolons.

CORRECT COLON USE

Colons are used before the beginning of a list and to separate two independent clauses when the second cause elaborates on the first clause and there is no transitional expression or coordinating conjunction. Use a colon to set apart hours and minutes in a description of the time, as in 8:20. Use a colon to divide the units in a ratio, as in, "Make a 1:5 dilution of sodium hypochlorite in water." Colons are used in lieu of commas in the salutation line of a business document. Legal letters and personal correspondence use a comma after the salutation. In the documents familiar to a medical assistant, a colon is found in the reference notations, attention lines, subject lines, enclosure notations, copy notations, and postscripts.

Colons can be used to draw attention to a certain part of a sentence. For instance, a colon might be used after the word *therefore* in order to emphasize the insight that is to follow. Colons can also be effectively used in cases where the anticipatory phrase is not explicit, as in "Red foxes are beautiful creatures: long tails, keen eyes, and sleek pelts." Avoid using a colon when the anticipatory expression is at the beginning of an extremely long sentence.

Copyright © Mometrix Media. You have been licensed one copy of this document for personal use only. Any other reproduction or redistribution is strictly prohibited. All rights reserved. This content is provided for test preparation purposes only and does not imply an endorsement by Mometrix of any particular political, scientific, or religious point of view.

CAPITALIZATION, PARENTHESES, AND QUOTATION MARKS

Capitalize the following words:

- First word in a sentence or list
- Independent questions within a sentence
- Proper nouns
- Adjectives derived from proper nouns
- Imaginative names and nicknames
- Each item in an outline
- The first word of a quoted sentence

Simple common nouns, like police officer or doctor, need not be capitalized.

Parentheses are used to set nonessential items apart, identify a citation, or to surround a brief explanation for example. Parentheses are often used for dates, references, authorities, or items on a list.

Quotation marks indicate the title of a piece of work. They may provide a special emphasis to certain words or phrases, or they may indicate that a person's exact words are being used. Any periods or commas at the end of a phrase inside quotation marks should be inside the quotation marks, though all semicolons and colons will go outside. Exclamation points and quotation marks should only go inside quotation marks when they are applied strictly to the quoted expression.

GREEK CHARACTERS AND MATHEMATICAL SYMBOLS AND EQUATIONS

To find Greek characters and mathematical symbols in Microsoft Word, choose *Insert > Symbol > More Symbols*. Scroll through the *Subsets*. To type the equation in Microsoft Word, choose *Insert > Equation >* and either *Built-In* or *Insert New Equation*.

Character	Pronunciation	Character	Pronunciation
α	alpha	ν	nu
β	beta	ξ	xi
γ	gamma	o	omicron
δ	delta	π	pi
ε	epsilon	ρ	rho
ζ	zeta	σ	sigma
η	eta	τ	tau
θ	theta	υ	upsilon
ι	iota	φ	phi
κ	kappa	χ	chi
λ	lambda	ψ	psi
μ	mu	ω	omega

Copyright © Mometrix Media. You have been licensed one copy of this document for personal use only. Any other reproduction or redistribution is strictly prohibited. All rights reserved. This content is provided for test preparation purposes only and does not imply an endorsement by Mometrix of any particular political, scientific, or religious point of view.

PROOFREADING ROUGH DRAFTS

To create accurate documents, a medical assistant must be adept at **proofreading**. The basic steps of proofreading a document are:

1. **Read backwards**: Three complete readings of a document are required. During the first reading, look for errors in punctuation and spelling, and word repetition with a software spellchecker. In the second reading, look for layout, grammar and style mistakes and add new words to the custom dictionary in the software's spellchecker. Here, it is helpful to read the document backwards, starting with the last sentence and working back up. This helps the author to see each sentence on its own. In the third reading, consider syntax. Ensure the document flows in logical sequence, and is easy to read and understand.
2. **Correct**: Check questionable words with the following references: Medical dictionary; English dictionary; drug compendium; spelling, grammar, and punctuation checking software; thesaurus; and directories (books or online) with the current addresses of relevant doctors, hospitals, and clinics.
3. **Revise**: Query the doctor in square or angle brackets or use Word's comment feature.
4. **Create an error analysis chart**: Keep a record of mistakes to save time in future.

TELEPHONE ETIQUETTE

Elements of appropriate telephone etiquette include the following:

- When starting work, ask the doctor which calls to put through immediately and which should be screened. Give messages to the doctor between appointments.
- Turn the lines over to a reliable answering service whenever out of the office. Record a detailed message (including where to go in an emergency and fax number for pharmacies) with music intervals whenever busy and check messages frequently.
- Get a landline number for the doctor when possible. Most hospitals forbid the use of cellular phones because they interfere with telemetry. They often permit pagers instead, but doctors cannot answer them in the OR.
- Write all telephone messages in a book with carbon copies, not on scrap paper. Include the caller's name, patient's name, phone number, a brief message, and the pharmacy or referring doctor's number.
- End personal calls immediately when a patient arrives. Acknowledge patients who arrive when on a medical call.

PRIORITIZING INCOMING TELEPHONE CALLS

The medical assistant answers the telephone within three rings. Identify oneself with, "Good morning/afternoon. Dr. Gentle's office, [your name] speaking." Record the caller's name, number, and detailed information in the day log. Do not put a call on hold until being certain that it is not an emergency.

Screen the call to determine if it is emergent, urgent, or routine. Do not interrupt the doctor, unless it is emergent or he or she instructs you to do so. If the doctor is occupied, instruct the emergent caller to go to the nearest emergency room. Phone 911 if the caller is unable to do so.

For routine and urgent calls, say, "The doctor is with a patient. May I give the doctor a message and ask him/her to return your call?" Most doctors allocate one hour per day to return phone calls and prepare prescriptions for the assistant to fax to pharmacies. The medical assistant must not give medical advice. Ask the routine or urgent caller to make an appointment. Do not release test results

Copyright © Mometrix Media. You have been licensed one copy of this document for personal use only. Any other reproduction or redistribution is strictly prohibited. All rights reserved. This content is provided for test preparation purposes only and does not imply an endorsement by Mometrix of any particular political, scientific, or religious point of view.

over the phone, unless instructed to do so by the doctor. Pass along urgent messages to the doctor before routine messages.

MANAGING EMERGENCY SITUATIONS VIA TELEPHONE

Some states have very specific guidelines as to which healthcare professional are able to screen patients by telephone or to give directions, so the certified medical assistant must be aware of state guidelines. Medical assistants, who are not trained or licensed to diagnose or give medical advice, can generally screen telephone calls but must be knowledgeable about the types of questions to ask and should follow a screening manual when taking calls to ensure consistency. The screening manual should list the appropriate questions to ask depending on the patient's complaints/issues and indicate which responses require intervention of other healthcare providers, such as emergency medical personnel or an RN. When using a screening manual, the medical assistant should not deviate from the manual and should immediately consult a nurse or physician if the patient's complaints are not in the manual or the medical assistant has concerns (such as the inability to make an immediate appointment for a patient in distress).

DISTRIBUTION OF TEST RESULTS

INFORMING PATIENTS OF TEST RESULTS

Patients should be informed of diagnostic procedure results as soon as possible, as patients are often anxious when awaiting results. Once test results are received and the date entered into the diagnostic procedure tracking log, the test should be reviewed by the ordering healthcare provider before the patient is notified of the results. The healthcare provider should indicate who should notify the patient. When test results are negative, the medical assistant may be tasked with notifying the patient either by letter (standard format is generally utilized) or telephone. If test results are positive and/or follow-up is required, then the ordering healthcare provider or a nurse usually contacts the patient. In some cases, the medical assistant may need to make a follow-up appointment for the healthcare provider to discuss test results with the patient. For serious results, such as a positive finding of cancer, the physician should speak directly to the patient, in person if possible.

HANDLING RESULTS RECEIVED FROM OUTSIDE PROVIDERS

Results from **outside providers** may include consultant reports and diagnostic test results. The physician should be immediately notified as per office protocol when a consultant report is received and a notation made in the patient's medical record. The diagnostic procedure tracking log is used to record all diagnostic procedures that are scheduled to ensure that no results are overlooked and that patients are informed of the results of all tests. Formats may vary somewhat. The diagnostic procedure tracking log should be filled out immediately when procedures are scheduled and again when results are received. The log should be checked every work day at the beginning of the day and again at the end so that calls to patients are made in a timely manner and recorded. The physician should be notified when diagnostic results are received and the results included in the patient's medical record.

Copyright © Mometrix Media. You have been licensed one copy of this document for personal use only. Any other reproduction or redistribution is strictly prohibited. All rights reserved. This content is provided for test preparation purposes only and does not imply an endorsement by Mometrix of any particular political, scientific, or religious point of view.

Medical Transcription

STANDARD SET-UP FOR MEDICAL TRANSCRIPTIONS

The standard set-up for any transcription includes the following:

- 8.5" x 11" white bond paper with black ink
- Margins at least 1" on all sides
- Portrait orientation
- Headings flush with the left margin, except for manuscripts, in which they are centered
- Double space between heading lines, paragraphs, and below the last line of the message
- Triple space before the memo, report, or chart message
- Most medical offices use full block style
- Double space drafts, with 5 spaces indented at the beginning of each paragraph
- Single space the body of the corrected message when it is ready to print and sign
- If the document is longer than one page, type the recipient's name, page number, date, and RE: Patient's Name at the top of each page.

Every document must contain:

- Date (and time if it is an Operating Room Report)
- Unique patient identifier (e.g., medical record number)
- Patient's name
- Dictator's name and credentials
- Typist's initials at the bottom left margin

TRANSCRIPTION ERRORS

The patient's health and life are at stake if a medical transcriptionist makes an **error**. One's reputation will be crippled if errors are discovered by accreditation surveyors or judges. Some of the most common errors found in medical records are incorrect usage, misspelling, added or omitted letters, grammatical errors, confusion of unfamiliar words, and confusion of similar-sounding words (homonyms). These errors can largely be avoided through careful proofreading and reference to the appropriate sources. Remember that the patient's health and life are also adversely impacted by transcription delays and slow turnaround time. Always find out which dictations are STAT before beginning the workday, and prioritize accordingly.

DIFFICULTIES FOR NOVICE TRANSCRIPTIONISTS

Novice transcriptionists often have a hard time learning to understand medical dictation, especially if the doctor has a foreign accent or a strong local dialect. Medical recordings are frequently made in a loud setting with many distractions, so they are choppy, disjointed, and bursting with jargon and medical terminology. A transcriptionist's income and reputation depend on productivity and accuracy. New transcriptionists need to make use of medical dictionaries and other references in order to make sense of medical dictation. They should familiarize themselves with the dictionary or reference format for quick and effective use. In most medical dictionaries, the most commonly used noun is listed as the main entry and any related terms are subentries.

Copyright © Mometrix Media. You have been licensed one copy of this document for personal use only. Any other reproduction or redistribution is strictly prohibited. All rights reserved. This content is provided for test preparation purposes only and does not imply an endorsement by Mometrix of any particular political, scientific, or religious point of view.

REFERENCE SOURCES FOR TRANSCRIPTIONS

The **Pharmaceutical Reference Guide** and **CPS** are alphabetical indices of all the drugs that have been approved for prescription by the Food and Drug Administration. The entry for each drug will include the drug's method of administration, recommended dosage, classification, indications and contraindications of use, generic name, and brand names. These books are expensive and released annually, so it is more cost effective to pay for an up-to-date online subscription or check the FDA Orange Book, available for free on the FDA's website. Other useful reference books include the *Taber's Cyclopedic Medical Dictionary*, and the *Medical Word Book* and *Surgical Word Book*, both available from Saunders. Word books contain an alphabetical list of all the words that are commonly associated with medical and surgical procedures but do not contain definitions. Users should find the closest sounding entry that makes sense when they cannot understand a dictated word.

TRANSCRIBING DOCTOR'S DICTATION

Time permitting, a medical transcriptionist should listen to the entire dictation tape before he or she begins to transcribe a document. This helps the transcriptionist to get a general idea of the structure of the dictation and have an opportunity to notice any areas of difficulty or complexity. Resources should be used to identify difficult words; similar documents transcribed by predecessors can be used for comparison. Once the initial listening is complete, the transcriptionist can begin listening to small portions of the tape and transcribing them electronically. After the entire tape has been transcribed, he or she can begin the process of proofreading. Institutional regulations should be followed to erase and reuse a tape.

OPERATIVE REPORT AND POSTOPERATIVE NOTES

Provided that surgery progressed well, the OR team transfers accountability for the patient to the recovery room team. The surgeon dictates a detailed **operative report**. The patient's physiological functioning generally returns to normal over 1-3 hours, depending on the type of surgery and anesthesia. The physician's assistant on the surgery usually dictates a brief **postoperative note**, which is not as detailed as a progress report, and can use abbreviations if the facility allows them. The following information should be included in the postoperative note:

- Date and time
- Unique patient identifier (e.g., medical record number)
- Patient's name
- Subjective symptoms (e.g., how the patient reports on the following: complaints of discomfort or anxiety, pain control, passing flatus, diet, comfort when ambulating)
- Objective signs (e.g., vital signs, edema, bowel sounds, chest sounds, incision status)
- Assessment (e.g., "The 42-year-old white female was alert and responsive after laparoscopic cholecystectomy...")
- Plan (e.g., remove Foley catheter, change from IV to oral pain control, advance to soft diet when flatus occurs, encourage ambulation)

Copyright © Mometrix Media. You have been licensed one copy of this document for personal use only. Any other reproduction or redistribution is strictly prohibited. All rights reserved. This content is provided for test preparation purposes only and does not imply an endorsement by Mometrix of any particular political, scientific, or religious point of view.

PROGRESS REPORTS

If the patient experienced complications during surgery or has difficulty recovering from anesthesia, he or she is transferred to the intensive care unit (ICU) for close monitoring. Vital signs (temperature, pulse, respirations, blood pressure, level of consciousness) are checked every 15-30 minutes. The interval increases as the patient's condition returns to baseline. The nurse may obtain central venous pressures and fluid balance (tracking all fluids that enter and exit the patient). The patient is stabilized before being moved to a step-down unit. The patient may move from step-down back to ICU or to an in-patient unit, according to his or her condition. The doctor, PA, or nurse practitioner dictates regular **progress reports** with more details than the Post Op Note. The progress report contains the following:

- Date and time
- Medical record number
- Patient's name
- Current level of functioning
- Amount of progress made
- Age appropriateness
- Assessments and plan
- The dictator's signature
- Avoid abbreviations and write in full sentences

DISCHARGE SUMMARY

The **discharge summary** is dictated at time of discharge. It contains the following:

- Admission and discharge dates
- Patient's name and medical record number
- Attending physician's name and contact information
- Chief complaint or reason(s) for admission
- History and physical examination
- Laboratory and x-ray findings
- Principal diagnosis
- Description of treatment
- Additional diagnoses
- Description of surgical procedure
- Disposition instructions given to the patient and/or caregivers (e.g., limit physical activity, medication timing, dietary restrictions, and follow-up appointment schedule)
- Prognosis for recovery
- Attending physician's signature and date

Documents required in the chart by law are the following:

- History and Physical Examination
- Operative Report
- Inpatient Progress Note
- Final Discharge Note

Discharge summaries are not required for routine births with a normal baby, including uncomplicated cesarean sections. If the patient's chart remains incomplete after 30 days, then the doctor's admitting privileges may be suspended.

Copyright © Mometrix Media. You have been licensed one copy of this document for personal use only. Any other reproduction or redistribution is strictly prohibited. All rights reserved. This content is provided for test preparation purposes only and does not imply an endorsement by Mometrix of any particular political, scientific, or religious point of view.

FINAL DISCHARGE NOTE

The intermediate recovery period follows the immediate postoperative period and continues until the patient's hospitalization is complete. The patient has totally recovered from anesthesia and the emphasis shifts to healing, maintaining a nutritious diet, and regaining independence. The case manager arranges therapy with the rehabilitation team and home care with visiting nurses. The doctor dictates a **final discharge note** for any patient hospitalized longer than 24 hours. Do not use abbreviations in the final discharge note. It is not as detailed as the discharge summary. Include this information:

- Date and time
- Principal diagnosis that required hospital admission
- Complications that developed during hospitalization and extended length of stay
- Comorbidities present prior to admission that require follow-up and additional resources (e.g., diabetes)
- Principle procedure related to the diagnosis
- Discharge plan, including available resources for home care or community care
- Signature of attending physician

Copyright © Mometrix Media. You have been licensed one copy of this document for personal use only. Any other reproduction or redistribution is strictly prohibited. All rights reserved. This content is provided for test preparation purposes only and does not imply an endorsement by Mometrix of any particular political, scientific, or religious point of view.

Business Practices

OFFICE EQUIPMENT

The medical assistant operates the following standard office equipment:

- Calculator
- Photocopier
- Computer
- Fax
- Telephone
- Scanner

In larger facilities, engineering welds an identification tag to each piece of equipment. The facilities manager (CHFM) tracks its whereabouts. Security investigates theft and vandalism. Security controls traffic, access, identification of personnel, and creates an environment that is reassuring to persons with a legitimate reason for being at the facility. In a small office environment, the medical assistant records all serial numbers and photographs each piece of equipment for insurance purposes. The medical assistant creates a sign-out log to keep track of borrowed equipment, asks local police and fire officials to perform a review of office security and fire safety, and reports theft and vandalism to local police.

MANAGING EQUIPMENT WITH A TICKLER FILE

File the manufacturer's recommendations for a preventative maintenance schedule when buying a new piece of equipment, and put the suggested date in the **tickler file** as a reminder. If there is no instruction guide provided when a second-hand machine was purchased, ask the vendor to provide one, or ask a biomedical engineer to write a manual as a resource for less skilled workers. Start a maintenance log for each new machine purchased, and keep it for the life of the machine or until its tax depreciation is finished, whichever comes later. Update the log with a description of each maintenance item performed, the name of the maintenance worker, the date and duration of maintenance, along with possible problems and feedback from the maintenance worker. Keep the log readily available with any relevant publications, such as service and operation manuals, and specialized tools for workers' use. Inspection and repair records, inspection schedules, and "as-built" drawings are also among the resources that should be available.

PROCESSING OF WORK ORDERS WHEN EQUIPMENT FAILS OR MUST BE MOVED

The medical assistant sends a **work order** to the maintenance department secretary by internal mail, fax, email, or phone. The maintenance secretary logs and time stamps the work order. The secretary alerts the supervisor if there are duplicate requests for the same work, and may phone the medical assistant to obtain clarification for the maintenance supervisor and to get the cost center number (if applicable). The supervisor reviews the work order to prioritize it. Work orders are not performed on a first-come-first-served basis. Work orders are prioritized as emergency (something that must be done at once), routine (something that should be done as quickly and efficiently as possible), and backlogged (something that must wait for parts, replacement, or cannot be done right away for some other reason). The supervisor may investigate who can do the work at the lowest cost. The supervisor signs the work order to authorize the work to begin as requested, and follows up to ensure it was completed.

MAINTENANCE AND REPAIRS OF MEDICAL AND OFFICE EQUIPMENT

In larger facilities, the facilities manager (CHFM) is responsible for equipment in all departments. In a small medical office, the medical assistant is responsible for ensuring the terms of a warranty or

170

Copyright © Mometrix Media. You have been licensed one copy of this document for personal use only. Any other reproduction or redistribution is strictly prohibited. All rights reserved. This content is provided for test preparation purposes only and does not imply an endorsement by Mometrix of any particular political, scientific, or religious point of view.

guarantee are fulfilled. The medical assistant deals with vendors and ensures that delivery dates and other specifications of purchase contracts are met. Careful record keeping lowers the risk of a warranty being voided based on poor maintenance. File all warranty records.

A large facility may have a **computerized maintenance management system (CMMS)** that contains illustrations and instructions for use of each piece of equipment. Scan the warranty into the facility's CMMS. In a small office, a manual **tickler file** is kept to prompt the medical assistant to schedule equipment maintenance on time. The tickler file helps reduce the costs associated with a piece of equipment by ensuring it is serviced according to the terms of its warranty. Include the expiration date of the warranty on the CMMS or tickler card.

MAIL

TYPES OF INCOMING MAIL

Types of incoming mail include the following:

Type of Mail	Example Carrier/Client
Routine letters and packages	United States Postal Service
Electronic money transfers	Western Union, chartered banks
Urgent letters and packages	Couriers such as DHL, FedEx, UPS; bike messengers
STAT specimens and drugs	Taxi-cab; armored vehicle (Brinks); Bus Express
Fax (facsimile)	Private offices, pharmacies, copy shops, postal outlets, hotels
Interoffice mail	Mailroom, porters, runners

HANDLING INCOMING MAIL

The modern medical assistant handles less paper today because email and voicemail have replaced most surface mail. The medical assistant can expedite processing so the doctor can deal with incoming mail efficiently by doing the following:

- Sign for insured or couriered mail and pay postage due from petty cash.
- Sort according to urgency the letters, bills, statements, interoffice, personal, newspapers and periodicals, ads and catalogs, and parcels.
- Open all mail except that marked "Personal and Confidential." If the addressee no longer works for the company, it goes to the successor if it is business-related. Forward personal mail to the last known home address.
- Inspect all business contents. If a date, signature, enclosure, or return address is missing, staple the envelope to the letter and annotate it. Tape torn letters. Discard most ads.
- Date and time stamp all mail for legal protection.
- Read and annotate each piece of mail, especially if it mentions an appointment date, a report being mailed separately, confirmation of a phone conversation, or requests a decision requiring more information.
- Present the doctor's mail to him or her covered in a folder to maintain confidentiality, with the most urgent on top.
- Distribute, route, or answer the remaining mail, as required.

Copyright © Mometrix Media. You have been licensed one copy of this document for personal use only. Any other reproduction or redistribution is strictly prohibited. All rights reserved. This content is provided for test preparation purposes only and does not imply an endorsement by Mometrix of any particular political, scientific, or religious point of view.

PREVENTING MAIL FROM GETTING DELAYED OR LOST

The following are the five tools the medical assistant uses to prevent mail from getting delayed or lost on another employee's desk:

- **Expected mail record**: If the medical assistant reads in the incoming mail that a report or other item will arrive separately, he or she should make note of it. When the expected item arrives, retrieve the original correspondence and attach it behind the new mail.
- **Annotation**: If there is a discrepancy or problem with the letter, write a note to the addressee in the margin. Examples:
  - The amount on an enclosed check does not match the amount stated in the letter.
  - The writer asks for a specific appointment time that conflicts with an existing booking.
- **Routing slip**: If the manager wants everyone in the office to read an item, attach a slip listing all their names, the reading sequence, and the date by which they need the item returned. Instruct the readers to initial and date the routing slip when they read the item.
- **Action requested slip**: Give informal directions to the reader, such as, "Please handle this for Marie while she is on vacation."
- **Digest of incoming mail**: When the manager is away for more than two days, log mail by date, sender, content, and the action taken, such as forwarding a request for employment verification to Human Resources.

PROCESSING OUTGOING MAIL

Cover outgoing mail at the desk with a folder or satchel to keep the addressee confidential. Delivery price is determined by size, weight, shape, urgency, destination, route (air or surface), insurance, signature verification, and contents. Price changes frequently, so check the USPS rate calculator on the USPS website. If insufficient postage is applied, then the item will be returned. If a return address is not included, then USPS will collect postage due from the recipient. Buy correct stamps and envelopes online at the USPS website.

Send items over 70 lb by freight carrier. The Department of Transportation (DOT) regulates shipping of diagnostic and biological specimens, infectious substances, and anything shipped on dry ice. Follow standards set by the International Air Transport Association (IATA), regardless of the distance the package is being shipped, or the transportation method (truck, rail, air, boat). The medical assistant needs the IATA Blue Pages to fill out the shipping manifest with the IATA shipping name, class, subsidiary risk, and UN codes. A Class 6.2 DOT sticker is also required, and if the biological is preserved with dry ice, a Class 9 DOT sticker.

Copyright © Mometrix Media. You have been licensed one copy of this document for personal use only. Any other reproduction or redistribution is strictly prohibited. All rights reserved. This content is provided for test preparation purposes only and does not imply an endorsement by Mometrix of any particular political, scientific, or religious point of view.

MEDICAL INVENTORY

The doctor and specialists inform the medical assistant which medical supply companies they purchase from routinely. Produce a list of required supplies, known as a **medical inventory**, including the following:

- Item name
- Size
- Color
- Number
- Units
- Cost
- Supplier's name
- Supplier's address
- Supplier's phone and fax numbers

This list tells the medical assistant how long an item lasts, when to reorder, and cost comparisons. Prescription pads and drug samples are available free from drug company sales reps.

Check the drug and supply cupboards against the supply list daily and weekly. Ensure the office always has adequate supplies available, but remember that reagents and drugs expire. Reorder before supplies are exhausted from the authorized suppliers only. Do not order large quantities without the doctor's authorization, as they may stale-date. Include the price quote on the purchase order (PO). Keep a copy of the PO in a pending file until the supplies arrive, for comparison to the packing slip.

Always lock the supply and drug cupboards. Drug addicts target painkillers, sleeping pills, tranquilizers, and syringes, so consult Pharmacy and Security about safe storage. Do not flush expired drugs down the toilet because they cause environmental harm. Call the hospital Pharmacy or drug rep to have the expired drugs incinerated.

OPERATING SYSTEMS AND SOFTWARE USED IN MEDICAL OFFICES

Most private medical offices use Windows **operating systems** on networked PCs. Most medical offices use Microsoft Office software, including Word, Outlook, Excel, Access, and PowerPoint. Common billing software packages are ABLEMed, EMR, Lytec, or Medisoft. The advantages of prepackaged software are that it is relatively cheap and many healthcare providers are already familiar with them. However, they are not customizable. The facility may hire programmers to write customized, proprietary software. Web-based scheduling and billing packages, such as Medical Office Online, are often much more expensive than prepackaged software.

If the clinic cannot afford prepackaged software, free alternatives to many of them are available, such as OpenOffice, an open-source software package that is largely compatible with Microsoft Office.

SAFEGUARDING PATIENT DATA

Medical office computers must comply with 1996 HIPAA Security Standards for the Protection of Electronic Protected Information. It is important for the medical assistant to recognize potential fraud and abuse. An unscrupulous user may sell a patient's information to a journalist or detective,

Copyright © Mometrix Media. You have been licensed one copy of this document for personal use only. Any other reproduction or redistribution is strictly prohibited. All rights reserved. This content is provided for test preparation purposes only and does not imply an endorsement by Mometrix of any particular political, scientific, or religious point of view.

or use it to stalk the patient, or alter the record to hide wrongdoing. **Safeguarding of patient data** includes the following:

- The medical assistant safeguards against computer viruses and hackers with regular antivirus and firewall updates.
- The supervisor ensures only authorized personnel access electronic health records (EHR) through an audit trail. The supervisor asks the IT Dept. to restrict access to a patient's EHR. The computer alerts the supervisor to a security breach (when someone attempts unauthorized access to the patient's EHR). The supervisor follows Standard ASTM E2147-01, which lists the specifications for audit trails in manual and EHR environments. Investigators will see who accessed a record, when, where, and previous versions.
- The IT programmer can restore the previous information through **versioning**, so that any tampering or falsification is not permanent.

SECURING ELECTRONIC APPLICATIONS CONTAINING PATIENT INFORMATION

Measures to ensure the security of electronic applications containing patient information include:

- **Password**: Passwords should be strong but not so complex that users write them down because that increases risk of unauthorized access. Passwords should be changed on a regularly scheduled basis, such as monthly. Passwords should not be birthdates, anniversary dates, or names of children or pets.
- **Screen saver**: Medical screensavers should be set to automatically launch after a specified period of time to protect any information that may be left on the screen.
- **Encryption**: All information entered into the application or transmitted must be encrypted (protected by converting to code) so that it cannot be accessed without the proper password.
- **Firewall**: A computer application or hardware that blocks unauthorized access to computer programs and data and monitors incoming data to ensure its safety. Firewalls can also block internet users from accessing private networks (such as medical networks).

PROTOCOLS FOR USING SOCIAL MEDIA

Some medical practices/organizations utilize **social media**, such as blogs, social networks, and websites, to communicate with patients and allow patients to set up appointments, obtain lab results, send messages, and receive messages. Strict protocols should be established for use of social media by healthcare professionals, including who has access, how access is obtained, the types of responses that are appropriate, and methods of dealing with inappropriate comments (such as from an angry patient). Personal social media, such as a personal Facebook account or Twitter account, should never be used to discuss any patient, patient care, or other healthcare-related issues associated with employment as this may violate HIPAA regulations regarding privacy and security and could place the practice/organization at risk for liability. Some healthcare organizations do not permit employees to even mention the place of employment on social media, so the medical assistant must review employment policies.

Copyright © Mometrix Media. You have been licensed one copy of this document for personal use only. Any other reproduction or redistribution is strictly prohibited. All rights reserved. This content is provided for test preparation purposes only and does not imply an endorsement by Mometrix of any particular political, scientific, or religious point of view.

PRINCIPLES OF ERGONOMICS AND PROPER BODY MECHANICS

Ergonomics is the study of how to design work and products according to principles of body mechanics to avoid injury, especially in the workplace. **Proper body mechanics** include the following as it relates to lifting and carrying heavy objects:

- Avoid reaching for prolonged periods of time, overhead, or more than 20 inches
- Avoid pulling—push, roll, or slide instead
- Avoid lifting—pull, push, roll, or slide instead
- Lift with leg muscles, not back
- Hold weight close to body rather than at arm's length
- Flex at hips and knees, not waist
- Maintain a straight back and avoid twisting
- Assess weight and recognize limitations in lifting/carrying
- Get help when necessary and communicate every step with partner ("Lift on the count of three")
- Maintain firm base of support with feet apart (shoulder width) to stabilize stance
- Maintain line of gravity (imaginary line between center of gravity and ground) within the base of support
- Position oneself close to the object that is to be lifted or carried

PREVENTING REPETITIVE STRAIN INJURIES THROUGH COMPUTER WORK

Supporting the principles of ergonomics includes designing a work environment that promotes comfortable, safe, and injury-free work. Because some of a medical assistant's responsibilities require time behind the computer, the **set-up of the computer and desk** must be done so in a manner that encourages proper body mechanics, and therefore **prevents repetitive strain injuries**. Consider the following:

- The work area must allow for full range of motion, including sufficient knee and leg room.
- An ideal chair has five castors, an adjustable seat and back, a broad base, a foot bar and lumbar supports, armrests low enough that they are not used during keyboarding, and a shallow seat to permit leaning backwards.
- The medical assistant should sit with the thighs at or just above the knees, feet firmly planted on the floor, and head directly over the shoulders.
- Position the monitor with the top just below eye level and at a slightly backward incline.
- Position the keyboard at a height that allows for relaxed shoulders and forearms parallel to the floor.
- Protect oneself from eyestrain with an anti-glare screen and by looking away from the computer for 10 minutes every hour.
- Use more lighting for dark walls and paper handling than for light walls and working with computer monitors.
- Use a mouse pad with a gel wrist support.

Copyright © Mometrix Media. You have been licensed one copy of this document for personal use only. Any other reproduction or redistribution is strictly prohibited. All rights reserved. This content is provided for test preparation purposes only and does not imply an endorsement by Mometrix of any particular political, scientific, or religious point of view.

Scheduling

SCHEDULE TYPES

Multiple schedule types are used in the medical office setting, including the following:

- **Stream**: The standard booking method, where patients are slotted in 15-minute intervals. A patient with a complex procedure takes two or three slots.
- **Double-booking**: Two patients are booked simultaneously. Staff take the history, vital signs, weight, height, and any standard tests (e.g., visual acuity, urinalysis, PFT). The physician performs a short exam and prescribes medications. Long wait times can result.
- **Wave**: A booking method for dealing with late arrivals. Schedule three patients simultaneously, at the beginning of each half hour. The doctor sees them in the order of their arrival. If one patient is late, it does not affect the other two. The longest wait is 20 minutes.
- **Modified wave**: Two to three patients are scheduled at the top of each hour, and all other call-ins may come in and wait their turns.
- **Open booking**: First-come, first-served. A booking method for dealing with no-shows and emergencies. Give the patient an appointment on the same day he or she calls. Used by walk-in clinics.
- **Clustering**: All patients of one type only are seen in a clinic on predetermined days/parts of days to increase efficiency, such as diabetics, pregnant mothers, or arthritics. Also called **categorization**.

APPOINTMENT MATRIX

An appointment matrix is the template on which the appointment schedule is recorded (on paper or in the computer). Typically, the matrix lists the physicians and nurse practitioners, and the times of day (usually in 10 minute-increments and the days of the week). The appointment matrix may be quite simple (as below) or complex. Any time that a physician or nurse practitioner is not available, that time slot is blocked out so that no appointments will be made at those times. If the physician or nurse practitioner sets aside certain days or times for extended visits, such as for admission history and physical, these times may be color-coded or otherwise noted. Example:

Dr. Smith	Hr.	May 15	May 16
	8:00	Mrs. Jones—BP check	Staff meeting
	8:10	Mr. Brown—Glucose	" "
	8:20	Miss White—UTI	" "
	8:30	" "	Mr. Smythe – Ulcer exam
	8:40	Telephone calls	" "

* " " indicates that the schedule block is a continuation of what is mentioned above. This is used for appointments or meetings that run over the 10-minute increment used in this example.

Copyright © Mometrix Media. You have been licensed one copy of this document for personal use only. Any other reproduction or redistribution is strictly prohibited. All rights reserved. This content is provided for test preparation purposes only and does not imply an endorsement by Mometrix of any particular political, scientific, or religious point of view.

SCHEDULING CONSIDERATIONS

Depending on the appointment being scheduled, the medical assistant must consider the following elements:

- **Scheduling a first appointment**: Necessary information includes the patient's name, date of birth, address, telephone number or other contact information as well as the purpose of the visit, name of referring physician/healthcare provider, and the patient's insurance company. Insurance information should include primary and secondary insurers as well as ID numbers and group numbers and a contact number necessary for preauthorization or referrals.
- **Scheduling subsequent appointments**: The patient's name and birthdate should be obtained to verify status, and the patient should be asked the purpose of the visit and the physician/nurse practitioner the patient wants to see. Confirm that there have been no changes to insurance since the last appointment.
- **Legal aspects of scheduling**: Patients may be charged for missed appointments only if a protocol is in place that applies to all patients. The patients must be advised at the time the appointment is made of the charge for missing the appointment or failing to notify the office within 24 hours. Medicare and many insurers don't pay for these charges.

HANDLING NO-SHOWS, CANCELLATIONS, DELAYS, AND EMERGENCIES

Remind patients the day before an appointment is scheduled. If a patient misses an appointment, notify a doctor and the referring doctor. If missing an appointment could compromise the patient's care (e.g., a suicidal patient), the medical assistant may be required to follow up. **No-shows and cancellations** that notify the medical office in less than 24 hours before an appointment may be charged a fine to cover the doctor's lost fees.

Always have patients' contact numbers handy in the scheduler. If the doctor is delayed, ensure urgent patients are seen by the *locum tenens* (doctor-on-call). Never leave an urgent case unattended. Rebook routine appointments. If a routine patient shows up anyway: Apologize, explain the absence (e.g., delivering a baby), estimate how long the wait will be, suggest rebooking, and offer hospitality if the patient decides to wait.

Always consider calls with complaints of chest pain, high fever, and earache an emergency. Ignoring or delaying emergency calls can result in legal action against the medical assistant and the doctor. Leave at least 20 minutes per day open on the schedule to handle emergent patients.

REFERRALS
COMPLETING A REQUISITION TO REFER PATIENT FOR OUTSIDE SERVICES

After the doctor finishes the consultation with a patient, review the written Physician's Orders in the chart before the patient leaves the office. The medical assistant may be required to book an appointment with a specialist, such as a dietitian, physiotherapist, or psychiatrist. The assistant may be required to arrange outside tests, such as audiology, bloodwork, ultrasound, or allergy screening. Call the outside service to book an appointment on the patient's behalf. Remember that a debilitated patient is unable to tolerate more than one invasive test per day. Obtain the correct requisitions for the tests from the outside services. Complete them by accurately transcribing information from the patient's chart into the requisition form. The medical assistant will find the patient's prescribed drugs on the nursing history chart. Send the requisition with the patient to the appointment. Remind the patient that most hospital operating rooms are booked several months in advance. The doctor may also dictate a referral letter to the specialist, which is typed later, and send it by fax or surface mail so that it arrives well before the appointment.

Copyright © Mometrix Media. You have been licensed one copy of this document for personal use only. Any other reproduction or redistribution is strictly prohibited. All rights reserved. This content is provided for test preparation purposes only and does not imply an endorsement by Mometrix of any particular political, scientific, or religious point of view.

RECEIVING REFERRED PATIENTS

Because referrals are an important source of new patients, patients that are referred are often given priority in scheduling, according to practice policy and depending on the urgency of the referral. If the referral is made directly, as per telephone, then the medical assistant should ask about urgency and obtain as much information as possible, including a request for medical records to save time later. In some cases, the patient calls after being advised to do so by a referring healthcare provider. In that case, medical records should generally be obtained in order to assess urgency before making the appointment. Three **types of referrals** are most common:

- **Consultation**: Usually these patients are referred to a specialist for diagnostic testing, surgery, or additional treatment. Some types of testing and treatment may require preauthorization for insurance companies.
- **Therapy/Treatments**: These may include psychological therapy, physical therapy, occupational therapy, or speech therapy. The therapy may require preauthorization for insurance companies.
- **Community resources**: These include home health agencies, meals programs, and respite care.

PREAUTHORIZATION PROCESS

Insurance carriers may require preauthorization for diagnostic procedures, hospitalization, and surgical procedures. Managed care programs often also require preauthorization for referrals. For this reason, determining the need for preauthorization should be part of verification of insurance benefits. Insurance cards often list a telephone number, fax number, or other contact information for preauthorization. The medical assistant should gather necessary information before contacting the insurance company and fill out the **preauthorization/referral form** with the following information:

- Patient's name and demographic information
- Healthcare provider's name, provider identification number, address, and telephone number
- Name of the insurance plan, address, and contact information (telephone, fax, secure email)
- Patient's preliminary diagnosis, including diagnostic codes
- Planned procedure/referral, including procedure codes
- Name, address and telephone number or other contact information for referrals
- Amount of patient's copayment and/or deductible
- Hospital benefits (inpatient and outpatient)
- Healthcare providers within the network (if applicable)

The preauthorization/referral form is usually faxed to the insurance company although in emergency situations preauthorization may be obtained by telephone.

SCHEDULING HOSPITAL ADMISSIONS

When scheduling **in-patient hospitalization** for a patient, the medical assistant should first gather all necessary information before calling the admitting department and should obtain preauthorization from insurance companies as needed. In the case of a non-emergent admission, the medical assistant should determine both the patient's and the physician's availability prior to scheduling. Information that the admitting department needs includes the patient's name, address, date of birth, admitting diagnosis, insurance information (primary and secondary), preauthorization number (if appropriate), and purpose of hospitalization. The medical assistant should also inform the admitting department when the admitting physician plans to see the patient,

178

Copyright © Mometrix Media. You have been licensed one copy of this document for personal use only. Any other reproduction or redistribution is strictly prohibited. All rights reserved. This content is provided for test preparation purposes only and does not imply an endorsement by Mometrix of any particular political, scientific, or religious point of view.

as the patient must be seen by his or her physician within 24 hours. In some cases, care of the patient is assumed by a hospitalist upon admission and not by the patient's personal physician. The patient must be informed of any prehospitalization testing, restrictions, and other special instructions.

SCHEDULING DIAGNOSTIC TESTS

To schedule diagnostic procedures, the medical assistant should gather information about the patient, and then determine the diagnostic test to be scheduled and the appropriate time frame within which the test must be conducted. Steps include:

1. Select a diagnostic center/laboratory and verify that services are covered under the patient's insurance plan.
2. Obtain the appropriate preauthorization necessary, or check with the insurance company if unsure of the need for preauthorization.
3. Discuss availability and time/date preferences with patient.
4. Call the diagnostic center/laboratory to schedule appointment.
5. Provide information to the patient regarding the place, date, and time of the diagnostic procedure.
6. Provide any pre- or post-test instructions (such as dietary restrictions or special preparation) to the patient and review with the patient to make sure the patient understands.
7. Record the scheduled procedure in the patient's medical record.
8. Record the scheduled procedure in the diagnostic procedure tracking log.

SCHEDULING SURGERIES

When scheduling surgical procedures, which may be done as an inpatient or in an outpatient surgery center, the medical assistant should first gather all necessary information: The location where the surgery is to be performed, the patient's name, the telephone number, the date of birth, the type of surgery that is to be scheduled, the timeframe, and the name of the surgeon and any assistants as well as the anesthesiologist. Additionally, the medical assistant should contact the insurance company for preauthorization and obtain the preauthorization number that the surgical center will need. If preauthorization testing (PAT), such as CBC, chem-panel, chest x-ray, or ECG, is required, the medical assistant must know who is to perform the testing and may need to schedule the tests as well. Patients must be provided pre-surgical instructions, such as the need to be NPO for a certain number of hours prior to surgery and whether or not to take medications the day of or in the days prior to surgery.

Copyright © Mometrix Media. You have been licensed one copy of this document for personal use only. Any other reproduction or redistribution is strictly prohibited. All rights reserved. This content is provided for test preparation purposes only and does not imply an endorsement by Mometrix of any particular political, scientific, or religious point of view.

Medical Records

RETENTION OF HEALTH INFORMATION

Health information is retained for predetermined periods of time, depending on the type of information:

Type of Information	AHIMA Recommended Retention Period
Adult medical record	10 years after the most recent encounter
Birth register	Permanently
Child (minor) medical record	Age of majority + statute of limitations
Death register	Permanently
Diagnostic images and x-rays	5 years
Disease index	10 years
Fetal heart monitor record	10 years after child reaches age of majority
Master patient index	Permanently
Operative index	10 years
Physician index	10 years
Surgical procedures register	Permanently

Consider federal and state statutes and regulations, the organization's policy, and the amount of storage space available before making a decision to purge. State and federal statutes of limitations determine the maximum of amount of time after an event that a lawsuit can be filed.

PERMANENTLY RETAINED PATIENT INFORMATION

Collaborate with the Medical Records manager on a retention and destruction schedule. Retain the following patient information permanently:

- Dates of admission, discharge, and encounters
- Physician names
- Diagnoses and procedures
- History and physical reports
- Operative and pathology reports
- Discharge summaries

DISPENSATION OF MEDICAL RECORDS WHEN A FACILITY CLOSES

In the event the medical facility closes, the medical assistant must carefully plan and articulate the **transfer of medical records**. If the facility is sold to another healthcare provider, then the records usually go to the new provider. If the employer is retiring and his or her practice will not be assumed by a successor, then arrange a storage contract with:

- Another healthcare provider
- The facility's attorney
- An appropriate storage facility

Scan the records so they remain accessible electronically. The State Department provides other options for dispensation of records. The medical assistant is responsible for ensuring that:

- The records are as complete as possible before transfer
- Living patients are kept informed if records are transferred

Copyright © Mometrix Media. You have been licensed one copy of this document for personal use only. Any other reproduction or redistribution is strictly prohibited. All rights reserved. This content is provided for test preparation purposes only and does not imply an endorsement by Mometrix of any particular political, scientific, or religious point of view.

IDENTIFYING THEFT PREVENTION

Elements of identity theft prevention include the following:

- **Answering machines/voicemail**: Never play messages aloud where they can be overheard. Use the receiver or earphones.
- **Fax**: Only dedicated lines should be used for faxes, and messages should be removed from the machine and properly filed immediately to prevent unauthorized access.
- **Email**: Never use emails to transmit information that should remain confidential.
- **Patient admission**: Greet patients in private if possible, but if the admission desk is in an open area, move the patient to a different area if personal questions must be asked, such as date of birth and Medicare number, or ask for the information needed in writing.
- **Computer**: All information should be password protected (with password changed frequently) and access limited to only those records the healthcare provider is authorized to use.
- **Telephone**: Conversations should be in private if possible. If not, care should be taken to avoid stating any identifying information that may be overheard.

SOURCE-ORIENTED AND PROBLEM-ORIENTED MEDICAL RECORDS

Source-oriented medical records are as follows:

- They are paper-based.
- They are organized by practitioner.
- Source-oriented records keep information in reverse chronological order in each section, with the latest information at the beginning.
- If a record is kept in the same order during and after care, it has "universal" chart order.

Advantage: Particular aspects of patient care can be readily accessed, such as lab reports or patient response to medication

Disadvantage: Does not allow easy access to particular patient problems or the contributions of each department to a specific problem

Problem-oriented medical records are as follows:

- They are paper-based.
- Problem-oriented records contain four sections: A database of standard checklists, a problem list, an initial plan, and progress notes.
- The problems are numbered, and the plans and progress notes are numbered to match the problem.

Advantage: Provides holistic patient information by problem

Disadvantage: Difficult to maintain

Copyright © Mometrix Media. You have been licensed one copy of this document for personal use only. Any other reproduction or redistribution is strictly prohibited. All rights reserved. This content is provided for test preparation purposes only and does not imply an endorsement by Mometrix of any particular political, scientific, or religious point of view.

INTEGRATED VS. ELECTRONIC HEALTH RECORDS

Integrated health records are paper-based and primarily kept in reverse chronological order. Each episode of care is defined by date, with the latest information at the beginning.

- **Advantages**: Integrated medical records provide easy access to current information, and the chronology of patient care is quickly apparent.
- **Disadvantage**: Integrated medical records do not allow easy access to particular aspects of patient care, by problem or by practitioner.
- **Note**: Some integrated medical records do divide lab reports from Progress Notes, making them more user-friendly.

Electronic health records are computer-based. Any chart order format can be the default in an electronic health record, with other formats available through data manipulation.

- **Advantages**: Electronic health records up less storage space, and can be parsed (arranged and rearranged) for specific kinds of access.
- **Disadvantages**: Software and hardware may become obsolete, so a paper back-up is legally required, expensive equipment and training are required, and stringent security is required to protect from hackers.

ELECTRONIC HEALTH RECORDS

The healthcare industry developed a foundational technology infrastructure with plans for expansion with added technological developments. Its primary component is the electronic health record (EHR), developed to share medical information easily among patients, providers, payers/insurers, and government agencies. The EHR includes:

- **Electronic medical records (EMRs)** generated by healthcare providers for individual patients
- **Point-of-care clinical information systems**, which allow caregivers to collect and input data at the bedside or service area on monitors and electronically transmit it by modem
- A **Decision Support System (DSS)**, a computerized system that gathers information from various sources and uses analytical models to assist providers in clinical decision-making

HIPAA requires standardized data formats for easy, secure information transfer.

DATA TYPES AND DATA INTERFACE STANDARDS

The following represent the basic types of data included in an electronic health record (EHR) and the sort of information that might typically be expressed by these types:

- **Text**: Reports, such as discharge summary, history and physical, and operative
- **Numbers**: ICD-10-CM codes, CFI codes, and blood pressure values
- **Voice**: Stored dictation accessed by phone or personal computer, voice recognition, or radiology images
- **Images**: Radiology film and document images
- **Video**: Echocardiograms
- **Drawings**: Rule of 9s charts showing burn distribution on the patient's skin surface
- **Signal**: EEG or EKG tracings

Copyright © Mometrix Media. You have been licensed one copy of this document for personal use only. Any other reproduction or redistribution is strictly prohibited. All rights reserved. This content is provided for test preparation purposes only and does not imply an endorsement by Mometrix of any particular political, scientific, or religious point of view.

Data-interface standards, such as those developed by X12 and HL7 standard development organizations, are standardized data formats that allow data to be transferred between units or facilities. HIPAA legislation imposes standards on data exchange of billing data to reduce administrative costs associated with the billing process. Certain coding systems and an X12 schema for data transfer are required.

PRIVACY, CONFIDENTIALITY, AND SECURITY

Privacy refers to the rights of individuals to control disclosure of their personal information. It is the principle behind HIPAA, mandated confidentiality requirements, and responding data security measures.

Confidentiality is endorsed by health professionals as a legal and ethical obligation to meet the expectation of privacy from patients.

Data security refers to the technical and procedural methods that manage and control confidential information.

Medical assistants oversee confidentiality matters and update organizational policies and procedures. It is important to review policies and procedures in light of the health record system, particularly if procedures have been developed around a paper-based environment, but the facility is moving to an electronic environment. Remember that the protection of confidentiality and patient privacy is not only a systems issue, but also a personnel issue in that training and oversight of facility personnel provide a distinguishing measure of security above and beyond system security.

THINNING PAPER RECORDS AND CODING HEALTH RECORDS

In a paper-based environment, hard copy health records must be thinned during a patient's long-term stay when the file has become too cumbersome to handle on a regular basis. **The thinned portions** are not destroyed but are returned to the main file room and should still be accessible.

Health records must be **coded**, which is the process of applying facility and professional coding, usually for billing purposes. In an electronic health record (EHR) environment, coding is done in the EHR on an ongoing basis and should be available when needed. In a paper or partial-paper environment, hospital information management (HIM) departments must be diligent about getting codes applied to paper records; paper records arrive in HIM for coding a period of time after the patient is discharged. HIM professionals also need to develop procedures for a combined environment, using electronic and hand coding.

AUTHENTICATION OF PATIENT RECORDS

The Joint Commission requires the following health records to be **authenticated with a date and signature**: History and physical (H&P), operative reports, consultations, and discharge summaries. Individual facilities may require authentication of additional records. All records requiring authentication must be signed by the original author, not a delegate. Some require

Copyright © Mometrix Media. You have been licensed one copy of this document for personal use only. Any other reproduction or redistribution is strictly prohibited. All rights reserved. This content is provided for test preparation purposes only and does not imply an endorsement by Mometrix of any particular political, scientific, or religious point of view.

countersignatures (e.g., the department head or admitting cashier). Consult federal, state, and facility regulations for authentication policies. The following considerations must be made:

- Basic authentication requires only an initial and a last name. Eliminate error by using full first names for staff with similar or duplicate last names.
- Keep a historical legend accessible in the facility to match initials and signatures with names, because staff rotate, quit, or retire.
- Signature stamps are unsafe. Keep a disclaimer on file, stating the doctor/owner takes legal responsibility for the stamp's use and storage.
- Electronic signatures may include an email signature; a digitized image of the signature; a unique PIN number; a biometric identifier, such as a fingerprint; and/or an encryption.

LOOK BACK

A look back refers to record checking, often on microfilm or microfiche, to find old contacts and disease vectors. For example, when a patient tests positive for HIV, the doctor is responsible for notifying public health authorities, which then check blood transfusion records to find out if the patient was a blood donor. If the patient did donate blood, those authorities attempt to find the recipients. Many years can elapse between donation and HIV diagnosis. The medical assistant may be required to "look back" through the patient's chart for clues to assist in this process.

To make the chart useful for a look back, document the following:

- A copy of all lab requisitions and test results, including the date and time
- Any no-shows
- Name and contact information of translators used to explain tests, if any
- Signed and witnessed consent forms
- Copies of any patient preparation or aftercare instructions
- Adverse reactions
- Patient refusal of tests and person in authority that was notified
- When and to whom the results were reported

PROCEDURES FOR DISASTER RECOVERY OF MEDICAL DOCUMENTS AND SUPPLIES

Disaster recovery refers to the salvaging of medical records, equipment, and insurance papers. Most disasters affecting medical records are water-based, like leaks and floods. Before using machinery to test or treat patients, ensure that a qualified Biomedical Engineer checks it for safety. Most supplies (blankets, gloves, bandages, medications, and needles) are unsalvageable. Arrange for their safe disposal.

Prevent disaster-induced record damage by training staff where sprinkler shut-off valves are located and how to close them. Take these post-damage steps:

1. For small amounts of paper, simply separate and dry out in a confidential area.
2. For larger amounts, contact a disaster recovery specialist through the Association of Specialists in Cleaning and Restoration (ASCR). Outside service providers need to know what kinds of paper are involved, such as printer paper or coated paper for electrocardiograms.
3. Reduce the chance of mildew by keeping the temperature down and the air as dry as possible.
4. Develop a reasonable estimate for the amount of time needed for recovery, and plan accordingly.

Copyright © Mometrix Media. You have been licensed one copy of this document for personal use only. Any other reproduction or redistribution is strictly prohibited. All rights reserved. This content is provided for test preparation purposes only and does not imply an endorsement by Mometrix of any particular political, scientific, or religious point of view.

Professionalism

TRAITS IMPORTANT TO DISPLAY IN PROFESSIONAL SITUATIONS

The following traits are important to display in professional situations:

- **Tact**: Speaking in such a manner to avoid giving offense. Being tactful can mean addressing issues in private rather than public, choosing the best time to address an issue, and softening criticisms by choosing words carefully.
- **Diplomacy**: Having skills in handling people and negotiating. Diplomacy usually includes keeping an end-goal in mind. For example, a medical assistant may need to use diplomacy if advocating for different work benefits for staff members.
- **Courtesy**: Being thoughtful and polite. Courteous behavior includes always remembering to say *please*, *thank you*, and *excuse me*, and treating others with respect and consideration.
- **Integrity**: Being honest and having high moral standards. This includes admitting errors, reporting errors, and acknowledging the need for more education/knowledge.

RESPONDING PROFESSIONALLY TO CRITICISM

Responding professionally to criticism includes:

- **Avoiding an emotional response**: Whether criticism is good or bad, responding with anger or enthusiasm should be avoided. If the criticism seems unfair, the best thing may be to take a deep breath and avoid responding right away, to allow time to calm down.
- **Accepting benefits of feedback**: Consider how the criticism can help to improve skills or relationships with others.
- **Understanding the message**: The medical assistant should listen attentively and ask clarifying questions that show that they are interested in what the person is saying. Ask for specific examples of any problems discussed and ask for suggestions as to how the situations might have been handled differently.
- **Asking about follow-up**: Be sure to understand what is expected, when, and how. If there is a timeframe or deadline, it should be clearly outlined.
- **Expressing appreciation**: Thank the person for providing feedback (even if you don't agree with the feedback). Always react with tact and courtesy.

JOB SEARCHING

The methods of job searching include the following:

- Personal contacts
- School career planning and placement offices
- Cold-calling employers
- Classified advertisements
- Internet job sites and message boards
- Professional associations
- Labor unions
- State employment service offices
- US Office of Personnel Management (OPM)
- Community agencies
- Private employment agencies and career consultants
- Internships

Copyright © Mometrix Media. You have been licensed one copy of this document for personal use only. Any other reproduction or redistribution is strictly prohibited. All rights reserved. This content is provided for test preparation purposes only and does not imply an endorsement by Mometrix of any particular political, scientific, or religious point of view.

The essentials of a good resume and cover letter include the following:

- An objective tailored to the target job
- Correct spelling and grammar
- Relevant skills, experience, education, and training
- Highlights of accomplishments and qualifications
- Truthfulness
- Chronological work history

The essentials of a good interview include the following:

- Research and rehearse
- Dress appropriately
- Stay calm
- Address the interviewer's concerns effectively
- If it is a behavioral interview, answer in a STAR pattern, stating the <u>s</u>ituation, <u>t</u>ask, <u>a</u>ction, and <u>r</u>esults achieved.

PERFORMANCE APPRAISAL

The supervisor conducts a performance appraisal (PA) with a staff member to:

- Confirm hiring
- Promote
- Schedule training or remediation
- Reward
- Refer to the Employee Assistance program
- Discipline

A human resources representative or the union shop steward may be present, particularly if discipline may result. The employee's first PA occurs at the end of the probationary period (3 months or 6 months) and annually thereafter. The written appraisal may include a rating scale, checklist, productivity studies, and narrative.

The supervisor must be acquainted with the employee and observe him or her at work. The PA is based on objective data from performance improvement measures. The employee must comply with published standards. The job description should include expectations and goals related to performance. The written PA should indicate compliance with performance expectations. The supervisor discusses the PA results with the employee and allows him or her to respond with new goals, based on findings from performance improvement measures and related to the organization's strategic plans.

Copyright © Mometrix Media. You have been licensed one copy of this document for personal use only. Any other reproduction or redistribution is strictly prohibited. All rights reserved. This content is provided for test preparation purposes only and does not imply an endorsement by Mometrix of any particular political, scientific, or religious point of view.

Medical Office Management

Medical Office General Management

COMFORTABLE AND SAFE MEDICAL RECEPTION AREA

Considerations regarding situating the medical reception area to provide comfort and safety include the following:

- **Traffic pattern**: The entrance and exit should be clear and layout such that patients can avoid crossing each other's paths.
- **Desk**: The reception desk should be clearly seen on entrance and the focal point of the room. The counter should be low enough to accommodate wheelchairs and chairs should be available for patients who need to sit. If in an open area, an adjacent area should be available for private conversations with patients.
- **Lighting**: Harsh artificial light, such as fluorescent, should be avoided. Windows with natural light are ideal.
- **Furniture/chairs**: Vinyl and manufactured fabrics can be more easily cleaned and usually hold up better than natural fibers. Chairs should be comfortable and large enough to accommodate patients who are obese.

OUTFITTING A RECEPTION AREA

To outfit a reception area optimally, consider the following:

- **Choose colors** to modulate patients' moods. Greens, blues, and pinks are calming and suitable for psychiatric areas. Yellows, oranges, and reds are energizing and suitable for children's areas.
- Keep the area **well ventilated**, regularly vacuumed, well-lit with as much window light as possible, and cool to discourage the growth of pathogens.
- Choose **washable fabrics** and surfaces that are easy to disinfect.
- **Small chairs, tables, and toys for children** help them pass the time easily. Choose large, hard toys with no small parts that can be swallowed and laminated books, which can be wiped with disinfectant every day to prevent the spread of infection.
- **Plants** help to calm and screen patients to give them privacy. Make sure they are not toxic, heavily scented, or parasite carriers.
- **Classical music** and news programs help mask private conversations. Magazines should be current and not contain perfume inserts.
- **Keep absorbent, rubber-backed rugs and boot trays** in the entrance and tile floors in the examining areas.

187

Copyright © Mometrix Media. You have been licensed one copy of this document for personal use only. Any other reproduction or redistribution is strictly prohibited. All rights reserved.
This content is provided for test preparation purposes only and does not imply an endorsement by Mometrix of any particular political, scientific, or religious point of view.

MAINTAINING A MEDICAL OFFICE ACCORDING TO GOVERNMENT ASEPSIS STANDARDS

OSHA requires that medical offices use good aseptic technique to reduce the spread of disease. Disinfection means cleaning objects to eliminate most pathogenic (disease-causing) microorganisms, such as bacteria, viruses, molds, and parasites. Disinfection and sanitization (washing) do not eliminate spores, which are dormant (sleeping) bacteria waiting for more hospitable growing conditions, or the seeds of algae, fungi, plants, and a few protozoans. The only way to kill spores is by autoclave oven. Autoclaving is appropriate for small instruments but not furniture or other large surfaces. To **maintain the office according to OSHA recommendations**:

- Prepare a fresh solution of germicidal detergent daily. Use the detergent to wipe down soiled walls, mattress covers, furniture, and any equipment that is not the responsibility of Central Sterile Supply (CSS). Mop the floors or wet-vacuum them if there is no housekeeping service.
- Post the appropriate signs outside isolation rooms. Keep the necessary isolation equipment outside of the isolation room for staff and visitors to don and doff.
- Keep a pump bottle of 70-80% alcohol cleanser at the entrance to each exam room and at the front desk.

RECEPTION TASKS

The **medical assistant at the reception** desk is responsible for the following:

- Directing outpatient traffic and salespeople
- Accepting drop-off specimens and courier deliveries
- Scheduling appointments
- Collecting insurance information
- Answering the switchboard
- Responding to emergencies

Reputable medical sales representatives sell innovative drugs and equipment that keep doctors current; arrange for the doctor to make additional money as a researcher, lecturer, or demonstrator; and provide important training materials. Representatives book appointments well in advance. Allow only one sales representative on the premises at a time, and do not allow them to touch patients. Ensure a staff member accompanies them to the stockroom and that they do not open sterile supplies or remove a competitor's products. Ask the doctor if staff is allowed to accept gifts or samples from medical companies. When any non-patient visitor is on the premises, do not allow him or her to film or access patient and financial files without a legal search warrant. If a salesperson or reporter arrives unannounced, explain that patient care is paramount, and an appointment is required. Have police wait away from reception, accompanied by staff, until the doctor is available.

Copyright © Mometrix Media. You have been licensed one copy of this document for personal use only. Any other reproduction or redistribution is strictly prohibited. All rights reserved. This content is provided for test preparation purposes only and does not imply an endorsement by Mometrix of any particular political, scientific, or religious point of view.

FILING SYSTEMS

The following are types of filing systems:

- **Alphabetic**: Indexing files from A to Z, in the same sequence as the letters of the alphabet. It is less accurate than numeric filing.
- **Numeric/terminal digit**: Indexing by numbers, especially the last unit. It is more accurate than alphabetical filing.
- **Subject**: Classifying, coding, and storing documents according to their topic, such as *Sales Receipts* or *Surgical Inventory*.
- **Tickler**: Also called a suspense file. Indexing files according to upcoming actions or unconcluded transactions, such as arranging an annual service check by a mechanic before the warranty expires.
- **EDP** (**E**lectronic **D**ata **P**rocessing): Use of a computer to record, classify arrange, summarize, and report information.
- **Cross-reference**: A direction to the reader to check another section for a more complete explanation or related information.
- **Master**: A computer file that contains long-term information, such as a patient database or payroll records. The master is updated regularly and workers refer to it as the most reliable source of information.
- **Color-coded**: Placing colored stickers on files to identify them quickly, usually so they can be purged easily. For example, medical files more than 10 years old can be legally purged; if all 10-year-old files have purple stickers, then the purging job can be safely delegated to a junior clerk.

Copyright © Mometrix Media. You have been licensed one copy of this document for personal use only. Any other reproduction or redistribution is strictly prohibited. All rights reserved. This content is provided for test preparation purposes only and does not imply an endorsement by Mometrix of any particular political, scientific, or religious point of view.

Coding, Billing, and Third-Party Payments

CODING SYSTEMS

The most commonly used coding systems are:

- The International Classification of Diseases, 10th Edition, Clinical Modification (ICD-10-CM)
- Healthcare Common Procedure Coding Systems (HCPCS) Level II
- Current Procedural Terminology 4th Edition (CPT-4)
- Systematized Nomenclature of Medicine (SNOMED CT) by the College of American Pathologists

Some coding systems are classification systems, and some are nomenclatures. Most healthcare organization use multiple coding systems.

ICD-10-CM

International Classification of Diseases, 10th Edition, Clinical Modifications, (ICD-10-CM) is a coding system used to code diagnoses. The ICD-10-CM codes are used for billing purposes to ensure that procedure codes match appropriate diagnoses. The codes all have at least three characters but may have up to four additional sub-categories. Diagnoses are classified by type of disease or system involved. For example, main categories include neoplasms and diseases of the respiratory systems. With ICD-10-CM, injuries are grouped by body part rather than category of injury.

HCPCS LEVEL II

Healthcare Common Procedure Coding Systems (HCPCS) Level II codes are used when filing claims for equipment, supplies and services that are not covered by CPT codes, including durable medical equipment ambulance services, laboratory service, orthotics, and prosthetics:

- D codes: procedures
- E codes: durable medical equipment, such as bedside commodes
- L codes: orthotic and prosthetic procedures and devices, such as orthopedic shoes
- P codes: pathology and laboratory services

CPT CODES

Current Procedural Terminology 4th Edition (CPT-4) codes were developed by the American Medical Association (AMA) and used to define those licensed to provide services and to describe medical and surgical treatments, diagnostics, and procedures. CPT codes specify procedures as well as typical times required for treatment. CPT codes are usually updated each October with revisions (additions, deletions) to coding. The use of CPT codes is mandated by both CMS and HIPAA to provide a uniform language and to aid research. These codes are used primarily for billing purposes for insurances (public and private). Under HIPAA, HHS has designed CPT codes as part of the national standard for electronic healthcare transactions:

- **Category I codes** are used to identify a procedure or service.
- **Category II codes** are used to identify performance measures, including diagnostic procedures.
- **Category III codes** identify temporary codes for technology and data collection.

SNOMED CT

SNOMED CT is the nomenclature system with the most potential to handle the complex data represented in electronic health records (EHRs). **SNOMED** (Systematized Nomenclature of

Copyright © Mometrix Media. You have been licensed one copy of this document for personal use only. Any other reproduction or redistribution is strictly prohibited. All rights reserved.
This content is provided for test preparation purposes only and does not imply an endorsement by Mometrix of any particular political, scientific, or religious point of view.

Medicine) offers comprehensive international clinical reference terminology, used worldwide. The CT suffix stands for *clinical terms*. Designed for computers, SNOMED CT offers a consistent language for capturing, sharing, and aggregating health data across specialties and sites of care. SNOMED links synonyms to a single concept. For instance, SNOMED recognizes appendicitis as an inflammatory and GI disease. SNOMED includes domain-specific vocabularies, such as those for nursing. SNOMED maps to interface with other clinical terminologies, such as ICD-10.

DIAGNOSTIC-RELATED GROUPS (DRGs)

Diagnostic-related groups (DRGs) were instituted in 1982 as a way to classify patients who shared similar diseases and treatments for billing purposes, under the assumption that patients who shared symptoms and/or diseases use the same number of resources and, therefore, should be billed the same amount. There are approximately 500 different DRGs, and patients are placed into specific DRGs using International Classification of Disease (ICD-10-CM) codes, along with specific patient information such as sex, age, and the presence of comorbidities. By placing patients into DRGs, Medicare is able to determine how much the hospital should be reimbursed for patient care. The institution of DRGs has changed the health care system from one that was provider-driven (meaning the individual clinician determined the billable amount) into one that is payer-driven (meaning that Medicare determines reimbursement).

HEALTHCARE FINANCING METHODS

Healthcare financing involves complex options. The payment methods are self-pay (also called direct pay or out-of-pocket payment), which entails the patient paying directly for his or her own health costs, and indirect pay, which involves a third party paying for the health costs. Third-party payers can be the government, insurance companies, managed-care programs, or self-insured companies. A common third-party payer is an insurance company. Insurance providers essentially have a contractual arrangement with individuals and/or companies to cover all or part of health costs incurred for a monthly fee, called a premium. Coinsurance means the insurer is partially responsible for the debt, and the patient is usually responsible for the remainder. Insurance companies generally pay for health costs after they have been incurred through a reimbursement arrangement with the healthcare provider.

HEALTHCARE REIMBURSEMENT ARRANGEMENTS

Healthcare reimbursement is ubiquitous across healthcare providers, in that most healthcare costs are covered by third parties after the costs have been incurred. Often this reimbursement involves several parties, but the general **arrangements** fall into a few key categories called reimbursement formulas or contracted amounts:

- **Retrospective payment systems** encompass several formulas, in which healthcare costs are determined after the healthcare has been provided.
- **Fee-for-service costs** are based on the provider's cost for each service, such as lab tests, and hospitals are paid on a per-diem basis.
- **Usual, customary, and reasonable charges** are based on what is normally charged for physician care or what is reasonable for the service provided.
- **Sliding scale fees** apply in low-income or public health programs, where cost is based on the patient's ability to pay.
- **Capitation** pays a prepaid amount to the provider, based on a predetermined per-person or per-capita amount.

Copyright © Mometrix Media. You have been licensed one copy of this document for personal use only. Any other reproduction or redistribution is strictly prohibited. All rights reserved. This content is provided for test preparation purposes only and does not imply an endorsement by Mometrix of any particular political, scientific, or religious point of view.

MANAGED CARE

Managed care encompasses various types of plans designed to effectively deliver healthcare by containing costs and use of services, while providing quality healthcare to its subscribers. Managed care organizations (MCOs) contract with employers, unions, individuals, and other purchasers to provide comprehensive healthcare to people who voluntarily enroll in the plan. Providers who participate in managed-care plans may be paid employees or may provide services on a per capita (capitation) arrangement, a fee-for-services arrangement, or other types of payment arrangement. There are many types of managed care programs, but the most common are health maintenance organizations (HMOs) and preferred provider organizations (PPOs). Some models integrate health insurance, delivery, and payment within one organization, and exercise control over utilization. MCOs generate complex information needs, affecting the responsibilities of the medical assistant.

HMO

HMO stands for **Health Maintenance Organization**. An HMO is a collection of doctors, allied healthcare providers, and hospitals that receive fixed monthly payments from the government to care for Medicaid patients or from an employer for its workers, rather than fee-for-service. Cost control is of major importance to the HMO. There are variations of HMOs, called preferred provider organizations (PPO) or point-of-service plans (POS).

Up until the 1980s, most patients had indemnity insurance that was fee-for service. The patient would co-pay for medical care with an insurance company, and had the option of visiting any licensed care provider. Today, more than 50% of Americans deal with HMOs as a cost-saving measure for the government, insurers, and employers. Care at an HMO costs a fraction of that with traditional providers, but the patient can only see providers and get tests that are in-network. Patients do not have to pay up front, fill out claim forms, or wait to be reimbursed at an HMO.

VARIATIONS AND COMPONENTS

PPOs, POS plans, case management, and utilization management are all variations or components of HMOs:

- **Preferred Provider Organization (PPO)**: A network of physicians and/or healthcare organizations that provide healthcare at a discounted rate in return for patient volume. PPOs contract with payers or employers.
- **Point of Service (POS) Plan**: An arrangement in a managed-care organization (MCO) whereby the patient chooses a provider each time a healthcare service is required. A point of enrollment plan refers to one in which the patient chooses a provider at the time of enrollment.
- **Case Management**: The overview and coordination of costs and resources for an MCO. An individual, such as a primary care provider, is designated as a case manager or gatekeeper. Case management is usually employed when a patient is suffering from a chronic, progressive, and/or terminal illness that requires several types of healthcare services.
- **Utilization Management**: The oversight/management of healthcare costs, usually required by the payer. Utilization review is the process of evaluation for healthcare cost/service efficiency.

Copyright © Mometrix Media. You have been licensed one copy of this document for personal use only. Any other reproduction or redistribution is strictly prohibited. All rights reserved. This content is provided for test preparation purposes only and does not imply an endorsement by Mometrix of any particular political, scientific, or religious point of view.

Federal and/or State Mandated Insurance Options

Medicaid, Tricare, CHAMPVA, and workers' compensation are federal and/or state mandated insurance provided to specific demographics:

- **Medicaid**: The program through which the federal and state governments help low-income individuals by paying for those medical services that are deemed to be absolutely necessary. Medicaid is covered by Social Security Act Title XIX. Medicaid is available to Federal Supplemental Security income recipients, low-income children under 6 years of age, pregnant women, individuals older than 65 with a disability, and individuals deemed categorically needy by their state.
- **TRICARE**: The Department of Defense provides healthcare for active and retired military personnel and their families through the TRICARE program, previously CHAMPUS.
- **CHAMPVA**: Civilian Health and Medical Program of the Department of Veterans Affairs. It is always the secondary payer, after Medicare, to minimize out-of-pocket expenses. CHAMPVA covers the families of veterans who were killed or permanently disabled in the line of duty, who are ineligible for Tricare.
- **Workers' Compensation**: Insurance provided under laws generated by each state, to cover medical expenses and lost income for workers injured on the job, or to their survivors if the injury results in death.

Medicare Part A

Medicare Part A is no-cost hospital insurance for the following individuals:

- Social Security recipients over 65 years old
- Patients receiving disability benefits for a minimum of 24 months
- Patients with renal failure (requiring dialysis or transplant)

Medicare Part A covers care in the following **facilities**:

- Critical access hospitals
- Home care
- Inpatient hospitals
- Hospice
- Skilled nursing facilities

Medicare Part A is financed primarily through payroll tax, and is unavailable to beneficiaries who are ineligible for federal retirement benefits.

193

Copyright © Mometrix Media. You have been licensed one copy of this document for personal use only. Any other reproduction or redistribution is strictly prohibited. All rights reserved. This content is provided for test preparation purposes only and does not imply an endorsement by Mometrix of any particular political, scientific, or religious point of view.

MEDICARE PART B

Medicare Part B insurance covers outpatient treatment for necessary and preventative services including the following:

- Blood transfusion
- Diagnostic tests like glaucoma, Pap smears, mammograms, and prostate exams
- Doctors' office visits
- Durable assistive devices, like beds, oxygen, walkers, and wheelchairs
- Laboratory tests
- One physical exam in the first 6 months
- Outpatient clinics for mental health, occupational therapy, and physiotherapy
- Outpatient surgery
- Vaccines, such as Hepatitis B and Pneumococcus

Part B is financed by federal appropriations with monthly premiums paid by the beneficiary, who also pays some deductibles and copayments.

MEDICARE C AND D

Medicare Part C is also known as **Medicare Advantage**. It is available to beneficiaries enrolled in Parts A and B (hospital and outpatient insurance coverage). Part C offers various managed-care plans, including HMO, POS, and PPO plans. Medicare Part D is a recently added option to be bundled into Medicare Advantage that provides prescription drug coverage. There are several plans available, but the beneficiary always pays a monthly premium and part of the drug cost. Medicare providers are reimbursed through an insurance company contracted by the federal government as a fiscal intermediary. Congress passed the *Tax Equity and Fiscal Responsibility Act* (TERFA) in 1983 to combat spiraling medical costs. TERFA created the Prospective Payment System (PPS), a method whereby reimbursement amounts are predetermined based on the services rendered. CMS annually reviews standardized rates, represented by classifications called Diagnosis-related Groups (DRGs) for inpatient care, and Resource-based Relative Value Scale (RSBRVS) for physician services.

> **Review Video: Medicare and Medicaid**
> Visit mometrix.com/academy and enter code: 507454

REQUESTING THIRD-PARTY PAYER REIMBURSEMENT

Third-party payers are insurance companies or employers that use patient care data as the basis for claims processing to pay for healthcare services provided. Many third-party payers encourage the use of ambulatory care by providing financial incentives. It is very time-consuming for the physician to qualify a claim for third-party reimbursement because he or she must specify diagnoses and provide exact details (e.g., a surgical procedure must document the reason for surgery, lesion length, layers of fascia involved, etc.). The medical assistant reduces the time the physician spends on documentation by reviewing the patient's record the day before an appointment and isolating the pertinent information. The patient must authorize disclosure of his or her information to third-party recipients. The third-party payer will probably redisclose the patient's information to the Medical Information Bureau (MIB), which allows access to other potential insurers for up to 7 years. Only drug or alcohol abuse cases are exempt. Third-party payers require a Progress Note for each visit billed.

Copyright © Mometrix Media. You have been licensed one copy of this document for personal use only. Any other reproduction or redistribution is strictly prohibited. All rights reserved. This content is provided for test preparation purposes only and does not imply an endorsement by Mometrix of any particular political, scientific, or religious point of view.

SENDING INFORMATION TO THIRD-PARTY PAYERS

The medical assistant deals with occasional third-party payers through surface mail, and with regular third-party payers through a virtual private network (VPN), or Extranet. One component of the VPN is a demilitarized zone (DMZ), which sits between the internal network and the VPN. It allows outside access to a third-party portion of the network, while protecting the Intranet, or internal, information.

ENROLLING DOCTOR AS PARTICIPATING PROVIDER

In order for a doctor to be considered a participating provider, they must produce specific documentation to payers to obtain billing privileges, for example:

- A doctor must meet **credentialing standards** established by the National Committee for Quality Assurance (NCQA).
- Individual healthcare providers and business owners must supply the payer with a **tax identification number** for the IRS.

MASTER CHARGE LISTS

Master charge lists delineate how much can be charged for each service, as identified by a CPT-4 code. These lists are also known as charge master, charge description master (CDM), or fee schedule. Charges are impacted by clinical modifiers, which affect reimbursement. Modifiers are given numeric or alphabetical codes. Either the medical assistant or the HIM manager is responsible for monitoring the accurate and timely coding of all services rendered, and regularly analyzing contracted reimbursement rates and expenses associated with services or product costing.

Copyright © Mometrix Media. You have been licensed one copy of this document for personal use only. Any other reproduction or redistribution is strictly prohibited. All rights reserved. This content is provided for test preparation purposes only and does not imply an endorsement by Mometrix of any particular political, scientific, or religious point of view.

Financial Bookkeeping

BOOKKEEPING

The medical assistant should understand the following elements of bookkeeping:

- Petty cash
- Single-entry bookkeeping
- Bank deposits, checking, and reconciliations
- Patient accounts and statements
- Payroll

The medical assistant completes the financial records when the office is not busy. Usually, a certified accountant (CPA) sets up the doctor's accounting records and provides instructions for how the medical assistant is to record transactions. For purchases, the medical assistant records the following:

- Date of purchase
- Reason for payment in the "explanation" column
- Check number used to pay for the purchase
- Amount

The accountant calculates the annual income tax and completes the financial statements through double-entry bookkeeping. The medical assistant is not typically involved with a practice's taxes or financial statements.

PETTY CASH ACCOUNTS

Petty cash is a small amount of cash (usually no more than $100) that is kept on hand to pay for miscellaneous costs, such as for overdue postage, tips for delivery, parking costs, and supplies, such as coffee or tea, for a break room. Petty cash should be kept in a locked, secure drawer or container. Money placed into petty cash should come from a practice account but never directly from cash payments directly received from a patient. That money should be kept separate. A petty cash record should be maintained and should include a record of any disbursement and replenishment. The date and purpose of disbursements must be recorded along with the signature of the person withdrawing funds. Additionally, petty cash receipts should be filled out each time a person receives money from petty cash, such as when a person withdraws money to purchase breakroom supplies.

DATA ENTRY PROCEDURES

Data entry procedures include posting the following:

- **Charges**: If the physician or nurse practitioner manually checks off services, print out a charge slip from the computer program and later use the information on the form to enter data into the computer application. In the charge posting screen, post the patient's name, identification number, date of service, the service provided (office visit, ECG, injection), the CPT code, the ICD-10-CM diagnostic codes, HCPCS Level II codes, and the charge for the service. The application may require co-payments and payments to be entered as well. Diagnostic codes must match the service provided.
- **Payments**: Access the payment posting screen, which should list the procedure charge history. Then post the correct date, payment type (cash, check, credit card), and amount and check the balance (view ledger).

Copyright © Mometrix Media. You have been licensed one copy of this document for personal use only. Any other reproduction or redistribution is strictly prohibited. All rights reserved. This content is provided for test preparation purposes only and does not imply an endorsement by Mometrix of any particular political, scientific, or religious point of view.

- **Adjustments**: Discounts, such as for Medicare or insurance, are usually entered in the charge posting screen, but this may vary from one application to another. The adjustment is to the balance owed.

REVENUE CYCLE, FRONT-END AND BACK-END ACTIVITIES, AND PAYER CONTRACTS

The **revenue cycle** begins when the patient enters the healthcare system for diagnosis, treatment, and follow-up services. It includes the flow of patient and financial information and ends with reimbursement for services rendered.

Front-end activities take place before a patient receives treatment, such as collection and verification of demographics, billing, and insurance information. **Back-end activities** involve billing and claims processing after admission, and even after discharge, if applicable.

Payer contracts are legally binding documents describing the obligations of both providers and payers. Healthcare billing adheres to industry standards of language and service codes, as noted by the Common Procedure Coding System (HCPCS) of the Healthcare Financing Administration (HCFA). A provider who contracts with a payer is considered a participating provider. If no contract exists, then the provider is considered a non-participating provider. He or she may be reimbursed less by a third-party payer. Non-participating providers usually obtain additional co-payment from the patient. This is especially true of mental healthcare providers, such as counselors and psychologists.

CLAIMS PROCESSING

Claims processing requires accurate, complete information and must meet standard formats. Denials of claims based on incomplete or inaccurate information can be avoided by monitoring for correct patient information and medical codes. Primary and secondary billing is generated for patients covered by multiple insurance plans. Insurance payments are accompanied by either a remittance advice (RA) or explanation of benefits (EOB), indicating the billed amount, allowable amount by insurance coverage, payment amount, patient liability, and the amount disallowed by insurance. Review accounts to ensure that the correct payment was made according to the individual payer's contract, which may be based on a percentage, per unit, DRG rate, or another fee schedule. A case mix analysis results in a "case mix index" or average, which is then multiplied by the number of cases.

IRS

The **Internal Revenue Service (IRS)** is the federal government agency responsible for tax collection and tax law enforcement. Often, the medical assistant is responsible for payroll in a small office and must be familiar with IRS withholding requirements. For example, Medicare A is financed primarily through payroll tax. The medical assistant must learn to prepare paychecks and deduct income tax, pension, unemployment insurance, and healthcare premiums. The medical assistant can obtain IRS forms from the IRS website. The medical assistant enters payroll records on a master sheet, which is a computer file that contains long-term information that changes infrequently, such as employees' names and addresses. The master is updated regularly, and the medical assistant refers to it as the most reliable source of information. The medical assistant must keep the payroll master entirely separate from accounts payable. An IRS auditor may ask to review the payroll master, and the medical assistant is obliged to show it.

TRUTH IN LENDING ACT

The federal *Truth in Lending Act* (Regulation Z) (1968) is part of the *Consumer Protection Act* and is enforced by the Federal Trade Commission. When a healthcare provider engages in a credit

Copyright © Mometrix Media. You have been licensed one copy of this document for personal use only. Any other reproduction or redistribution is strictly prohibited. All rights reserved.
This content is provided for test preparation purposes only and does not imply an endorsement by Mometrix of any particular political, scientific, or religious point of view.

agreement, a truth-in-lending statement must be provided to the patient/guardian/payor at the time the credit agreement is made. The statement must be easily understood by the payor. The credit agreement includes the total amount owed and the payment schedule and amounts that have been agreed upon (usually monthly payments). When applicable, the truth-in-lending statement must include the maximum dollar amount that can be charged to the account, the interest rate, the method used to calculate the interest rate, and the method used to determine the minimum monthly payment. If a party pays in four or fewer installments without a specific agreement, the provisions of the *Truth in Lending Act* do not apply.

ACCOUNTS RECEIVABLE AGING REPORTS

The accounts receivable aging report is used to track insurance payments, including those that are past due. The aging of accounts is done by 30-day increments (0-30, 31-60, etc.). Unless a payment agreement has been agreed upon in advance, all payments are considered past due after 30 days. Those that exceed 120 days are usually referred to a collection agency or written off by the practice. In some cases, the practice may send a letter asking for payment and indicating plans to take the matter to small claims court if payment is not received and the amount due is within the small claims court limits.

COLLECTIONS PROCESS

IDENTIFYING DELINQUENT ACCOUNTS

The turn-around time for a claim submitted to an insurance company is usually 30–60 days if submitted on paper and 10–15 days if submitted electronically. Payments received after this time are considered delinquent. If a claim is **delinquent**, then the usual policy is to send a tracer within a few days to determine if there is a problem with the claim or if the insurance company requires more information. The insurance claim register should be checked routinely to ensure that delinquent claims are not overlooked. The tracer form should include:

- Name and address of insurance company
- Patient's and insured's names
- Employer's name (if applicable)
- Date claim was initially submitted and the amount of the claim
- Note indicating excess time has passed with no word from insurance company or request for further information
- Area for the insurance company to explain reason for delay (pending, processing, denied)
- Physician's name, address, and telephone number

FAIR DEBT COLLECTION PRACTICES ACT

The federal *Fair Debt Collection Practices Act* (1977) is intended to protect debtors from third-party collection agencies or others acting on behalf of another (such as an attorney) regarding consumer debts (medical bills) and to ensure debtors are treated fairly. The regulations, however, do not apply to a healthcare provider attempting to collect his or her own debts. Third party agents are prohibited from harassing debtors, making false statements or threats in order to gain payments, or being in any way frightening or verbally abusive. Third parties may not make threats that they cannot legally follow through on, such as threatening to have a debtor arrested. Additionally, third parties are prohibited from calling or contacting debtors before 8 AM or after 8 PM. The debtor must receive appropriate notices, and third parties must identify themselves as debt collectors. If requested to cease communication, they must do so, and they cannot attempt to collect from those who have filed for bankruptcy.

Copyright © Mometrix Media. You have been licensed one copy of this document for personal use only. Any other reproduction or redistribution is strictly prohibited. All rights reserved. This content is provided for test preparation purposes only and does not imply an endorsement by Mometrix of any particular political, scientific, or religious point of view.

OPERATING BUDGET

The operating budget for a facility is a summary of all projected income and expenses for a specific time period. Operating budgets are often constructed on a monthly basis and include projections for the year. Seasonal expenses, such as lawn mowing and snow removal, must be included. Fluctuations in such items as payroll, administrative expenses, prices for materiel and supplies, taxes, insurance, and general costs should be forecast as accurately as possible. The budget should be reviewed monthly by the facility manager and accounting and at least quarterly by a member of upper management. Discrepancies between the budgeted amount of a line item and the actual cost should be investigated and revisions made as necessary.

FORMULATION OF OPERATING BUDGET

Senior management and departmental managers negotiate and prepare the operating budget. The **operating budget team** considers both corporate guidelines and forecasts of departmental activity. Each department estimates the demand for its services, but the priorities that must be met are primary care, hospitalizations, surgeries, births, and emergency care. The management team creates forecasts based on market trends, past history, and executive judgment. The team evaluates trends in resource prices and the cost of in-house personnel versus contractors. Purchasing and human resources provide the statistics for these forecasts. The operating budget affects the medical assistant most directly. The capital budget concerns the actual building, and the utilities budget concerns how the building is heated, cooled, and lit.

FINANCIAL MATHEMATICS

Financial mathematics related to patient and practice accounts require primarily a basic knowledge of addition and subtraction, but the medical assistant needs to have an understanding of financial documents, such as invoices, which are essentially billing forms that describe a purchase/service and the amount due to pay for the purchase/service. Additionally, the medical assistant should be familiar with single-entry bookkeeping, which is often utilized to record income and expenses:

Date	Description	Income	Expense	Balance
Jan 1	Balance			500.00
Jan 12	Printer cartridges		126.00	374.00
Jan 15	Vitamin supplements		50.00	324.00
Jan 16	Cash deposit	220.00		544.00

IMPORTANT TERMS

Important finance and bookkeeping-related terms for the medical assistant to understand include the following:

- **Relative value studies**: A schedule that assigns a unit value to a medical procedure to compare costs.
- **Resource-based relative value scale (RSBRVS)**: The Center for Medicare and Medicaid (CMS) reviews its standardized rates every year. Resource-based Relative Value Scale (RBRVS) are standardized rates the CMS pays providers for physician services.
- **Contracted fees**: The participating provider agrees to accept a list of specific fees from the payer. A fee is the total the provider can charge. This benefit plan prohibits extra billing.
- **Accounts receivable (A/R)**: Money owed to the practice by a patient for services and products the provider sold on credit and for which the patient has been invoiced. Enter A/R as a current asset on the balance sheet.

Copyright © Mometrix Media. You have been licensed one copy of this document for personal use only. Any other reproduction or redistribution is strictly prohibited. All rights reserved. This content is provided for test preparation purposes only and does not imply an endorsement by Mometrix of any particular political, scientific, or religious point of view.

- **Accounts payable (A/P)**: Unpaid bills the practice owes to suppliers. A/P does not include payroll, rent, taxes, or accrued interest. Enter A/P as current liabilities (short-term) on the balance sheet.
- **Billing cycle**: The period between billing for services and products, which is usually one month in most practices.
- **Aging of accounts**: Classifying the accounts according to risk by the number of days that have elapsed since the due date or billing date. Most practices have an aging schedule of 1-30 days, 31-60 days, 61-90 days, and more than 90 days. The longer an account is unpaid, the greater the risk that the patient will default.
- **Collections**: The medical assistant transfers a delinquent account more than 90 days overdue to the collection department or a private collection agency. It is cheaper for the medical assistant to negotiate with the patient than it is to accept 10% of recovered money from the collection agency or risk that no money will be recovered if the patient files for bankruptcy.
- **Itemization**: The medical assistant prepares a bill for the payer with a detailed list of all procedures performed and products used during one visit for a particular patient. The supplier prepares a bill for the practice listing all products sold in detail (size, shape, quantity, color, material, etc.).
- **Consumer Protection Act**: A legal statute that prohibits deceptive marketing, encourages the seller to give the consumer information, and enforces product safety standards.
- **Ordering**: The medical assistant issues a Purchase Order (PO) Number to the supplier to confirm a request for goods or services. When the medical assistant accepts receipt of the goods or services, the PO becomes a binding legal agreement for the practice to pay the supplier.
- **Invoice**: A bill of sale or contract that identifies the practice and patient, or the seller and buyer. This lists the quantity of products or services sold and describes them. Invoices also show the date of service or shipment, delivery or transport mode, price, and payment terms, including discounts. When the medical assistant or doctor signs the invoice, it becomes a demand for payment. When the patient pays the invoice in full, it becomes a document of title.
- **Tracking**: The monitoring of performance or delivery. As a person or product passes through checkpoints, the medical assistant notes if there is deviation from a benchmark through tracking software.
- **Bank deposit**: The medical assistant deposits the takings for the practice at least once per week at a banking institution in one of these types of accounts: Current, checking, savings, money market, or time deposit account. The bank is liable to give the depositor (the practice) cash, less the transaction fees.

Copyright © Mometrix Media. You have been licensed one copy of this document for personal use only. Any other reproduction or redistribution is strictly prohibited. All rights reserved. This content is provided for test preparation purposes only and does not imply an endorsement by Mometrix of any particular political, scientific, or religious point of view.

Law and Ethics

Medical Laws/Regulatory Guidelines

ADVANCE DIRECTIVE, CODE BLUE, AND DNR ORDER

An **advance directive** is a legal document in which the patient communicates to his or her family and physician what kind of medical intervention he or she desires. A **living will** is a type of advance directive that terminally ill patients often make. Specific laws regarding advance directives vary by state, but the patient must always be competent.

A **"do not resuscitate" order** is a type of advance directive. A DNR order must be written in the patient's chart by the attending physician in order to be valid. All discussions with the patient and the family should be clearly documented in the chart. In the absence of a written DNR order, call a full Code Blue and proceed with resuscitation.

Code blue is a distress call that indicates a patient is in cardiac arrest. Call the resuscitation team immediately. Some patient rooms have code blue buttons that can be pushed to activate the code blue. Additional codes exist for respiratory distress, patient/family violence, elopement, or the abduction of a newborn or child.

INFORMED CONSENT

Informed consent protects patients by ensuring that they or those legally responsible for them are fully educated about tests, treatments, and procedures. The patient has the legal right to know about his or her own condition. The exceptions are life-threatening emergencies and legal incompetence. Informed consent protects healthcare professionals from battery lawsuits. Informed consent is obtained when the patient is given written information in regards to the treatment plan, risks, benefits, and alternative treatment options, the provider truthfully answers any questions, and the patient/parent/guardian comprehends the discussion. The patient or legal guardian then voluntarily signs the consent form, without duress or coercion. The medical assistant must obtain signed consent from the patient/guardian before treatment commences. Moreover, it is advisable to obtain the minor patient's assent prior to the procedure. Always keep the original informed consent form in the patient's chart. Assent should also be recorded in the medical record.

MEDICAL JURISPRUDENCE, CIVIL LAWS, AND CRIMINAL LAWS

Jurisprudence is the legal system set up and enforced at various governmental levels. Civil and criminal laws that pertain to medical situations are referred to as **medical jurisprudence**. Medical jurisprudence also involves applying the science of medicine to legal issues such as forensics or paternity testing.

Civil laws are more often invoked in the medical setting, as they pertain to either contracts or torts.

- A **contract** is an enforceable covenant between two or more competent individuals. An agreement between a doctor and his or her patient is a contract. It can be an expressed contract, with written or verbal terms, or it can be an implied contract, where actions create the contract.
- **Tort law** governs the other branch of civil law. Torts relate to standards of care and wrongful actions that cause injury to a patient.

Copyright © Mometrix Media. You have been licensed one copy of this document for personal use only. Any other reproduction or redistribution is strictly prohibited. All rights reserved. This content is provided for test preparation purposes only and does not imply an endorsement by Mometrix of any particular political, scientific, or religious point of view.

Criminal laws speak to crimes that endanger society in general. There are occasions when criminal law may apply to medicine, usually resulting in fines, incarceration, and discipline by the state medical board.

CONTRACT LAW

There is an expressed or an implied contract between the doctor and patient. The medical assistant and other personnel are the doctor's agents. The doctor is ultimately responsible for breach of contract under the *Doctrine of Respondeat Superior. Respondeat Superior* is Latin for "let the master answer." The *Doctrine of Respondeat Superior* means if a medical assistant is involved in a legal action resulting from work, then the doctor is ultimately responsible for the medical assistant's actions or losses incurred. However, the medical assistant employee is also held accountable for due diligence.

Breach of contract is failure to fulfill and complete the terms of the contract. There are four situations where a contract can be legally abandoned:

- The patient releases the doctor by failure to return for treatment. Ideally, the patient sends the doctor a certified letter of discharge, but this is not required.
- The patient/guardian does not comply with specific instructions from the doctor regarding care.
- The patient no longer requires treatment.
- The doctor formally withdraws from the case by sending a certified letter to the patient explaining the situation, to preclude any charges of patient abandonment.

TERMINATING PATIENT'S CARE

Regardless of the medical assistant's personal opinion, it is his or her responsibility as a healthcare professional to support and respect the choices made by the patient and family. If the family's choices conflict with the medical assistant's strong personal opinions related to care, then the medical assistant must **terminate care**, after giving adequate written notice to the patient and physician to avoid charges of patient abandonment. The medical assistant is legally required to wait until relieved by another member of the healthcare team who has equal or greater training. Examples of common conflicts that arise are:

- Parents refuse blood transfusions, pain relief, and treatments for minors
- Safety hazards (e.g., a dangerous dog, sexual harassment, or threats)
- Patient will not or cannot pay bills because of insurance problems
- Patient is unruly and obnoxious

REPORTABLE INCIDENTS

A reportable incident is a dangerous event that must be reported to the supervisor or Safety Officer within a specific time frame, usually 24 hours to 5 days. Reportable incidents include:

- Medication errors
- Failure to assess and treat a patient according to state protocols, especially if it results in serious injury or death
- Injuries or death while in care (e.g., attempted suicide)
- Inappropriate use of a device or drug that results in death or injury
- Motor vehicle accident resulting in death or injury
- Suspicion of drug or alcohol abuse by a healthcare provider
- Acts or omissions that threaten public safety or result in poor patient outcome

Copyright © Mometrix Media. You have been licensed one copy of this document for personal use only. Any other reproduction or redistribution is strictly prohibited. All rights reserved.
This content is provided for test preparation purposes only and does not imply an endorsement by Mometrix of any particular political, scientific, or religious point of view.

ANATOMICAL GIFT

The *Uniform Anatomical Gift Act* of 1968 facilitates organ transplantation under one standard, which is important when organs are transported across state lines. The Act was revised in 1987 and 2006 to cover transplants from cadavers and fetuses only through the national Organ Procurement and Transplantation Network (OPTN). Organ donations from living donors have many ethical and legal pitfalls, and are addressed in separate laws by each state.

OSHA AND THE FDA

The U.S. Department of Labor's **Occupational Safety and Health Administration (OSHA)** sets standards for:

- Proper hand washing
- Wearing gloves and other personal protective equipment (PPE)
- Bagging specimens in biohazard bags
- Disposing of needles and lancets in a sharps container
- Cleaning up spills to prevent spread of bloodborne pathogens
- Harmful chemical control
- Safe equipment use
- Adequate work space

Check for updates regularly at OSHA's website at http://www.osha.gov. These updates are required to be adopted as part of the facility's standards of practice.

The U.S. **Food & Drug Administration (FDA)**:

- Assigns the official (generic) name for drugs when it approves them
- Reports recalls and adverse events through *MedWatch*
- Publishes a free, downloadable *Orange Book* of approved drugs
- Divides drugs into five schedules, based on their potential for abuse, numbered Schedule I (generally illegal) to Schedule V (generally benign)
- Sets the temperature regulations for dish sanitization

HIPAA

HIPAA stands for **Health Insurance Portability and Accountability Act** of 1996. HIPAA's Title I regulates healthcare accessibility, especially in the cases of job change and loss; Title II regulates patient privacy rights. HIPAA requires the following:

- Every patient's medical record must bear a unique identifier to prevent misidentification
- Patients must be given access to their protected health information (medical records) at any time, upon request
- Only relevant health information can be disclosed to authorized parties
- A record must be kept of every disclosure
- Every patient or the parents/guardian must receive a *Notice of Privacy Practices*, outlining how the protected health information will be used
- Physical access to protected health information must be limited (including electronic files via password protection or swipe cards, firewall, and SSL encryption)
- Retired electronic equipment must have all data records wiped clean

> **Review Video: What is HIPAA?**
> Visit mometrix.com/academy and enter code: 412009

203

Copyright © Mometrix Media. You have been licensed one copy of this document for personal use only. Any other reproduction or redistribution is strictly prohibited. All rights reserved.
This content is provided for test preparation purposes only and does not imply an endorsement by Mometrix of any particular political, scientific, or religious point of view.

ADA

Americans with Disabilities Act (ADA) of 1990 provides the following protections for individuals with disabilities:

- Prevention of discrimination in employment
- Access to public services, accommodations, and goods
- Sophisticated telecommunication services to facilitate the hearing and speech impaired
- Requires medical offices to have ramps, entryways, and at least one treatment room that provides access and accommodates the needs of the disabled
- Applies to facilities with more than 15 employees, but all medical offices should strive to comply with ADA

DEA

DEA stands for **Drug Enforcement Agency**. Medical offices are targeted by drug addicts for syringes and narcotics, so the assistant may need to contact the DEA and local police. Medical assistants must be familiar with government sites that list drugs, so they can stay up-to-date with the industry, and spell and classify drugs correctly.

- US Drug Enforcement Agency Drug Scheduling: https://www.dea.gov/drug-scheduling
- FDA Electronic Orange Book: http://www.fda.gov/cder/ob/default.htm
- FDA National Drug Code Directory: https://www.fda.gov/drugs/drug-approvals-and-databases/national-drug-code-directory
- US National Library of Medicine (Medline): http://www.nlm.nih.gov/medlineplus/druginformation.html
- US Pharmacopeia: http://www.usp.org/aboutUSP/

HITECH ACT

The American Recovery and Reinvestment Act (2009) (ARRA) included the **Health Information Technology for Economic and Clinical Health Act (HITECH),** which provided incentives for healthcare providers to switch to electronic health records and allowed patients greater access to their electronic health records. Security provisions include:

- Individuals and HHS must be notified of breach in security of personal health information.
- Business partners must meet security regulations or face penalties.
- The sale/marketing of personal health information is restricted.
- Individuals must have electronic access to electronic health information, although the law doesn't specify the form that the disclosed information must take (email, CD, web portal). Copies must be in a format that is readable if the individual requests it, and the healthcare provider may charge a fee.
- Individuals must be informed of disclosures of personal health information.
- Individual can direct healthcare providers to transmit a copy of their health records to individuals or entities of their choosing.

Copyright © Mometrix Media. You have been licensed one copy of this document for personal use only. Any other reproduction or redistribution is strictly prohibited. All rights reserved. This content is provided for test preparation purposes only and does not imply an endorsement by Mometrix of any particular political, scientific, or religious point of view.

PUBLIC HEALTH STATUTES RELATED TO PUBLIC HEALTH AND WELFARE DISCLOSURE

Public health statutes related to public health and welfare disclosure include:

- **Communicable diseases**: Title 42 (The Public Health and Welfare) and each state's regulations control reporting requirements for communicable diseases and for quarantine. Diseases that must be reported to the CDC include cholera, giardiasis, hepatitis, salmonellosis, shigellosis, cryptosporidiosis, and COVID-19. State requirements vary, but generally include influenza and measles.
- **Vital statistics**: Each state has a department of vital statistics that compiles birth and death records.
- **Abuse/Neglect against children/older adults**: All states have laws regarding abuse/neglect, and all healthcare providers are mandatory reporters. Reporting agencies may differ from one state to another.
- **Wounds of violence**: All states have laws regarding which types of wounds of violence (usually knife and gunshot wounds) must be reported to the police.

SUBPOENA DUCES TECUM

Subpoena duces tecum literally means "bring [it] with you under penalty of punishment." It is a court order for a witness to produce documents. The judge must carefully consider if *subpoena duces tecum* transgresses the patient's HIPAA rights.

The physician and other health professionals must report to authorities:

- Gunshot wounds
- Possible terrorist incidents, especially if they involve the spread of disease
- Known or suspected abuse of a child, senior, or disabled person
- Sexual assault of a juvenile or disabled person
- Poisoning
- Wounds intentionally caused by knives and sharp objects
- Criminal violence, including domestic violence
- Client-specific information for the central cancer registry
- Specific contagious diseases determined by each state

The medical assistant must keep a written record of the patient's information that was disclosed to authorities.

GOOD SAMARITAN ACT

There are two kinds of Good Samaritan Acts:

- A first aider who provides unpaid assistance to the injured in an emergency and acts as "a reasonable man" up to his or her level of training is protected by state law from unfair prosecution for death, disability, or disfigurement. A judge would dismiss assault and battery charges.
- A living donor who offers a non-directed donation of an organ to the transplant center is a Good Samaritan. The following organs can be donated by a living donor: kidneys, liver lobes, lung lobes, pancreas segments, and small bowel segments. Non-direct donors do not have anyone particular in mind whom they would like to receive their donated organ. The donation is usually anonymous and the Good Samaritan is blameless for complications the recipient suffers.

Copyright © Mometrix Media. You have been licensed one copy of this document for personal use only. Any other reproduction or redistribution is strictly prohibited. All rights reserved.
This content is provided for test preparation purposes only and does not imply an endorsement by Mometrix of any particular political, scientific, or religious point of view.

AMERICAN ASSOCIATION OF MEDICAL ASSISTANTS

The professional organization that certifies medical assistants is the **American Association of Medical Assistants.** Candidates must complete an accredited medical assistant training program and write an exam. Topics covered include anatomy, physiology, terminology, law, medical records, finance, diagnostics, medication, nutrition, and communication. The test consultant for the medical assistant national certification exam is the National Board of Medical Examiners, which examines physicians. Therefore, employers consider the certification results reliable and valid.

IMPORTANT LEGAL TERMS

Important legal terms for the medical assistant to understand include the following:

- **Consent to treatment**: Required for all treatment, unless the patient is unconscious or an unaccompanied minor in an emergency. Patient agrees to receive basic, routine services, diagnostic procedures, and medical care.
- **Consent to release information**: Patient's signature authorizes release of health information between provider and other entities, such as third-party payers. Design of this form should be carefully considered, and may include language translation (verbal and/or written).
- **Subpoena**: A legal writ (order) requiring a person to come to court, to testify in court, and/or to produce documents or evidence. Failure to do so may result in fine or jailing.
- **Res ipsa loquitur ("the thing speaks for itself")**: The principle of law that allows the use of circumstantial evidence as proof.
- **Locum tenens ("to substitute for")**: Allows one medical professional to serve temporarily in place of another. For example, a physician's practice may be covered by another physician usually for a few days up to 6 months when the first goes on vacation or takes leave. Companies specialize in providing *locum* physicians to work on a contract basis.
- **Deposition**: This is a sworn out-of-court witness statement taken under oath, usually in an attorney's office prior to a court case to document what the witness knows and to preserve the statements for use in court.
- **Statute of limitations**: A law defining the maximum period the complainant or appellant can wait before filing a lawsuit. The limitation date varies according to the type of case and if it falls within state or federal jurisdiction. Usually, the limitation is 1-6 years. Homicide has no limitation. If the complainant misses the deadline, then the right to sue is "stats barred" (dead). Rarely, a judge will "toll" (extend) the deadline if the injury was discovered late or a trusted person hid misuse of funds or failure to pay. Minors' rights to bring negligence charges are tolled until the age of 18.
- **Assumption of risk**: (A.) A defense against an accusation of negligence. The defendant states the situation was obviously hazardous, so the complainant should have realized injury could result. (B.) An insurance company takes the risk of extending coverage, realizing the policyholder might make a claim, but it is statistically more likely to make a profit from the premiums.
- **Arbitration agreement**: The patient agrees to give up the right to sue the doctor. An arbiter (arbitrator) awards damages if injury results. Settlement is faster for the patient, and the doctor gets a malpractice insurance discount. Both parties save on legal fees.
- **Negligence**: Taking an unreasonable, careless action that could foreseeably cause harm. Failing to exercise due care for others that a prudent, reasonable person would do. Negligence is accidental. Negligence is not an intentional tort, such as trespass or assault. Business errors, miscalculations, and failure to act can be negligent.

Copyright © Mometrix Media. You have been licensed one copy of this document for personal use only. Any other reproduction or redistribution is strictly prohibited. All rights reserved. This content is provided for test preparation purposes only and does not imply an endorsement by Mometrix of any particular political, scientific, or religious point of view.

- **Contributory negligence**: If a person is injured partially because of his or her own negligence—even if it is slight—then the person who caused the accident does not pay any damages (money) to the injured person. Forty-four states recognize that applying the rule of contributory negligence could lead to unfair acquittal of genuinely negligent defendants, so they now use a comparative negligence test as a more balanced approach. In the 6 states that still have contributory negligence rules, juries tend to ignore it as unfair.
- **Comparative negligence**: A rule used in accident cases to calculate the percentage of responsibility of each person (joint tortfeasors) directly involved in the accident. Damages (money compensation) are awarded based on a complex formula.
- **Defamation**: Defaming a person exposes him or her to public ridicule or tarnishes his or her memory through untrue and malicious statements. The defamed person can lose business due to loss of his or her good name.
- **Slander**: Oral statements that damage someone's reputation. It is a form of defamation.
- **Libel**: A written statement that harms an individual's character, name, or reputation. A defamatory libel statement may be true, but is published maliciously (without just cause).
- **Invasion of privacy**: Unsolicited or unauthorized exposure of patient information.
- **Malpractice**: Professional misconduct, resulting in failure to provide due care. Most malpractice lawsuits are related to professional negligence, the failure to perform what is considered standard care.
- **Fraud**: Intentional dishonesty for unfair or illegal gain.
- **Assault and battery**: Assault is declaring or threatening an intent to touch a patient inappropriately or to cause physical harm. Battery is the actual act of inappropriate touching.

Copyright © Mometrix Media. You have been licensed one copy of this document for personal use only. Any other reproduction or redistribution is strictly prohibited. All rights reserved. This content is provided for test preparation purposes only and does not imply an endorsement by Mometrix of any particular political, scientific, or religious point of view.

Medical Ethics

CORE ETHICAL PRINCIPLES FOR MEDICAL ASSISTANT PRACTICE

Core ethical principles include:

- **Beneficence**: Performing actions that are for the purpose of benefitting another person. In the care of a patient, any procedure or treatment should be done with the ultimate goal of benefitting the patient.
- **Nonmaleficence**: Providing care in a manner that does not cause direct intentional harm to the patient. Care must be intended only for good effect, and good effects must have more benefit than bad effects that result.
- **Autonomy**: The right of the individual to make decisions about his or her own care. In the case of children, the child cannot make autonomous decisions, so the parents serve as the legal decision maker.
- **Justice**: Relates to the distribution of the limited resources of healthcare benefits to the members of society. Resources must be distributed fairly and decisions made according to what is most just.
- **Privacy/Confidentiality**: Protecting information (conversations, assessments) and body (close door, pull curtains, use drapes to avoid exposing patient) and protecting personal information about a patient and the patient's health condition.

PATIENTS' RIGHTS

The Advisory Commission on Consumer Protection and Quality on Health Care Industry, an initiative under President Clinton, outlined eight **rights and responsibilities of American patients**, as follows:

- The right to information
- The right to choose
- The right to access emergency services
- The right to fully participate in decisions regarding one's own health care
- The right to care without discrimination
- The right to privacy
- The right to speedy complaint resolution
- The responsibility for maintaining one's health to retain those rights

The American Hospital Association replaced its *Patients' Bill of Rights* in April 2008 with a brochure called *The Patient Care Partnership*, available in many languages. Obtain a free copy for the patient at http://www.aha.org. Additionally, the Health Insurance Portability and Accountability Act (HIPAA) include provisions for patient's rights. Information can be found at http://www.hhs.gov/ocr/.

Copyright © Mometrix Media. You have been licensed one copy of this document for personal use only. Any other reproduction or redistribution is strictly prohibited. All rights reserved. This content is provided for test preparation purposes only and does not imply an endorsement by Mometrix of any particular political, scientific, or religious point of view.

Medical Assistant Practice Test #1

Want to take this practice test in an online interactive format?
Check out the bonus page, which includes interactive practice questions and
much more: **https://www.mometrix.com/bonus948/ncctncma**

1. Title I of the Americans with Disabilities Act (ADA) mandates that individuals with disabilities are

  a.   to be provided access to public services
  b.   to be given opportunities for public housing
  c.   not be discriminated against in obtaining employment
  d.   to be provided means of telecommunication

2. Which of the following health care issues is NOT covered under the Health Insurance Portability and Accountability Act (HIPAA)?

  a.   Increasing the portability of health insurance
  b.   Addressing health care fraud and abuse
  c.   Standardizing the electronic transmission of health data
  d.   Outlining payment of Medicare and Medicaid

3. Which of the following constitutes a breach of contract by a health care provider?

  a.   Discontinuing treatment because the patient did not pay in a timely manner
  b.   Discontinuing treatment because it is no longer needed
  c.   Being formally discharged by the patient
  d.   Withdrawing from the case due to patient noncompliance or an inability to serve the patient

4. Under the doctrine of respondeat superior, which of the following CANNOT potentially be held legally responsible for an act of negligence by a medical assistant?

  a.   The medical assistant
  b.   The medical assistant's supervisor
  c.   The medical assistant's education provider
  d.   The medical assistant's employer

5. Touching a patient in a manner to which they have not consented is considered a tort of

  a.   invasion of privacy
  b.   battery
  c.   libel
  d.   slander

6. All of the following minors (under age 18) are considered emancipated EXCEPT a minor who is

  a.   a member of the armed forces
  b.   financially responsible and no longer under parental care
  c.   married
  d.   being treated for a sexually transmitted disease

Copyright © Mometrix Media. You have been licensed one copy of this document for personal use only. Any other reproduction or redistribution is strictly prohibited. All rights reserved.
This content is provided for test preparation purposes only and does not imply an endorsement by Mometrix of any particular political, scientific, or religious point of view.

7. Unless public safety is involved, what is required in all cases to release patient medical records after a subpoena is issued?

a.   The patient's written consent
b.   A court order
c.   A deposition
d.   An interrogatory

8. According to typical statutes of limitations involving negligence or malpractice, which of the following time points is NOT used as a starting point?

a.   When the negligent act occurred
b.   When the negligent act was revealed
c.   When the litigant filed a claim
d.   When treatment was terminated

9. What normal patient right is suspended upon discovery of child abuse?

a.   Privacy
b.   Confidentiality
c.   Documentation
d.   Standard of care

10. A POLST form is a type of

a.   document declaring durable power of attorney for health care
b.   document releasing a provider from liability under Good Samaritan laws
c.   living will or advance directive
d.   PSDA

11. Generally, medical assistants are permitted to do certain clinical procedures only under the supervision of an employer/provider because they are NOT

a.   certified
b.   registered
c.   licensed
d.   certified, registered, or licensed

12. Which of the following best describes ethics?

a.   Individual choices relating to conduct
b.   Personal values governing an individual's perceptions of right and wrong
c.   Laws defining acceptable behavior
d.   Creeds to live by

13. Bioethics is defined as

a.   any ethical matter that pertains to life and/or health care
b.   issues regarding abortion and the use of fetal tissue
c.   dealings with individuals who have committed sexual abuse or exploitation
d.   dealings with individuals who have committed physical or emotional abuse

Copyright © Mometrix Media. You have been licensed one copy of this document for personal use only. Any other reproduction or redistribution is strictly prohibited. All rights reserved. This content is provided for test preparation purposes only and does not imply an endorsement by Mometrix of any particular political, scientific, or religious point of view.

14. Which of the following principles for a medical assistant is NOT set forth by the American Association of Medical Assistants (AAMA) Code of Ethics?

  a. Respect for the confidentiality of patient information
  b. Performance of service while respecting all patients
  c. Continuous professional improvement
  d. Specific ways of dealing with certain situations

15. At present, what is the main difference between reporting child abuse and reporting elder or intimate partner abuse?

  a. Child abuse must be reported to authorities in all 50 states while other types of abuse do not always need to be reported
  b. Sexual abuse is the main offense related to child abuse, but not to elder or intimate partner abuse
  c. Physical abuse is more predominant in elder and intimate partner abuse than in child abuse
  d. Child abuse is more likely to involve a reportable criminal act

16. A provider is dealing with a patient with HIV or AIDS. Which of the following statements regarding the provider's legal or ethical requirements is NOT TRUE?

  a. The provider cannot withhold treatment to the HIV-positive patient
  b. The provider should protect the patient's confidentiality
  c. The provider can ethically deny treatment
  d. The patient's intimate partner should be notified by the patient, the provider, or authorities

17. What is the time frame during which an abortion can be legally performed in all states?

  a. There is no universal time frame for all states
  b. Abortion can be performed during the first trimester
  c. Abortion can be performed during the first trimester only in cases of rape
  d. Abortion can be performed during the first and second trimesters

18. Therapeutic communication interjects what element into communication?

  a. Empathy
  b. Advice
  c. Recommendations
  d. Knowledge of the process of communication

19. Which of the following adequately describes the qualities necessary for active listening?

  a. being alert and interested in what the other person is saying
  b. maintaining eye contact with the other person
  c. being attuned to what is said and what is communicated nonverbally
  d. being able to respond quickly with a corrective action

20. In order for verbal communication between two people to be effective, the sender's message must be

  a. complete
  b. clear and concise
  c. cohesive
  d. all of the above

Copyright © Mometrix Media. You have been licensed one copy of this document for personal use only. Any other reproduction or redistribution is strictly prohibited. All rights reserved. This content is provided for test preparation purposes only and does not imply an endorsement by Mometrix of any particular political, scientific, or religious point of view.

21. In the United States, what do most people consider a comfortable personal space for dealing on a personal (not intimate) level with another individual?

    a. In contact to 1-1/2 feet
    b. Between 1-1/2 and 4 feet
    c. Between 4 and 12 feet
    d. Between 12 and 15 feet

22. The use of a defense mechanism in which a person unconsciously ascribes their own undesirable acts or impulses to someone else is known as

    a. sublimation
    b. repression
    c. projection
    d. compensation

23. According to Maslow's hierarchy of needs, what is the first level of need that people must satisfy before all others?

    a. Physiological and survival needs
    b. Necessities for safety and security
    c. Needs related to loving and belonging
    d. Conditions promoting prestige and esteem

24. A cultural broker is someone who

    a. acts as a medical interpreter for a family member
    b. is responsible for a non-English-speaking relative
    c. acts as an intermediary or advocate for another person or cultural group within the health care community
    d. interviews non-English-speaking patients and later conveys the information to a medical professional

25. When interviewing a patient, which of the following types of question prompts only a yes or no response?

    a. Indirect statement
    b. Closed question
    c. Open-ended question
    d. Active question

26. Which of the following does NOT initially occur when a person is exposed to an acute stressor?

    a. Triggering of the parasympathetic nervous system
    b. Activation of the fight-or-flight response
    c. Releasing of adrenaline and other hormones into the bloodstream
    d. Increased respiration rate

27. In order, what are the four stages of job burnout?

    a. Value, ambiguity, overload, conflict
    b. Value, reality, dissatisfaction, detachment
    c. Honeymoon, dissatisfaction, reality, a sad state
    d. Honeymoon, reality, dissatisfaction, a sad state

Copyright © Mometrix Media. You have been licensed one copy of this document for personal use only. Any other reproduction or redistribution is strictly prohibited. All rights reserved.
This content is provided for test preparation purposes only and does not imply an endorsement by Mometrix of any particular political, scientific, or religious point of view.

28. Which of the following activities does NOT relieve stress?

a. Goal setting
b. Meditation
c. Gladly accepting all assigned work
d. Taking time off for lunch or a break

29. The symptoms lethargy and weight loss can be associated with which of the following conditions?

a. AIDS
b. Cancer
c. End-stage renal disease
d. All of the above

30. According to Dr. Kubler-Ross, what are the most likely stages of grief experienced by a patient with a life-threatening illness, in order?

a. Denial, bargaining, anger, depression, acceptance
b. Denial, anger, bargaining, depression, acceptance
c. Acceptance of reality, experience of pain, adjustment, development of a new reality
d. Denial followed by any number of stages leading to acceptance in the end

31. Which of the following management styles offers rewards to subordinates in terms of teamwork, recognition by other workers, and self-actualization?

a. Authoritarian management
b. Micromanagement
c. Participatory management
d. Management by walking around

32. If an office manager is using a teamwork approach, what is the first step in getting the team started?

a. Brainstorming with the team
b. Developing a work statement with the team
c. Looking at benchmarks from other institutions
d. Developing a time frame and standards for goal achievement

33. As an office manager, when is the best time to carry out a salary review for employees?

a. At the same time as their performance evaluation
b. When the employee asks for a salary review
c. At the beginning of each year
d. When the office experiences changes in funding

34. A medical assistant who functions as a human resources manager is responsible for developing and updating which of the following documents?

a. Office policy manual
b. Office procedure manual
c. HIPAA manual
d. Safety data sheets

Copyright © Mometrix Media. You have been licensed one copy of this document for personal use only. Any other reproduction or redistribution is strictly prohibited. All rights reserved.
This content is provided for test preparation purposes only and does not imply an endorsement by Mometrix of any particular political, scientific, or religious point of view.

35. **Which of the following actions during an initial employment interview is discouraged?**

    a. Providing a time frame for decisions on hiring or additional interviews
    b. Using predetermined questions during the interview
    c. Providing a quiet and private environment for the interview
    d. Offering the applicant the job on the spot

36. **The standard rate of overtime pay for administrative or clinical medical assistants is generally**

    a. twice the regular hourly rate for each hour over 40 in a week
    b. at least one-and-one-half times the regular hourly rate for each hour over 40 in a week
    c. not applicable because most medical assistants are considered exempt employees
    d. only applicable in terms of increasing benefits outside pay

37. **Medical assistants and other individuals who handle finances in the medical office should**

    a. be bonded
    b. maintain liability insurance
    c. be registered
    d. be licensed

38. **When must a medical assistant functioning as an office manager pay federal and state taxes related to employee wages?**

    a. Monthly
    b. Quarterly
    c. At the end of the year
    d. Upon filing of W-2 form

39. **What types of nutrients can be converted into energy?**

    a. Carbohydrates
    b. Fats
    c. Proteins
    d. All of the above

40. **Unhealthy trans unsaturated fatty acids are found in**

    a. olive and canola oils
    b. linoleic acid
    c. stick margarine
    d. unhydrogenated oils

41. **Which of the following statements is NOT true regarding a person's basal metabolic rate (BMR)?**

    a. It is the level of energy needed when the body is resting
    b. It is higher in people who have a large percentage of body fat
    c. It is elevated in children during growth spurts
    d. It is increased when a woman is pregnant

Copyright © Mometrix Media. You have been licensed one copy of this document for personal use only. Any other reproduction or redistribution is strictly prohibited. All rights reserved. This content is provided for test preparation purposes only and does not imply an endorsement by Mometrix of any particular political, scientific, or religious point of view.

42. **Which of the following summarizes the symbol through which the U.S. Department of Agriculture makes dietary recommendations?**

   a. Recommendations are divided by category with recommended intake of each category in the form of a food pyramid
   b. Recommendations are divided by a plate diagram that represents the proportion of each food group that should make up every meal
   c. Statements of recommended intake for each food group based on age, weight and comorbidities are presented in the form of a color-coded chart
   d. Statements of recommended intake are divided into four sections of a box diagram based on age and gender

43. **What are the main inorganic nutrients that act as antioxidants?**

   a. Vitamin K and folic acid
   b. Vitamin D and the minerals calcium and phosphorus
   c. Vitamins A, C, and E, and the mineral selenium
   d. Several B-complex vitamins and the minerals phosphorus, magnesium, and sulfur

44. **What type of diabetes mellitus requires the individual to take insulin regularly throughout life?**

   a. Type I only
   b. Type II only
   c. Types I and II
   d. Gestational

45. **What is the cardiovascular disease in which arteries narrow due to inner deposition of cholesterol and fat?**

   a. Hypertension
   b. Atherosclerosis
   c. Arteriosclerosis
   d. Myocardial infarction

46. **Cancerous cells that are derived from epithelial cells are known as**

   a. carcinomas
   b. sarcomas
   c. lymphomas
   d. germ cell tumors

47. **Which of the following characteristics does NOT distinguish a virus from other types of microorganisms?**

   a. A virus can only reproduce within another type of living cell
   b. Viruses are pathogenic
   c. Viruses produce spores
   d. Viruses cannot be observed directly under light microscope

215

Copyright © Mometrix Media. You have been licensed one copy of this document for personal use only. Any other reproduction or redistribution is strictly prohibited. All rights reserved.
This content is provided for test preparation purposes only and does not imply an endorsement by Mometrix of any particular political, scientific, or religious point of view.

48. An organism that serves as a carrier of a disease to another organism such as a human is known as a(n)

    a. fomite
    b. vector
    c. bloodborne carrier
    d. exudate

49. Which of the following currently available vaccines are contraindicated in pregnant women, immunocompromised patients, and those with active AIDS?

    a. Measles, mumps, rubella (MMR)
    b. MMR and influenza
    c. MMR, varicella, and zoster
    d. Hepatitis A and B

50. Pathogenic microorganisms, cancer cells, and transplanted tissues are initially recognized as foreign by

    a. macrophages and helper T cells
    b. B cells
    c. memory and killer T cells
    d. immunoglobulins

51. The biggest concern regarding the infectious diseases methicillin-resistant Staphylococcus aureus (MRSA) and tuberculosis is that

    a. identification of the infectious agent is difficult
    b. they are highly drug-resistant, limiting antibiotic treatment options
    c. they are viral and cannot be cured
    d. symptoms are hard to identify

52. Which of the following is NOT a characteristic of Hepatitis A infection?

    a. It is spread via the oral-fecal route
    b. It can be prevented by an available vaccine
    c. Patients usually develop jaundice, dark urine, and flu-like symptoms
    d. It becomes a chronic infection

53. Which of the following is a progressive neurologic disorder in which brain cells degenerate due to an absence of dopamine in the brain, causing rigid muscles and akinesia?

    a. Multiple sclerosis
    b. Meningitis
    c. Parkinson's disease
    d. Sciatica

54. Which of the following is the neurotransmitter released at the neuromuscular junction between axons of motor neurons and the motor end plate?

    a. Acetylcholine
    b. GABA
    c. Serotonin
    d. Dopamine

Copyright © Mometrix Media. You have been licensed one copy of this document for personal use only. Any other reproduction or redistribution is strictly prohibited. All rights reserved.
This content is provided for test preparation purposes only and does not imply an endorsement by Mometrix of any particular political, scientific, or religious point of view.

55. A streptococcal infection might be linked to all of the following circulatory disorders, EXCEPT

    a.   rheumatic fever
    b.   mitral valve stenosis
    c.   congestive heart failure
    d.   varicose veins

56. Which of the following types of anemia can be controlled by injecting the patient with vitamin B_{12}?

    a.   Iron deficiency anemia
    b.   Pernicious anemia
    c.   Sickle cell anemia
    d.   Hodgkin disease

57. What layer of the skin contains blood vessels, nerve endings, and glands?

    a.   Epidermis
    b.   Dermis
    c.   Hypodermis
    d.   Integumentary

58. Which of the following is a contagious skin disorder characterized by pustules and caused by staphylococci and/or streptococci?

    a.   Dermatitis
    b.   Dermatophytosis
    c.   Impetigo
    d.   Psoriasis

59. Which of the following statements is NOT true regarding herpes zoster infection?

    a.   It is caused by the same virus associated with varicella or chicken pox in children
    b.   It usually presents as a linear area of a skin rash
    c.   A later symptom can be post-herpetic neuralgia
    d.   Since it is caused by a virus, there is no available vaccine

60. The purpose of immunotherapy for allergies is to use extracts of allergens to

    a.   induce production of blocking IgG class antibodies toward the allergens
    b.   induce production of IgE class antibodies toward the allergens
    c.   generally build up the immune system
    d.   use immunomodulation to suppress the immune system

61. Which of the following urinary tract disorders should be suspected if a patient has chills, fever, abrupt back pain, and tenderness in the suprapubic region?

    a.   Cystitis
    b.   Glomerulonephritis
    c.   Pyelonephritis
    d.   Renal calculi

Copyright © Mometrix Media. You have been licensed one copy of this document for personal use only. Any other reproduction or redistribution is strictly prohibited. All rights reserved.
This content is provided for test preparation purposes only and does not imply an endorsement by Mometrix of any particular political, scientific, or religious point of view.

62. **Which of the following functions is NOT performed by the kidneys?**
    a. Regulation of water and acid-base balance
    b. Filtration of the blood to remove waste
    c. Regulation of blood pressure
    d. Collection and storage prior to urinary excretion

63. **Gastroesophageal reflux disease (GERD) is caused by**
    a. lesions in the mucous membranes in the stomach or duodenum
    b. return of stomach acid due to leakage of the valve leading to the stomach
    c. inflammation of diverticula
    d. inflammation of the ileum

64. **Which of the following statements about the pancreas is FALSE?**
    a. It functions as both an endocrine and an exocrine gland
    b. It is involved in the secretion of insulin
    c. It can develop stones, causing pain.
    d. It can become inflamed, which can be life-threatening

65. **In order, the large intestine is comprised of the**
    a. cecum, colon, and rectum
    b. duodenum, jejunum, and ileum
    c. ascending, transverse, descending, and sigmoid colons
    d. liver, gall bladder, and pancreas

66. **What is the chief cause of blindness in the United States?**
    a. Retinal detachment
    b. Glaucoma
    c. Diabetic retinopathy
    d. Presbyopia

67. **The gel occupying space between the lens and retina of the eye is called the**
    a. fovea centralis
    b. vitreous body
    c. sclera
    d. aqueous humor

68. **In patients with myopia, light rays entering the eye focus**
    a. on several areas of the retina
    b. in front of the retina
    c. beyond the retina
    d. on the retina

69. **When a person moves their head, their equilibrium is usually maintained by**
    a. the vestibular system in the inner ear
    b. the tympanic cavity in the middle ear
    c. the auricle
    d. the cochlea

Copyright © Mometrix Media. You have been licensed one copy of this document for personal use only. Any other reproduction or redistribution is strictly prohibited. All rights reserved. This content is provided for test preparation purposes only and does not imply an endorsement by Mometrix of any particular political, scientific, or religious point of view.

70. **Hearing loss due to hardening of the stapes of the middle ear is known as**
    a. tinnitus
    b. otitis media
    c. otosclerosis
    d. Ménière disease

71. **Which of the following is NOT a possible cause of epistaxis?**
    a. Allergic rhinitis
    b. Blunt force
    c. Hypertension
    d. Childbirth

72. **In the respiratory system, gas exchange between oxygen breathed in and carbon dioxide to be removed takes place in the**
    a. pharynx
    b. trachea
    c. bronchi
    d. alveoli

73. **The main characteristic that distinguishes asthma from forms of chronic obstructive pulmonary disease (COPD) is that asthma**
    a. does not cause dyspnea
    b. is characterized by a permanent narrowing of the airways
    c. can usually be reversed either spontaneously or through use of agents such as bronchodilators
    d. is caused by a loss of elasticity of the alveoli

74. **Which of the following can cause pneumonia?**
    a. Bacteria
    b. Fungi
    c. Viruses
    d. All of the above

75. **Which of the following is a spinal defect in which there is a sideways curvature of the spine?**
    a. Lordosis
    b. Kyphosis
    c. Paget disease of bone
    d. Scoliosis

76. **A fracture in which the bone is broken into a number of fragments is described as**
    a. greenstick
    b. comminuted
    c. oblique
    d. transverse

Copyright © Mometrix Media. You have been licensed one copy of this document for personal use only. Any other reproduction or redistribution is strictly prohibited. All rights reserved.
This content is provided for test preparation purposes only and does not imply an endorsement by Mometrix of any particular political, scientific, or religious point of view.

77. The main type of arthritis or joint inflammation that is considered a systemic autoimmune disease is

    a. osteoarthritis
    b. rheumatoid arthritis
    c. gout
    d. psoriatic arthritis

78. Which of the following is NOT true of endochondral ossification?

    a. It is responsible for the growth in length of long bones
    b. The cell types involved are bone cells, their progenitors, and cartilage
    c. It begins during embryonic development and continues until the late teens and early twenties
    d. It is direct deposition of bone into the mesenchyme

79. The largest leg bone that connects the kneecap to the foot is the

    a. patella
    b. femur
    c. tibia
    d. fibula

80. The human vertebral column normally consists of

    a. 24 articulating vertebrae and the spinal cord
    b. 24 articulating vertebrae and nine fused vertebrae
    c. the vertebral body and the vertebral arch
    d. clearly separated regions

81. The cervical region of the spinal cord controls certain movement in the

    a. neck, diaphragm, shoulder, arm, wrist, and hand
    b. trunk and abdomen
    c. abdomen, thigh, leg, and toes
    d. leg, foot, and toes

82. Viral infections have been associated with which of the following neurologic disorders?

    a. Cerebral palsy
    b. Trigeminal neuralgia
    c. Reye syndrome
    d. Huntington's disease

83. Which of the following is NOT characteristic of cerebrovascular accident (CVA)?

    a. A loss of blood to the brain, depriving it of oxygen
    b. Direct impairment of cranial nerves
    c. Symptoms like loss of consciousness and paralysis
    d. Caused by hemorrhage or blockage of a blood vessel

Copyright © Mometrix Media. You have been licensed one copy of this document for personal use only. Any other reproduction or redistribution is strictly prohibited. All rights reserved. This content is provided for test preparation purposes only and does not imply an endorsement by Mometrix of any particular political, scientific, or religious point of view.

84. Which of the following portions of the brain is primarily responsible for maintaining homeostasis?

    a. Cerebellum
    b. Cerebral cortex
    c. Hypothalamus
    d. Pons

85. Which of the following injuries and conditions is NOT known to cause paralysis?

    a. Spinal cord injury
    b. Stroke
    c. Poliomyelitis
    d. De Quervain's syndrome

86. When a patient is covered by more than one insurance policy, the total amount paid is limited by policy language regarding

    a. preauthorization
    b. assignment of benefits
    c. coordination of benefits
    d. the deductible

87. What is capitation?

    a. A payment system in which the health care provider is paid a fixed fee per patient
    b. A payment system in which the health care provider is paid a specific fee for a particular service
    c. Payment for the full fee for health care services by the patient
    d. Payment for health care services by the government through Medicare

88. The Managed Care Organization model, in which a network of providers and hospitals sign agreements to provide patient services at a discount to the insurance company nonexclusively, is a

    a. Point-of-Service (POS) Plan
    b. Preferred Provider Organization (PPO)
    c. Exclusive Provider Organization (EPO)
    d. Integrated Delivery System (IDS)

89. What health care services are covered under Medicare, part B?

    a. Hospital stays, home health care, and hospice care
    b. Outpatient expenses
    c. Prescription drug coverage
    d. All of the above

90. The resource-based relative value scale (RBRVS) is used to

    a. coordinate with Medigap policies
    b. determine whether a Medicare payment is PAR or non-PAR
    c. calculate Medicare payments
    d. determine practice overhead

Copyright © Mometrix Media. You have been licensed one copy of this document for personal use only. Any other reproduction or redistribution is strictly prohibited. All rights reserved. This content is provided for test preparation purposes only and does not imply an endorsement by Mometrix of any particular political, scientific, or religious point of view.

91. Which of the following groups is NOT a mandatory eligibility group to receive medical care under the Medicaid program?

    a. Low-income families
    b. Individuals with tuberculosis
    c. Individuals receiving supplemental security income
    d. Disabled adult children

92. Which of the following is the medical insurance program that covers active-duty soldiers?

    a. CHAMPVA
    b. TRICARE Prime
    c. TRICARE Extra
    d. TRICARE Standard

93. Workers' compensation insurance covers which of the following expenses for a person injured on the job?

    a. All medical expenses
    b. All medical expenses plus lost wages
    c. All medical expenses plus lost wages, and an automatic settlement for pain, suffering, and other punitive damages
    d. Some medical expenses and lost wages, as determined by state laws

94. If a usual, customary, and reasonable (UCR) fee structure is used for billing, an insurance carrier that pays fees that are considered customary will pay the provider

    a. the top fee in the customary range for that region
    b. the full fee as long as it falls within the customary fee range
    c. the RBRVS-calculated fee
    d. an adjustment

95. When is patient health information that is transmitted via telephone call or fax subject to the security rule under the Health Insurance Portability and Accountability Act (HIPAA) regarding electronic transmission?

    a. Always
    b. Never
    c. When that information was derived from electronically stored information
    d. When the patient has signed a privacy agreement

96. The relative value units (RVUs) issued for a particular service fee under Medicare are computed using which of the following factors?

    a. The provider's rate for the service, practice expenses, and malpractice expenses
    b. All of the factors listed in response A plus adjustors like the geographic practice cost index and the Budget Neutrality Adjuster
    c. Standard national codes
    d. Sliding fees within an acceptable range

Copyright © Mometrix Media. You have been licensed one copy of this document for personal use only. Any other reproduction or redistribution is strictly prohibited. All rights reserved.
This content is provided for test preparation purposes only and does not imply an endorsement by Mometrix of any particular political, scientific, or religious point of view.

97. According to the Current Procedural Terminology (CPT) system, what is the procedure to change a code for billing a medical procedure to reflect that the service lasted longer than described?

a. Enter the code twice
b. Add a plus sign (+) before the code
c. Use an unlisted code and add a report
d. Use a Category III code

98. Under the Current Procedural Terminology (CPT) system of coding, what type of modifier should be added to a code to indicate a slight difference in the description (for example, using a surgical team instead of one surgeon)?

a. Indicate both the described code and 09999
b. Put a -99 after the described code
c. Use a code beginning with 099 and ending with the two-digit modifier
d. Add the modifier 09966

99. Which medical insurance coding system should be used when billing Medicare or Medicaid?

a. International Classification of Disease, 10th Revision, Clinical Modification (ICD-10-CM)
b. Current Procedural Terminology (CPT)
c. Healthcare Common Procedure Coding System (HCPCS)
d. V Codes

100. Which of the following is the general format for describing a diagnosis due to disease under the International Classification of Disease, 10th Revision, Clinical Modification (ICD-10-CM) system?

a. Three-character coding for the diagnosis, starting with a letter; may be followed by a decimal point with a one- or two-digit modifier
b. Three-digit coding for the diagnosis, followed by a decimal point, and then a one- or two-digit modifier
c. A five-digit numeric code plus two-digit modifiers if required
d. Seven-digit alphanumeric code

101. Which of the following is the standard claim form to be completed for situations such as inpatient admissions, emergency department services, and walk-in facilities?

a. CMS-1500 (08-05)
b. Uniform Bill 04 (UB-04)
c. Authorization for Release of Medical Information
d. Encounter form

102. When can Medicare patients be held responsible for paying out-of-pocket expenses in addition to what is paid by the government?

a. Never
b. If they sign a written waiver
c. If they sign an Advanced Beneficiary Notification (ABN)
d. In any situation that is beyond the scope of Medicare

Copyright © Mometrix Media. You have been licensed one copy of this document for personal use only. Any other reproduction or redistribution is strictly prohibited. All rights reserved. This content is provided for test preparation purposes only and does not imply an endorsement by Mometrix of any particular political, scientific, or religious point of view.

103. Which of the following is the most commonly used manual system of managing a patient's account?

a. Patient ledger
b. Encounter form
c. Posting system
d. Pegboard system

104. In a patient's account or ledger, what should be posted as a credit?

a. The services provided and the charges for each
b. Payments by the insurance company or patient
c. Payments by the insurance company or patient and adjustments
d. The difference between charges and payments

105. The primary reason to keep day sheets and month-end sheets is to maintain accurate records of

a. accounts receivable for the practice
b. accounts payable for the practice
c. individual patient accounts
d. receipts

106. Which of the following is NOT generally included in monthly billing statements generated in computerized account systems?

a. Contact information for both the practice and the patient
b. History of all past services performed
c. Aging of past due balances
d. Itemized charges, payments, and a running balance

107. Which of the following types of check endorsement will ensure safety against cashing by anyone else?

a. Rubber endorsement stamp
b. Daily depositing
c. Blank endorsement
d. Restrictive endorsement

108. In order to comply with the Truth in Lending Act, what must be done by a provider who allows a patient to pay using installment payments?

a. Always have the patient sign a written agreement outlining cost of services rendered and outstanding terms of the agreement, including interest
b. Have the patient sign a written agreement outlining cost of services rendered and outstanding terms of the agreement, including interest, only if there are at least five installments
c. Explain to the patient when payments are due and whether there will be interest charged if they do not comply
d. Explain to the patient at the time of service that they must pay any insurance-required co-pay at that time, and that further payments will be assessed after the insurance company pays their portion of the bill

Copyright © Mometrix Media. You have been licensed one copy of this document for personal use only. Any other reproduction or redistribution is strictly prohibited. All rights reserved. This content is provided for test preparation purposes only and does not imply an endorsement by Mometrix of any particular political, scientific, or religious point of view.

109. Which of the following tools is used to measure how rapidly patient accounts are being paid?

    a. Collection ratio
    b. Accounts receivable (A/R) ratio
    c. Account aging
    d. Number of accounts with balances over two months old

110. Which of the following is generally the last resort for collection of an overdue bill?

    a. Telephone collections
    b. Collection letters
    c. Outside collection firm
    d. Filing in small claims court

111. When a patient has declared bankruptcy under Chapter 7, what should the medical office do regarding their unpaid account?

    a. Write off the outstanding charges
    b. Send a proof-of-claim and a copy of the patient's debt to bankruptcy court
    c. File a claim to the individual's attorney as an outstanding unsecured debt
    d. File a claim in probate court

112. An accounting software package that computerizes every aspect of running a medical facility is known as a

    a. single-entry system
    b. double-entry system
    c. computer service bureau
    d. TPMS

113. Which of the following is an accounting system designed to generate information for governmental or other external organizations?

    a. Managerial accounting
    b. Cost accounting
    c. Cost analysis
    d. Financial accounting

114. If a practice uses an accrual basis for income reporting, when is the income is recorded?

    a. The date the money was collected
    b. The date the charges were accrued
    c. The completion date for treatment
    d. A convenient date every month

115. Which of the following is a fidelity bond purchased to guard against embezzlement or other financial loss caused by any employee of a practice?

    a. Position-schedule bond
    b. Personal bond
    c. Blanket-position bond
    d. Total practice bond

Copyright © Mometrix Media. You have been licensed one copy of this document for personal use only. Any other reproduction or redistribution is strictly prohibited. All rights reserved. This content is provided for test preparation purposes only and does not imply an endorsement by Mometrix of any particular political, scientific, or religious point of view.

116. When closing the facility, an administrative medical assistant should lock up

   a. cabinets used for record storage
   b. cabinets used for storage of drugs named under the Controlled Substances Act
   c. petty cash and the day's receipts
   d. all of the above

117. Which of the following is a good estimate of the number of chairs needed in a waiting room?

   a. As many as will fit
   b. One and a half seats per examination room
   c. Two seats per provider per their hourly turnover
   d. Two seats per appointment scheduled per hour

118. Which of the following is the type of internal computer memory that is used for temporary storage of data and programs until saved?

   a. Read-only memory (ROM)
   b. Random-access memory (RAM)
   c. Data storage memory
   d. Redundant array of independent disks (RAID) storage

119. Which of the following is a sign that an Internet site is secure?

   a. Site address that includes www
   b. Site address located on a .org domain
   c. Site address located on a .gov domain
   d. Site address beginning with https://

120. The combination of various sources into a comprehensive electronic database for a patient is known as a(n)

   a. electronic medical record (EMR)
   b. electronic health record (EHR)
   c. medical office simulation software (MOSS)
   d. total practice management system (TPMS)

121. Where is good place to position a computer monitor relative to incoming light from windows or artificial lighting?

   a. Such that the light is directed at a downward angle toward the top of the monitor
   b. Such that the light is directed at a downward angle toward the individual's face
   c. Such that the light is to the individual's side, parallel to the sight line to the monitor
   d. At the same height but an angle to the incoming light

122. Which of the following types of calls cannot be handled by the medical assistant and should be referred to the provider?

   a. Obtaining information such as date of birth and insurance carrier from a new patient
   b. Scheduling an appointment
   c. Scheduling patient tests
   d. Authorizing a prescription refill

Copyright © Mometrix Media. You have been licensed one copy of this document for personal use only. Any other reproduction or redistribution is strictly prohibited. All rights reserved. This content is provided for test preparation purposes only and does not imply an endorsement by Mometrix of any particular political, scientific, or religious point of view.

123. When needed for administrative or medical purposes, a medical assistant can always discuss information about a patient with their

    a.   parent or legal guardian
    b.   employer
    c.   insurance carriers
    d.   attorney

124. Which of the following is NOT true of encrypted email?

    a.   It is a good way to send medical data via email
    b.   It utilizes a virtual private network (VPN) for security
    c.   It requires a digital ID consisting of public and private keys and a digital signature
    d.   It ensures that the email is secure

125. The patient scheduling style in which several patients are scheduled in the first half hour of each hour and then seen on a first-come, first-served basis is

    a.   double booking
    b.   clustering
    c.   wave scheduling
    d.   stream scheduling

126. What should a medical assistant do when a patient cancels an appointment or is a no-show?

    a.   Cross out no-shows with a red X and cancellations with a red line on a paper appointment sheet
    b.   Keep a permanent record and count these up so the provider is aware
    c.   Input this information using computer scheduling software to remove the name and document the missed appointment
    d.   Do any of the above, depending on the system used

127. How should errors discovered shortly after entry be corrected when using an electronic medical record?

    a.   Draw a single line through the error in red, add the correction, indicate "Corr." or "Correction" above the error, and initial and date the area
    b.   Erase or white-out the error and put in the correct information
    c.   Set the computer software to track the error slot, line out the error with the dash key, make the correction to the right of the lined-out error, key in "Corr." or "Correction," and initial and date the error
    d.   Create a new citation identifying and correcting the error, sign and date it, and insert it into the original record

128. What is an accession record?

    a.   A cross-reference method used in a numeric filing system
    b.   A numeric filing system in which a journal or computer listing with predetermined numbers assigns patient or other records
    c.   The order of filing used in alphabetic filing
    d.   The rationale for the filing system used in subject filing

Copyright © Mometrix Media. You have been licensed one copy of this document for personal use only. Any other reproduction or redistribution is strictly prohibited. All rights reserved. This content is provided for test preparation purposes only and does not imply an endorsement by Mometrix of any particular political, scientific, or religious point of view.

129. Which of the following is the letter style in which all of the lines commence at the left margin except the date, complimentary closure, and keyed signature, which start near the center?

a. Simplified
b. Full block
c. Standard modified block
d. Indented modified block

130. Which of the following statements regarding mail sent under the postal class of bulk mail is FALSE?

a. Use of bulk mail requires the organization to pay an annual fee
b. Bulk mail can be sent by first-class mail, standard mail, parcel post mail, or as bound printed matter
c. Bulk mail can be picked up by the postal service at the medical facility
d. There are rules regarding the format of bulk mail

131. The turnaround time for transcription and return to the provider of a STAT report should be no more than

a. 12 hours
b. 24 hours
c. 48 hours
d. 72 hours

132. The Occupational Safety and Health Act (OSHA) Bloodborne Pathogen Standard applies to contact with

a. blood and all body fluids
b. blood and all body fluids, secretions, and excretions
c. the items in response B plus non-intact skin and mucous membranes
d. the items in response C plus unfixed human tissue and tissue culture, cells, or fluid known to be positive for HIV, HBV, or HCV

133. The Centers for Disease Control (CDC) guidelines for isolation of patients with highly transmissible diseases are to use

a. Standard Precautions
b. personal protective equipment (PPE)
c. Transmission-Based Precautions
d. Standard Precautions and the applicable type of Transmission-Based Precautions

134. The preferred method for disposal of sharps is to

a. use the scoop technique
b. put them into a puncture-proof sharps container marked "biohazard"
c. put them in a metal pan for later sterilization
d. recap the sharp and then put it in a sharps container

Copyright © Mometrix Media. You have been licensed one copy of this document for personal use only. Any other reproduction or redistribution is strictly prohibited. All rights reserved. This content is provided for test preparation purposes only and does not imply an endorsement by Mometrix of any particular political, scientific, or religious point of view.

135. According to the Occupational Safety and Health Act (OSHA) Bloodborne Pathogen Standard, what is required if an employee is accidentally exposed to blood or other potentially infectious materials?

a. The employer must conduct an immediate medical evaluation of the employee
b. The incident must be reported to a superior and documented within 48 hours
c. The employer must offer to test the employee for HBV, HCV, and HIV
d. The employer must submit an ISO 9001 form

136. Which of the following is NOT an acceptable method of hand-washing as part of infection control?

a. Medical asepsis hand wash using an antimicrobial soap
b. Medical asepsis hand wash using a non-antimicrobial soap
c. Antibacterial wipes
d. Alcohol-based hand rub

137. Which of the following best describes the use of chemical germicidal agents on surfaces to kill most microorganisms?

a. Sanitization
b. Disinfection
c. Sterilization
d. Antisepsis

138. What is the sequence for removing potentially contaminated personal protective equipment when exiting an isolation room?

a. Remove gown and gloves, remove goggles, remove mask, wash hands
b. Remove gown, remove goggles, remove mask, remove gloves, wash hands
c. Remove mask, remove goggles, remove gloves, remove gown
d. Remove gloves, wash hands, remove gown, remove mask

139. When applying sterile gloves or assisting in a sterile procedure, where should the hands and/or sterile objects be held?

a. In front, at a distance from the body
b. In front, at a distance from the body and above waist level
c. Above waist level
d. Toward the sterile field

140. Which statement regarding the differences between surgical hand cleansing and medical hand cleansing is NOT true?

a. Surgical hand washing takes longer
b. During rinsing, hands should be down for medical hand cleansing and up for surgical hand cleansing
c. Lotion can be applied after medical hand cleansing, but not after surgical hand cleansing
d. Medical hand cleansing includes the forearm to the elbow, while surgical hand cleansing focuses only on the hands

Copyright © Mometrix Media. You have been licensed one copy of this document for personal use only. Any other reproduction or redistribution is strictly prohibited. All rights reserved. This content is provided for test preparation purposes only and does not imply an endorsement by Mometrix of any particular political, scientific, or religious point of view.

141. Which of the following sterilization processes is most appropriate for a heat-sensitive item such as a fiber-optic endoscope?

    a. Gas sterilization
    b. Dry heat sterilization
    c. Chemical sterilization
    d. Steam sterilization.

142. When sterilizing instruments using an autoclave, what parameters should be achieved for wrapped instrument packages or trays?

    a. 212 °F, 15 psi, 30 min exposure
    b. 270 °F, 15 psi, 30 min exposure
    c. 270 °F, 15 psi, 15 min exposure
    d. 270 °F, 20 psi, 20 min exposure

143. Which of the following types of quality control is recommended by the Centers for Disease Control (CDC) for checking the effectiveness of steam sterilization by an autoclave?

    a. Autoclave tape
    b. Sterilization strips placed in the wrapped package
    c. Biological indicators with strips or ampules containing bacteria, which are later cultured
    d. Biological indicators with strips or ampules containing heat-resistant bacterial spores, which are later cultured

144. Which of the following chemicals is usually used to destroy tissues using cryosurgery?

    a. Silver nitrate
    b. Sodium hydroxide
    c. Liquid nitrogen
    d. Nitrous oxide

145. Which of the following designates the smallest suture material available?

    a. Swaged
    b. Gauge 6-0
    c. Gauge 0
    d. Gauge 4

146. Which of the following features on an instrument locks it closed and is situated between the handle rings?

    a. Serration
    b. Tooth
    c. Ratchet
    d. Serrated loop

147. How do Mayo dissecting scissors differ from all other types of surgical scissors?

    a. Their tips have beveled, not blunt or sharp, edges
    b. They are actually knives used to cut skin
    c. One of the tips has a notched blade
    d. Their blades are very delicate

Copyright © Mometrix Media. You have been licensed one copy of this document for personal use only. Any other reproduction or redistribution is strictly prohibited. All rights reserved.
This content is provided for test preparation purposes only and does not imply an endorsement by Mometrix of any particular political, scientific, or religious point of view.

148. All hemostatic forceps have which of the following features?

a. Straight tips and serrations
b. Ratchets and serrations
c. Ring handles and bent shape
d. Ratchets and teeth

149. Which of the following is NOT true of scopes?

a. They are lighted
b. They are used to visualize inside body orifices
c. They have parts that are disposable or must be disinfected instead of sterilized
d. They are long and narrow

150. Which of the following should NOT be done when using an ultrasonic cleaner to sanitize surgical instruments after use?

a. Put the instrument in an open position
b. Completely submerge the instruments
c. Mix stainless steel instruments with those composed of other metals
d. Process the instruments for at least five minutes

151. Which of the following is a sterile cream designed for topical application on burns and other abrasion wounds?

a. Povidone-iodine
b. Silver sulfadiazine
c. Chlorhexidine
d. Hydrogen peroxide

152. Which of the following bandage-wrapping techniques should be utilized at a joint where movement is necessary?

a. Spiral turns
b. Reverse spiral turns
c. Figure-eight turns
d. Circular turns

153. Epinephrine is often added to injectable anesthetics because it is a

a. vasoconstrictor
b. vasodilator
c. mild anesthetic
d. monitor of anesthesia effectiveness

154. Which of the following is a type of open wound in which skin structures are torn off or away?

a. Laceration
b. Avulsion
c. Puncture
d. Incision

Copyright © Mometrix Media. You have been licensed one copy of this document for personal use only. Any other reproduction or redistribution is strictly prohibited. All rights reserved. This content is provided for test preparation purposes only and does not imply an endorsement by Mometrix of any particular political, scientific, or religious point of view.

155. Which of the following types of gloves should be worn when changing a surgical dressing?

    a. Non-sterile gloves throughout

    b. Sterile gloves throughout

    c. Non-sterile gloves for removal and sterile gloves for cleaning of the wound and application of sterile cream and dressing

    d. The same procedure in response C, but with an ungloved hand-washing in between

156. In which of the following types of fever does the person's body temperature swing between being elevated and being at or below baseline?

    a. Continuous

    b. Intermittent

    c. Remittent

    d. Febrile

157. When using a temporal artery (TA) thermometer to measure a patient's temperature, how is the probe generally used?

    a. Used behind the earlobe

    b. Inserted into the ear

    c. Attached to an electronic thermometer and inserted orally or rectally

    d. Pressed against the forehead and then slid across the forehead to the temple area while scanning

158. How is a temperature in degrees Celsius converted into degrees Fahrenheit?

    a. Multiply by 9/5

    b. Multiply by 9/5 and then add 32

    c. Multiply by 5/9

    d. Subtract 32 and then multiply by 5/9

159. Which of the following pulse sites is normally used to take a pulse rate in emergencies?

    a. Radial pulse

    b. Brachial pulse

    c. Carotid pulse

    d. Apical pulse

160. An adult with a pulse rate of 70 beats per minute has

    a. a normal pulse rate

    b. bradycardia

    c. tachycardia

    d. arrhythmia

161. All of the following abnormalities of respiration are associated with a period of complete absence of breathing EXCEPT

    a. voluntarily holding one's breath

    b. orthopnea

    c. sleep apnea

    d. Cheyne-Stokes respiration

Copyright © Mometrix Media. You have been licensed one copy of this document for personal use only. Any other reproduction or redistribution is strictly prohibited. All rights reserved. This content is provided for test preparation purposes only and does not imply an endorsement by Mometrix of any particular political, scientific, or religious point of view.

162. Which of the following breath sounds should be documented when taking a respiration rate, occurs with many lung diseases, and sounds like rattling?

a. Stridor
b. Stertorous respiration
c. Rales
d. Wheezing

163. Blood pressure is a function of all of the following EXCEPT

a. how strong the heart muscle is
b. the elasticity of the arteries
c. the size of the lumen of the arteries
d. the ejection fraction

164. The major difference between electronic and other types of sphygmomanometers used to measure blood pressure is that electronic types

a. do not use a pressure cuff
b. do not require simultaneous use of a stethoscope
c. tend to lose calibration and accuracy
d. can only read systole or diastole measurements in one take

165. When using a mercury or aneroid sphygmomanometer for blood pressure reading on an adult, the systolic pressure reading is recorded

a. during the first phase of deflation when a sharp tapping sound is heard
b. during the auscultatory gap
c. as tapping and muffled sounds begin to fade
d. when all sounds cease

166. How should a blood pressure measurement be recorded on an adult patient's chart?

a. Systolic pressure/diastolic pressure
b. Systolic pressure/diastolic pressure, arm used, patient position
c. Diastolic pressure/systolic pressure
d. Diastolic pressure/systolic pressure, arm used, patient position

167. An adult whose blood pressure is 125/85 is considered to have

a. normal blood pressure
b. prehypertension
c. hypertension
d. secondary hypertension

168. A traditional beam balance scale includes a lower measuring bar, with stops set at 50-pound increments, and an upper measuring bar that slides freely between 0 and 50 pounds. To weigh a patient, the medical assistant begins by setting the lower bar to the closest 50-pound increment below the patient's weight, and then moves upper bar until the beam is centered. What additional steps are needed to find the patient's weight in kilograms?

a. Add the measurements on the upper and lower measuring bars
b. Subtract the measurement on the upper bar from the one on the lower bar
c. Add the measurements on the upper and lower bars, then multiply by 2.2
d. Add the measurements on the upper and lower bars, then divide by 2.2

Copyright © Mometrix Media. You have been licensed one copy of this document for personal use only. Any other reproduction or redistribution is strictly prohibited. All rights reserved.
This content is provided for test preparation purposes only and does not imply an endorsement by Mometrix of any particular political, scientific, or religious point of view.

169. In which of the following physical examination methods is a stethoscope used to listen for lung and heart sounds?

    a. Palpation
    b. Percussion
    c. Auscultation
    d. Mensuration

170. A patient with a probable cardiovascular or respiratory problem should be positioned on the examination table in what position?

    a. Dorsal recumbent or lithotomy
    b. Semi- or high-Fowler's
    c. Trendelenburg
    d. Sims'

171. During a physical examination, the provider may use a tongue depressor and light source to check for any of the following EXCEPT

    a. dental hygiene along the teeth and gums
    b. swelling of the tonsils and uvula
    c. functioning of cranial nerve XI
    d. functioning of cranial nerves IX and X

172. During examination of the abdomen, which of the following observations is NOT a cause for concern?

    a. Palpable liver or spleen
    b. Presence of bowel sounds
    c. Presence of masses
    d. Abdominal distention

173. During the prenatal visit, a woman's obstetrical history should be recorded as

    a. one number for gravidity, then one number for parity
    b. one number for gravidity, then four numbers separated by dashes under the FPAL system for parity
    c. either A or B
    d. one number for gravidity, then one number for total previous live births

174. Which of the following laboratory tests commonly done at the initial prenatal visit is NOT part of a urinalysis?

    a. Venereal disease research laboratory (VDRL)
    b. Human chorionic gonadotropin (HCG)
    c. Glucose
    d. White and red blood cell counts

175. The pregnancy disorder in which the placenta is positioned over the cervical opening and can potentially cause bleeding during labor and fetal anoxia and death is

    a. eclampsia
    b. placenta previa
    c. placenta abruptio
    d. incompatibility

Copyright © Mometrix Media. You have been licensed one copy of this document for personal use only. Any other reproduction or redistribution is strictly prohibited. All rights reserved. This content is provided for test preparation purposes only and does not imply an endorsement by Mometrix of any particular political, scientific, or religious point of view.

176. As part of assisting the provider in inserting an intrauterine device (IUD) for pregnancy prevention, the medical assistant might do all of the following EXCEPT

a. assist the patient into the lithotomy position and drape them
b. hand the speculum to the provider
c. swab the cervix with an antiseptic and inject a local anesthetic if needed
d. document the procedure in the patient's chart

177. Which of the following is NOT true of a breast self-examination (BSE)?

a. The examination should be done standing up
b. The three middle fingers should probe for lumps or abnormalities in the opposite breast
c. Each breast should be checked using an up-and-down pattern
d. The individual should also check for abnormalities or redness in the mirror

178. According to the Bethesda system of classifying Pap tests, how should potential malignancy, defined as squamous cell carcinoma, be classified?

a. CIN 3
b. Category 2, subgroup 1a
c. Category 2, subgroup 1c
d. Category 3

179. Wet preps/mounts and potassium hydroxide preps are performed in order to

a. screen for chlamydia and gonorrhea
b. ascertain the cause of vaginitis in women or urethritis in men
c. diagnose conditions such as endometriosis or fibroids
d. biopsy for malignancies

180. What is always administered to children who experience an allergic reaction to a vaccine?

a. Subcutaneous epinephrine once, at 1:1000 dilution and a dose of 0.01 mg/kg body weight for up to 0.3 mg
b. Epinephrine as described in response a, up to three times, in 10-20 minute intervals
c. Oral or intramuscular diphenhydramine, 1 mg/kg body weight for up to 30 mg
d. Cardiopulmonary resuscitation (CPR)

181. The preferred intramuscular vaccine injection site for toddlers, older children, adolescents, and adults is the

a. anterolateral aspect of the thigh
b. gluteal muscle
c. deltoid muscle
d. triceps muscle

182. Growth charts for newborns, infants, and toddlers are differentiated according to percentiles for

a. length or weight versus age in months
b. length and weight versus age in months, separated according to sex
c. length, weight, and chest circumference versus age in months
d. length, weight, and chest circumference versus age in months, separated according to sex

Copyright © Mometrix Media. You have been licensed one copy of this document for personal use only. Any other reproduction or redistribution is strictly prohibited. All rights reserved. This content is provided for test preparation purposes only and does not imply an endorsement by Mometrix of any particular political, scientific, or religious point of view.

183. When taking the pulse rate for child younger than 5 years old, which of the following is the preferred pulse site?

  a. Radial pulse
  b. Brachial pulse
  c. Apical pulse
  d. Dorsalis pedis pulse

184. When checking a patient for prostate cancer, which of the following tests is NOT typically performed?

  a. Prostatic MRI
  b. Prostatic ultrasound
  c. Biopsy
  d. Prostate-specific antigen (PSA)

185. When performing a urinary catheterization on a female patient, which of the following should NOT be done?

  a. Use sterile gloves to maintain sterility of both hands throughout
  b. Wipe each portion of the labia with antiseptic-soaked cotton balls in a front-to-back motion
  c. Have the patient in a dorsal lithotomy position during the procedure.
  d. Use sterile lubricant on the catheter tip prior to insertion

186. When developing a fecal occult blood test, a positive result is indicated by

  a. immediate appearance of a blue color around the periphery of the stool smear
  b. appearance of a blue color around the periphery of the stool smear as well as the positive control within 30-60 seconds
  c. immediate appearance of a red color around the periphery of the stool smear and all controls
  d. patches of red in the stool sample

187. Which of the following pulmonary function tests is a good indication of the extent of someone's asthma or other respiratory disorder?

  a. Forced vital capacity (FVC)
  b. Forced expiration volume at one second (FEV1)
  c. Mean expiration flow rate (MEF)
  d. Peak expiratory flow rate (PEFR)

188. Which of the following is NOT true of an erythrocyte sedimentation rate (ESR)?

  a. A value of 25 mm/hour is always considered abnormal
  b. An ethylenediaminetetraacetic acid (EDTA) or sodium citrate venous blood sample is used
  c. The test must be read at precisely 60 minutes
  d. The test should be performed within two hours of the blood draw

189. A patient who cannot walk or lift himself is to be transferred. He should be lifted

  a. by the arms
  b. under the armpits
  c. by gripping their gait belt from underneath and lifting
  d. by their waist

236

Copyright © Mometrix Media. You have been licensed one copy of this document for personal use only. Any other reproduction or redistribution is strictly prohibited. All rights reserved.
This content is provided for test preparation purposes only and does not imply an endorsement by Mometrix of any particular political, scientific, or religious point of view.

190. A patient can bear only partial weight on one leg. Which of the following types of gait should this patient use with a crutch?

    a. Two-point gait
    b. Three-point gait
    c. Four-point gait
    d. Swing-to gait

191. Which of the following is a range of motion (ROM) exercise that involves a motion directed away from the body's midline?

    a. Flexion
    b. Rotation
    c. Abduction
    d Adduction

192. Which of the following best describes the current American Heart Association guidelines for emergency cardiopulmonary resuscitation (CPR) on an adult?

    a. Perform rescue breathing using two breaths, and if obstructed, five abdominal thrusts
    b. For circulation, use a ratio of 30 fast compressions to two breaths
    c. Shock with an automated external defibrillator (AED) prior to CPR
    d. Perform all of the above

193. Under the Controlled Substance Act, a special Drug Enforcement Agency (DEA) form must be utilized to order which of the following types of drugs in a medical setting?

    a. Schedule I
    b. Schedule II
    c. Schedule III
    d. Schedule IV

194. Of the cardiac-related drugs that should be kept on hand in an ambulatory setting, which one is used for angina pectoris?

    a. Nitroglycerin
    b. Atropine
    c. Digoxin
    d. Isoproterenol

195. A provider must administer a drug available in units/mL. How should the number of mL be determined to obtain the dose ordered?

    a. Multiply the available dose in units/mL by 16
    b. Divide the dose ordered by the dose on hand
    c. Divide the dose on hand by the dose ordered
    d. Convert to mg for each, and then divide the dose ordered by the dose on hand

Copyright © Mometrix Media. You have been licensed one copy of this document for personal use only. Any other reproduction or redistribution is strictly prohibited. All rights reserved.
This content is provided for test preparation purposes only and does not imply an endorsement by Mometrix of any particular political, scientific, or religious point of view.

196. When taking a standard electrocardiograph (ECG), where should the bipolar leads be placed?

    a. Between the left and right arms, the left leg and right arm, and the left leg and left arm

    b. Between the middle of the left arm to left leg and the right arm, the middle of the right arm to left leg and the left arm, and the middle of the right arm to left arm and the left leg

    c. Between six different points on the chest and a point on the right arm to left leg lead

    d. Between six different points on the chest and the intersection of the left arm/right arm/left leg leads

197. An irregular electrocardiograph (ECG) characterized by closely spaced premature ventricular contractions (PVCs), a lack of P waves, and distorted QRS complexes indicates

    a. atrial fibrillation

    b. paroxysmal atrial tachycardia

    c. ventricular tachycardia

    d. ventricular fibrillation

198. A "3" in the blue diamond on a chemical label indicates that the chemical is

    a. a flammable liquid

    b. reactive with water

    c. a corrosive or toxic health hazard

    d. potentially explosive near a spark or if heated

199. A Centers for Medicare and Medicaid (CMS)-approved basic metabolic panel includes laboratory tests for

    a. carbon dioxide, potassium, chloride, and sodium

    b. the tests listed in response A plus blood urea nitrogen (BUN), total calcium, creatinine, and glucose

    c. the tests listed in response B plus albumin, total bilirubin, total protein, SGOT, and SGPT

    d. albumin, alkaline phosphatase, direct bilirubin, total bilirubin, total protein, SGOT, and SGPT

200. In which of the following color top tubes should a venipuncture specimen be collected if the laboratory tests to be performed require a serum sample?

    a. Red top or red-gray mottled top

    b. Lavender top or blue top

    c. Dark green top

    d. Light gray top

Copyright © Mometrix Media. You have been licensed one copy of this document for personal use only. Any other reproduction or redistribution is strictly prohibited. All rights reserved. This content is provided for test preparation purposes only and does not imply an endorsement by Mometrix of any particular political, scientific, or religious point of view.

Answer Key and Explanations for Test #1

1. C: There are five titles outlined in the ADA. Title I covers prohibition of discrimination in employment for those individuals with physical or mental disabilities. The other answers describe the content of Titles II, III, and IV. Title V covers insurance, defining exclusions, etc.

2. D: HIPAA covers all of the issues discussed in choices A through C as well as a number of others, such as tax breaks for medical savings accounts, in its seven titles. However, the only reference in the Act to Medicare type plans is that they must coordinate with other plans to prevent duplication of coverage.

3. A: Discontinuation of treatment by a health care provider merely because the patient has not paid in a timely manner would be considered a breach of contract. The other choices describe the three instances in which the provider can legally discontinue treatment. Choices C and D require the professional to send a notice describing the situation by certified mail with return receipt to the patient.

4. C: Under the doctrine of respondeat superior, both the medical assistant's employer and supervisor (usually a doctor, nurse, or some other licensed professional) is responsible for the employee's actions to a degree and can be sued in instances of negligence by the medical assistant. However, the medical assistant can also be sued, because they are considered responsible for providing a reasonable standard of care.

5. B: All of the given choices are types of torts, which are wrongful actions that culminate in injury to the other person (in this case, the patient). Battery is the touching of a patient in manner to which they have not consented. Invasion of privacy includes a number of situations in which a patient's privacy is invaded, such as releasing information about them without permission or failing to shield them properly during examination. Libel and slander are two types of defamation of character, which are false and malicious writing or speaking about someone, respectively.

6. D: The minors described in A, B, and C, as well as minors who are parents, are considered to be emancipated and are capable of signing their own consent. In most states, minors being treated for sexually transmitted diseases, as well as those who are pregnant or have a drug or alcohol addiction, can also sign their own consent, but in this case, they are considered mature (not emancipated) minors.

7. A: A subpoena is a court-issued request for access to part or all of a patient's medical record. Unless public safety is involved, the basic requirement for record release to anyone is the patient's written consent. A court order is sometimes also required when sensitive issues are involved, such as AIDS or other sexually transmitted diseases, mental illness, etc. Choices C and D refer to later processes during the discovery phase of litigation, dealing with oral and written testimony, respectively.

8. C: The time point most often used as the starting point for the statute of limitations on negligence is generally choice A, when the act occurred, but choices B and D are sometimes utilized. However, choice C, the date the litigant filed the claim, is not a valid starting point for the statute of limitations to apply.

9. B: When a health care provider or other professional observes an instance of suspected child abuse, they are legally required to report this to the police, social services agency, and parents; this

Copyright © Mometrix Media. You have been licensed one copy of this document for personal use only. Any other reproduction or redistribution is strictly prohibited. All rights reserved. This content is provided for test preparation purposes only and does not imply an endorsement by Mometrix of any particular political, scientific, or religious point of view.

suspends the normal patient right to confidentiality. The right to privacy is slightly different. The provider must still properly document the case and provide the expected standard of care.

10. C: POLST stands for the Physician Orders for Life-Sustaining Treatment form, which is available in some configuration in the majority of states and is a type of living will or advance directive for level of care in the near-death of a patient. This may also be referred to as a MOLST (Medical Orders for Life-Sustaining Treatment). A durable power of attorney designates another individual for decisions regarding the patient's health care. PSDA refers to the federal Patient Self-Determination Act, which is related in that it discusses Medicare/Medicaid payments and availability of advance directives in institutions. POLST forms are unrelated to the Good Samaritan laws.

11. C: Medical assistants are only allowed to do certain clinical procedures because they are not a licensed profession, like doctors and nurses, who must fulfill specified educational requirements and pass a state-administered examination. Many medical assistants choose to voluntarily become certified.

12. B: Ethics refers to the set of personal values that shape an individual's perceptions of right and wrong, which is different from morals. Ethics are not laws defining acceptable behavior or creeds to live by, although the latter generally are derived from ethics.

13. A: Bioethics is an overall term relating to all ethical matters pertaining to life and/or health care. The other responses describe particular situations in which bioethics might be invoked.

14. D: The AAMA Code of Ethics for medical assistants does not outline specific ways of dealing with certain situations, but it does expound five things that should be strived for. These five things include A, B, and C, as well as upholding the principles and disciplines of the profession, and taking part in further service activities related to the betterment of the community.

15. A: Not all states have legislation related to reporting of elder (60 years of age or older) or intimate partner abuse. All three types of abuse could potentially be sexual, physical, or emotional. Other types include neglect in cases of child or elder abuse, financial in cases of elder abuse, and sexual exploitation and incest in cases of child abuse. All types could also potentially involve a reportable criminal act, such as rape.

16. C: The provider cannot withhold treatment to an HIV-positive patient, so C is the correct answer. In addition, patient confidentiality should be maintained, and any intimate partners notified.

17. A: Nearly all of the states allow elective abortion during the first trimester. However, recent legislation prohibiting abortion once a heartbeat can be detected has passed in a handful of states, including Texas, though legal challenges are expected. It is important to know the law in the state in which you work. Regardless of the circumstances under which state law permits abortions, a health care provider is not required to perform or participate in an abortion procedure if he or she is ethically opposed.

18. A: Therapeutic communication is distinguished from normal social communication in that it interjects empathy toward the other person, not advice or recommendations. A person effective at therapeutic communication is often knowledgeable about the process of communication, but that is not required.

19. C: Active listening requires the receiver to be attuned not only to what the other person is saying, but also to what they may be hinting at through body language or nonverbal

Copyright © Mometrix Media. You have been licensed one copy of this document for personal use only. Any other reproduction or redistribution is strictly prohibited. All rights reserved. This content is provided for test preparation purposes only and does not imply an endorsement by Mometrix of any particular political, scientific, or religious point of view.

communication. Being alert and interested is helpful but does not in itself constitute active listening. Maintaining eye contact can be helpful at times but is neither essential nor sufficient. Making a quick response defining a corrective action is generally thought to be detrimental to communication.

20. D: According to references such as Legal Nurse Consulting Principles and Practice, effective verbal communication occurs when the message is complete, clear, concise, cohesive, and also courteously delivered.

21. B: There are cultural differences in what is considered a comfortable personal space, but generally in the United States between 1-1/2 and 4 feet is considered comfortable space for personal interaction with another individual. The other responses represent the personal spaces generally considered necessary for intimate communication, social communication, and in public spaces.

22. C: All of the listed responses are types of defense mechanisms, but C is the described mechanism. Sublimation is diverting a socially unacceptable behavior into one that is socially acceptable. Repression is subconsciously forgetting an event. Compensation is disguising a real or imagined undesirable trait by overemphasizing one that is considered healthy or acceptable. Other types of defense mechanisms include regression, denial, displacement, rationalization, and undoing.

23. A: The most basic needs on the base of Maslow's hierarchy are those related to physiology and survival such as food, water, and air. Maslow describes five levels of needs. The listed responses represent levels two, three, and four. The fifth and final level is self-actualization, the achievement of one's potential.

24. C: A cultural broker is an intermediary or advocate for another person or cultural group. A cultural broker can act as a medical interpreter, but generally a family member is not the best choice because they may not comprehend the medical terminology. In this role, the cultural broker should never interview the patient independently, but rather act as a direct interpreter.

25. B: A question that is designed to prompt only a yes or no response is a closed question. An open-ended question is one designed to prompt more information and therefore facilitate therapeutic communication. An indirect statement, which can also encourage therapeutic communication, is posed in a form such as "Tell me about..." Active listening is a good way of observing what a patient is communicating nonverbally.

26. A: When a person is exposed to an acute stressor, the sympathetic nervous system (not the parasympathetic) is initially triggered as the flight-or-fight response which includes things like release of hormones, increasing of respiration rate, short-term memory loss, etc. After the body is exhausted by these reactions, then the parasympathetic nervous system is triggered to allow the body to resume normal functions.

27. D: Response D describes, in order, the four stages a person goes through on the way to job burnout. The four characteristics in response A, when preceded by the word "role," are features associated with job burnout.

28. C: If a worker accepts a workload that is too heavy, beyond his/her skill level, or not clearly differentiated from work others are doing, he/she can experience frustration, stress, and potentially burnout. Activities A, B, and D are all good ways to relieve stress.

Copyright © Mometrix Media. You have been licensed one copy of this document for personal use only. Any other reproduction or redistribution is strictly prohibited. All rights reserved. This content is provided for test preparation purposes only and does not imply an endorsement by Mometrix of any particular political, scientific, or religious point of view.

29. D: AIDS, cancer, and end-stage renal disease are all potentially life-threatening illnesses that can result in lethargy and weight loss in addition to other symptoms.

30. B: Response B illustrates the most likely scenario, according to Dr. Kubler-Ross. Response C, called the TEAR acronym, is another way of looking at the stages of grief.

31. C: The type of management technique that offers subordinates these types of rewards is participatory management. Authoritarian management is essentially the same as micromanagement; managers practicing this style plan everything on their own and offer the subordinate only monetary return. Management by walking around (MBWA) is a style in which the manager visits employees to collect data about how smoothly the organization is running.

32. B: The first step as a manager in getting a team started is development of a work statement with the team, which should include mutually established (not pre-established) time frames and standards. Brainstorming should be done after development of the work statement, and it often includes looking at benchmarks from other institutions to determine feasibility. The later steps are planning, implementation, and recognition.

33. C: The best time to carry out a salary review for all employees is the beginning of each year because that ensures equality and continuity for each employee. This is fairer than waiting for the individual to ask for a salary review, which can result in much longer time periods, or at the time of their performance evaluation, to keep the two reviews separate. Practice funding is important, but it is more cost-effective to retain good employees than to hire new ones.

34. A: The only responsibility listed that applies strictly to a medical assistant who functions as a human resources manager is developing and updating the office policy manual. The other responsibilities apply to medical assistants acting as office managers.

35. D: The only response that is discouraged is D, offering the potential employee the job at the time of the initial interview, because the interviewer should review all candidates before making any decisions. The other responses are all suggested behaviors during the initial interview of a potential employee.

36. B: Although overtime may be paid at twice the regular hourly rate, the general standard rate is at least one-and-one-half times the regular hourly rate for each hour over 40 in a week. Some medical assistants (Mas) may be exempt employees, but those are usually MAs functioning in higher grade levels, such as managers.

37. A: The act that guarantees that a provider will get back any monies an employee embezzles is to buy a bond that covers losses in that employee's name. Professional liability insurance should be purchased by practicing medical assistants, but in that case things like malpractice are covered. Registration, while desirable, is not required for handling finances, and medical assistants are not licensed.

38. B: A medical assistant functioning as an office manager must pay federal and state taxes related to employee wages quarterly.

39. D: All these nutrients can be converted into energy, although carbohydrates are the primary source. Proteins are mainly used to generate amino acids, which can be utilized as building blocks of structural proteins, enzymes, and hormones.

Copyright © Mometrix Media. You have been licensed one copy of this document for personal use only. Any other reproduction or redistribution is strictly prohibited. All rights reserved.
This content is provided for test preparation purposes only and does not imply an endorsement by Mometrix of any particular political, scientific, or religious point of view.

40. C: Trans unsaturated fatty acids are hydrogenated. This occurs when substances like vegetable oil are heated, making them solid at room temperature in things like stick margarine. These fats elevate the bad type of cholesterol, low-density lipoprotein (LDL), and lower the good type of cholesterol, high-density lipoprotein (HDL). Olive and canola oils both have healthier types of unsaturated and saturated fats. Linoleic acid is the one essential fatty acid needed in the human diet.

41. B: All of the statements are true, except for B. BMR is actually higher in people with lean body mass or relatively more muscle because it takes more energy to fuel muscles than to store fat.

42. B: The USDA uses MyPlate as a symbol to present dietary recommendations. This graphic has replaced the formerly used food pyramid. In this diagram, fruits and vegetables take up half of the plate, with grains taking up one quarter, and protein taking up the other, with dairy include within a circular shape outside of the plate (like a cup). Rather than listing explicit amounts, this symbol is meant to provide a visual of the proportion each food group should make up for each meal.

43. C: Antioxidants attack free radicals in the body that can harm DNA and blood vessel cells. The main antioxidants are vitamins A, C, and E, and the mineral selenium. Vitamin K and folic acid contribute to blood clotting and formation of red blood cells and DNA. Vitamin D and the minerals calcium and phosphorus contribute to bone growth. Several B complex vitamins and the minerals phosphorus, magnesium, and sulfur contribute to energy metabolism.

44. A: People with type I diabetes mellitus are insulin-dependent because they do not produce insulin, a hormone needed to signal to cells that glucose is available for conversion to energy. If they do not receive insulin, carbohydrates will not be metabolized. People with type II diabetes are not insulin-dependent and can usually control their disease through diet because they produce insulin, but in insufficient quantities. Gestational diabetes is a temporary situation in which a woman develops glucose intolerance while pregnant.

45. B: Atherosclerosis is the correct answer, but all of these cardiovascular conditions can be interrelated. Hypertension is high blood pressure, which can be due to things like high bodily water levels due to high sodium intake, but can also occur with atherosclerosis. Arteriosclerosis is the hardening of the arteries due to reduced elasticity of the vessel, often as a result of atherosclerosis. Myocardial infarction or a heart attack is an interruption of the blood supply to a coronary artery due to eruption of an atherosclerotic plaque.

46. A: Cancer is the general term for unregulated cell growth. Cancers derived from epithelial cells are the most common type and are known as carcinomas. Cancers derived from connective tissues such as bone are called sarcomas. Cancers derived from blood-forming hematopoietic cells are called lymphomas and leukemias. Cancers derived from pluripotent stem cells are called germ cell tumors.

47. C: Viruses do not produce spores, but a number of other types of microorganisms do, including certain bacteria, fungi, and protozoa. Viruses can only reproduce within another type of living cell. They are pathogenic like most microorganisms (but not all bacteria are). They cannot be observed directly under light microscope, although their effects may be.

48. B: Vectors are disease carriers, such as ticks or mosquitoes, that carry a microorganism to ultimately infect a human or other organism; most are associated with transmission of rickettsiae, which are small, nonmotile bacteria that are intracellular parasites. The other answers are other modes of transmission for microorganisms. A fomite is an inanimate object, such as a piece of equipment, on which a microorganism lives until it is transmitted. Bloodborne transmission is a

243

Copyright © Mometrix Media. You have been licensed one copy of this document for personal use only. Any other reproduction or redistribution is strictly prohibited. All rights reserved. This content is provided for test preparation purposes only and does not imply an endorsement by Mometrix of any particular political, scientific, or religious point of view.

common mode in which infection occurs through exposure to blood. An exudate is wound drainage, which often transmits a microorganism through direct contact. Other transmission modes include airborne transmission and ingestion.

49. C: MMR, varicella, and zoster vaccines are all contraindicated in the described patient categories, because all of these vaccines contain live attenuated viruses and the patients have low immune responses. The other vaccines are safer because they contain either inactivated virus or only viral proteins.

50. A: Foreign invaders are initially recognized by macrophages and helper T cells. After they are recognized, the two types of immunity directed against specific antigens, cellular and humoral, are activated. Cellular immunity involves activation of helper T cells to develop memory and killer T cells; along with macrophages, the killer T cells surround and kill the foreign organism or cell. Humoral immunity involves activated B cells, which divide into memory B cells and plasma cells. These produce specific immunoglobulins called antibodies, which bind to the antigens.

51. B: MRSA, caused by methicillin-resistant Staphylococcus aureus, and tuberculosis, caused by Mycobacterium tuberculosis, are both highly drug-resistant bacterial infections, thus limiting antibiotic treatment options. There are a number of ways to diagnose each, and they are not viral.

52. D: All of the statements are true except for D. The other two major hepatitis virus infections, hepatitis B and C, usually become chronic, but hepatitis A is generally resolved within two months of contraction and patients do not become carriers of the virus.

53. C: This is a description of Parkinson's disease. Multiple sclerosis is demyelination of nerve fibers resulting in symptoms such as visual disruptions and muscle weakness. Meningitis is inflammation in the brain or spinal cord, caused by a viral or bacterial infection and resulting in symptoms like headache, fever, and stiff neck. Sciatica is sharp leg pain along the sciatic nerve due to its compression by a severed intervertebral disk or osteoarthritis.

54. A: These are all neurotransmitters of some type, but acetylcholine is the one released at the neuromuscular junction. Gamma aminobutyric acid (GABA), is an inhibitory transmitter in the brain. Serotonin is found primarily in the intestinal tract and central nervous system, and contributes to feelings of well-being. Dopamine activates a number of receptors in the brain. There are a number of other neurotransmitters as well.

55. D: The major circulatory disorder associated with a streptococcal infection is rheumatic fever. This can, in turn, cause narrowing or stenosis of the mitral value, thwarting blood flow between the atrium and ventricle of the heart. It can also cause carditis, or inflammation of the heart muscle, which could manifest as congestive heart failure or other heart conditions. The correct answer, varicose veins, is completely different; these enlarged veins are caused by impaired venous return.

56. B: The term "anemia" refers to any disorder characterized by low circulating red blood cells and hemoglobin, resulting in symptoms like pallor, weakness, and malaise. There are three variations: iron deficiency anemia due to decreased levels of iron; pernicious anemia, due to lack of intrinsic factor which results in an inability to absorb vitamin B_{12}; and sickle cell anemia, a hereditary disorder in which the red blood cells are shaped like sickles and often lyse and clump in blood vessels. Hodgkin disease is a type of cancer of the lymphatic system.

57. B: The skin consists of three layers: the outer epidermis, made up of squamous epithelium, keratin, and melanin; the middle dermis, which contains the blood vessels, nerve endings, glands, and some connective tissue; and the deepest hypodermis, with subcutaneous connective and

Copyright © Mometrix Media. You have been licensed one copy of this document for personal use only. Any other reproduction or redistribution is strictly prohibited. All rights reserved. This content is provided for test preparation purposes only and does not imply an endorsement by Mometrix of any particular political, scientific, or religious point of view.

adipose tissue. Integumentary is the inclusive name for the system of the skin and its connected structures like hair nails, nerve endings, and oil and sweat glands.

58. C: The contagious skin disorder described is impetigo. Dermatitis is erythema (redness) due to an irritant. Dermatophytosis is a contagious fungal infection causing skin to flake, scale, and itch, most often in the foot area (also called athlete's foot or tinea pedis). Psoriasis is a chronic autoimmune type of dermatitis, the most common presentation of which is red and white scaly patches.

59. D: All of these statements are true regarding herpes zoster infection or shingles, except for D. There is an available vaccine recommended for adults over 60.

60. A: There are various types of immunotherapy, including immunomodulation for instances such as cancer. However, when the term is applied to allergic diseases, it refers to the injection of increasing amounts of allergens (to which the patient is allergic) to induce production of blocking IgG class antibodies, not IgE class antibodies, which are the type causing the allergy in the first place. The goal is not general buildup of the immune system.

61. C: Pyelonephritis presents with these types of symptoms after a pyogenic bacterial infection. It is usually located in the bladder and kidneys. Pyelonephritis can occur due to pregnancy or renal calculi or kidney stones, the main symptom of which is excruciating pain when they are lodged in and move within the ureter. Cystitis is inflammation of the bladder due to a urinary tract infection. It is characterized by signs like urinary frequency and burning. People with glomerulonephritis also have chills, fever, and hypertension due to inflammation of the glomeruli or small blood vessels in the kidneys; streptococcal infection is one cause.

62. D: The bladder is the final part of the urinary system that collects and stores urine prior to excretion. The kidneys perform all of the functions listed in A, B, and C, as well as others, such as releasing certain hormones.

63. B: GERD occurs when there is valve leakage in the area between the esophagus and stomach, which brings up stomach acid and causes heartburn. Response A describes gastric (stomach) and duodenal ulcers, which can be caused by things like Helicobacter pylori, salicylates, alcohol, and too much secretion of hydrochloric acid. The other responses refer to diverticulitis in diverticula of the colon, and Crohn disease in the ileum or final section of the small intestine.

64. C: Pain due to stones is generally associated with the gall bladder. The other statements all pertain to the pancreas. Inflammation of the pancreas is pancreatitis, which can be life-threatening because pancreatic enzymes can cause the organ to necrose and hemorrhage.

65. A: Response A is the order in which parts of the digestive system comprise the large intestine, not just the parts of the colon. Response B is the order of structures within the small intestine. The structures described in D are organs that are associated with the digestive system.

66. C: Diabetic retinopathy, the chief cause of blindness in the United States, is injury to the retina in individuals with diabetes due to vascular changes. Retinal detachment, separation of the retina from the choroid layer, can also cause blindness. Untreated glaucoma, high intraocular pressure due to accumulation of aqueous humor, can impair vision significantly. Presbyopia is the loss of elasticity in the lens which occurs as people age, thus impairing close vision.

67. B: This gel between the lens and the retina on the inner surface of the eye is the vitreous body or vitreous humor, which differs from the aqueous humor, which is a watery substance occupying

Copyright © Mometrix Media. You have been licensed one copy of this document for personal use only. Any other reproduction or redistribution is strictly prohibited. All rights reserved. This content is provided for test preparation purposes only and does not imply an endorsement by Mometrix of any particular political, scientific, or religious point of view.

the space between the lens and the cornea on the front of the eye. The fovea centralis is the spot in the middle of the central macula region of the retina, which is responsible for sharp central vision. The sclera is the outer white layer of the eye.

68. B: Myopia, also known as near-sightedness, occurs because the eyeball is elongated, causing light rays to focus in front of the retina. Astigmatism is due to non-uniform lens curvature or cornea shape. Farsightedness is due to shortening of the eyeball, causing light rays to focus beyond the retina. Response D describes normal vision.

69. A: Equilibrium is maintained by the vestibular system in the inner ear. The cochlea is also in the inner ear, but it is associated with hearing. The middle ear is made up of three bones (malleus, incus, and stapes) carrying waves from the outer ear, and the hollow space called the tympanic cavity. The auricle is the external ear.

70. C: This is a description of hearing loss called otosclerosis. Tinnitus is hearing sound within the ear in the absence of external sound, which could be due to something like impacted cerumen (ear wax). Otitis media is a middle ear infection resulting in symptoms like pain, discharge, hearing loss, etc. Meniere disease is a composite of the symptoms of hearing loss, vertigo, tinnitus, and nausea, probably due to swelling of the labyrinth in the inner ear.

71. D: Epistaxis is another word for nosebleed. This could be caused by a variety of factors, including those listed in A, B, and C, as well as low humidity in the environment, nasal infections, and many others. Childbirth has nothing to do with this condition, but an episiotomy (which sounds similar) is sometimes done during childbirth. Hormones in pregnancy cause dilation of the blood vessels in the nose, increasing blood supply and pressure on the vessels, and at times causing epistaxis.

72. D: Gas exchange takes place in the alveoli, which are the tiniest air sacs in the lungs. When air is taken in during the inspiration phase of respiration, the order of intake is nose or mouth, pharynx, trachea, bronchi, bronchioles, and then the alveoli.

73. C: Asthma is usually reversible because it involves inflammation but not actual airway narrowing, whereas in the two types of COPD, emphysema and chronic bronchitis, there is permanent narrowing of the airways. Dyspnea, shortness of breath, is a common symptom of both asthma and COPD. Loss of elasticity of the alveoli (most commonly due to smoking) is the hallmark of emphysema.

74. D: Pneumonia is inflammation of the lungs resulting in symptoms like chills, fever, cough, and yellow sputum. It can be caused by various bacteria, fungi, viruses, and sometimes chemical irritants.

75. D: Three of the options are abnormal curvatures of the spine, with scoliosis being a sideway curvature to the right or left. Lordosis is an inward curve to the lower spine, resulting in swayback. Kyphosis is an outward curve to the upper portion, resulting in hunchback. Paget disease of bone is characterized by localized, irregularly shaped, weakened bones, resulting from relatively excessive bone destruction followed by their irregular repair.

76. B: Comminuted fractures involve splintering into a number of fragments; if those fragments are forced into another bone, they are said to be impacted. A greenstick fracture is a fracture in which the bone bends and partially breaks, usually found in soft, young bones. An oblique fracture is a fracture in which the break is diagonal to the bone's long axis. A transverse fracture is a fracture at a right angle to the bone's long axis.

Copyright © Mometrix Media. You have been licensed one copy of this document for personal use only. Any other reproduction or redistribution is strictly prohibited. All rights reserved.
This content is provided for test preparation purposes only and does not imply an endorsement by Mometrix of any particular political, scientific, or religious point of view.

77. B: There are many types of arthritis or joint inflammation. A number of these are either proven or suspected to be autoimmune diseases, the most prevalent being rheumatoid arthritis. Osteoarthritis is a chronic joint inflammation due to degeneration and overgrowth of bone and cartilage. Gout is joint inflammation due to deposition of uric acid crystals through a defect in purine metabolism. Psoriatic arthritis is joint inflammation in individuals with the skin condition psoriasis.

78. D: Direct deposition of bone cells into the primitive connective tissue mesenchyme is the other type of bone formation, intramembranous ossification. The other characteristics listed are associated with endochondral ossification.

79. C: There are two bones connecting the knee cap (the patella) to the foot; the larger is the tibia and the narrower one is the fibula. The femur is the thigh bone.

80. B: The vertebral column consists of 24 articulating vertebrae and nine fused vertebrae in the sacrum and coccyx. It does house and protect the spinal cord, but that is not part of it. Individual vertebrae are made up of the anterior vertebral body and the posterior vertebral arch. The vertebral column is continuous, not clearly separated into regions, although there is a characteristic curvature to the spine normally and the fused areas look different than the articulating ones.

81. A: The cervical region is the top portion of the spinal cord; it consists of eight levels (C1 to C8) and controls movements in the areas listed in response A. There is some overlap in the functions in other regions. However, essentially response B describes movements controlled by the next section, the thoracic (T1 to T12), response C describes those controlled by the next lower lumbar section (L1 to L5), and response D describes movements controlled by the even lower sacral region (S1 to S5).

82. C: Viral infections have been associated with neurological disorders such as Reye syndrome, meningitis, encephalitis, and shingles. Cerebral palsy is a developmental disorder. Trigeminal neuralgia is a pain disorder, believed to be caused by excess pressure on the trigeminal nerve. Huntington's disease is a genetic disorder.

83. B: All of the statements except B, direct impairment of cranial nerves, are true. Regarding response D, there are two types of CVA or stroke: hemorrhagic, caused by hemorrhage of a blood vessel in the brain, and ischemic, whose potential causes include obstruction by a blood clot (thrombosis) or embolus from somewhere else (embolism), systemic hypoperfusion, and venous thrombosis.

84. C: The hypothalamus is the brain portion primarily responsible for maintaining homeostasis, equilibrium of the internal environment. The pons is involved in these functions also, but it is in the brainstem. The cerebellum modulates things like motor function and cognition, and the cerebral cortex or gray matter controls functions such as memory and language.

85. D: Paralysis can be caused by spinal cord injury, stroke, and poliomyelitis, as well as a number of other means of interfering with nerve function, such as the drug curare, and conditions like multiple sclerosis, spina bifida, meningitis and Guillain-Barré syndrome. De Quervain's syndrome is a musculoskeletal disorder that does not cause paralysis.

86. C: Coordination of benefits (COB) refers to policy language that describes how multiple applicable policies will be coordinated to limit the amount paid to no more than 100% of the fee. This is different than assignment of benefits, which means the signing over of benefits to someone else. Preauthorization is the carrier's consent prior to care, which, depending on the policy, may or

Copyright © Mometrix Media. You have been licensed one copy of this document for personal use only. Any other reproduction or redistribution is strictly prohibited. All rights reserved.
This content is provided for test preparation purposes only and does not imply an endorsement by Mometrix of any particular political, scientific, or religious point of view.

may not be required. The deductible is the amount of out-of-pocket medical expenses a person must pay before the policy starts to pay, generally on a yearly basis.

87. A: Capitation is a payment system in which the health care provider is paid a fixed fee per patient, a common method used by Managed Care Organizations, as opposed to a specific fee for a particular service, which is more common with traditional insurance.

88. B: This is a description of the PPO model of a Managed Care Organization. Health Maintenance Organizations (HMOs) are similar but usually require use of only physicians in the system and selection of a primary care provider for payment as well. A POS plan allows the patient to use HMO provider services or non-HMO providers at higher rates. An EPO consists of providers and facilities under exclusive contract. An IDS uses associated service providers that work together to reduce cost.

89. B: Medicare Part B covers outpatient expenses, such as provider charges, laboratory tests, and durable medical equipment. Hospital stays and home health and hospice care are covered to an extent under Medicare Part A, and prescription drug coverage is the essence of Medicare Part D, if purchased. Medicare Part C or Medicare Advantage plans are private plans approved by Medicare that usually cover the same things as Parts A, B, and sometimes C.

90. C: RBRVS, which is a comprehensive regional scale of fees for Medicare services, is used to calculate Medicare payments. Response B is a related answer in that PAR and non-PAR signifies whether the provider is a regular Medicare provider or not, which influences how Medicare payments are determined. Medigap policies, which are supplemental insurance policies addressing non-covered fees, are not taken into account.

91. B: Mandatory eligibility groups are those identified by the federal law as qualifying for Medicaid. Examples include low-income families, individual receiving supplemental security income (SSI), and disabled adult children. Each state has the option to expand coverage to optional categorically needy groups such as individuals with tuberculosis.

92. B: The TRICARE program offers 3 levels of medical insurance for active-duty soldiers, national guardsmen, reserves, military retirees, their families, and survivors. TRICARE Prime is the level for active soldiers and is administered mostly in military hospital facilities. TRICARE Extra uses civilian preferred providers, and TRICARE Standard uses fee-for-service providers. CHAMPVA stands for Civilian Health and Medical Program of the Veterans Administration, which provides insurance to spouses and dependents of veterans who were disabled or killed in the line of duty.

93. B: Workers' compensation insurance always covers all medical expenses and lost wages as defined by state minimum standards. The company may pay a settlement at a later date as well, but that is not part of workers' compensation per se.

94. B: When using a customary fee system, the insurance carrier will pay the full fee the provider charges, providing it falls within the customary fee range charged in that geographical region. Anything above that range will have to be written off by the provider as an adjustment. The top fee is not automatically paid. The RBRVS-calculated fee, as determined relative to Medicare, may be the actual fee paid, but not necessarily.

95. C: HIPAA laws govern patient health information that is generated, transmitted, received, or stored electronically. Therefore, when information in an electronic record is transmitted via phone or fax, it becomes subject to the HIPAA security rule.

Copyright © Mometrix Media. You have been licensed one copy of this document for personal use only. Any other reproduction or redistribution is strictly prohibited. All rights reserved. This content is provided for test preparation purposes only and does not imply an endorsement by Mometrix of any particular political, scientific, or religious point of view.

96. B: RVUs are computed using a complex equation involving all of these factors, which is then multiplied by a conversion factor to convert the RVU into dollars.

97. B: The addition of a plus sign before the code indicates the service lasted longer than described in the original code. The provider should not enter the code twice, use an unlisted code with an attached report (which is used for services for which a code cannot be clearly identified), or use a Category III code (which is temporary and designed for emerging technologies).

98. C: While the correct modifier for use of a surgical team would be 09966, the question asks for the general method of determining the modifier. This is described in response C, using a code beginning with 099 and ending with the appropriate two-digit modifier. The other responses describe coding options if multiple modifiers are required.

99. C: When billing for Medicare or Medicaid patients, HCPCS codes should be used. ICD-10-CM codes are widely used but they are not specific to Medicare/Medicaid; V codes are part of this system. The CPT coding system is also widely used.

100. A: Response A is the general format for an ICD-10-CM description of the disease diagnosis. The format in response B was the format used under ICD-9-CM. Response C describes the general format used for coding under the Current Procedural Terminology (CPT) or Healthcare Common Procedure Coding System (HCPCS) systems. Seven-digit alphanumeric codes are used for the International Classification of Disease, 10th Revision, Procedure Coding System (ICD-10-PCS).

101. B: The correct answer in this case is the UB-04 form. The claim form generally used for office visits is A, the CMS-1500 (08-05), which derives information from the initially completed encounter form. The Authorization for Release of Medical Information form is usually signed by a patient to allow for transmission of medical information.

102. C: Medicare patients can be held responsible for some out-of-pocket expenses if they have signed an ABN. A written waiver is the same type of document as referred to for Medicaid.

103. D: Although the majority of facilities now use computerized financial systems, the most commonly used manual system is the pegboard system, also called the write-it-once method. This system incorporates the patient ledger, the encounter form, and other things like charge and deposit slips, day sheets, and checks. Posting is the term for the recording of financial transactions into the bookkeeping system.

104. C: All payments by the insurance company or patient, as well as adjustments, which include discounts and write-offs, should be posted as credits. The ledger should also include all debits and a running balance.

105. A: In a manual pegboard-type system, day sheets and month-end sheets are used to reconcile practice balances with patient ledgers. Accounts payable are promises to pay suppliers for expenses incurred and are not part of day or month-end sheets. Receipts are given to patients to record their payments.

106. B: Typically, computerized account systems will generate bills that include contact information for both the practice and the patient, itemized charges for recent services, payments, running balance, and aging of how long past due balances have accrued, as well as the account number, date of billing, and possibly other information. A history of all past services performed is not generally included.

Copyright © Mometrix Media. You have been licensed one copy of this document for personal use only. Any other reproduction or redistribution is strictly prohibited. All rights reserved.
This content is provided for test preparation purposes only and does not imply an endorsement by Mometrix of any particular political, scientific, or religious point of view.

107. D: The only way to ensure against cashing of a check by anyone else is restrictive endorsement, which means that in addition to a signature, the words "for deposit only" or "pay to the order of..." are added. Further information, such as the account number for deposit, should also be included. A blank endorsement is the signature alone, which does not ensure safety. Daily depositing of a practice's checks is a good idea, but not sufficient.

108. B: All of these practices are good ways of guaranteeing payment, but response B describes what is required under the Truth in Lending Act for making installment payments.

109. B: Rapidity of patient account payment is calculated by the accounts-receivable ratio, which is defined as: current accounts receivable/average monthly gross charges = A/R or turnaround time in months. Many feel a good ratio is two or less, meaning that, on average, practice account balances are past due by two months or less. Aging is similar, but it refers to a specific patient account. The collection ratio is an indication of the effectiveness of billing procedures, and is defined as: current month collections/total monthly charges minus adjustments.

110. C: Generally, the order of attempting to settle overdue bills is telephone collections, followed by one or more collection letters, and then use of an outside collection firm. Occasionally, a tactic might be filing in small claims court, but only small claims can be brought and the process is time-consuming.

111. B: There are two types of bankruptcy that can be declared. Under Chapter 7, the debtor is cleared of all debts, so the office may need to write-off the charges; however, the required procedures are outlined in response B. Answer C describes what should be done if the patient has declared Chapter 13 bankruptcy, in which they come up with a plan to pay off some of their debt; unfortunately, a medical provider is low on the list of payees because their services are unsecured debt. Probate court is the court that deals with debt related to an estate.

112. D: An accounting software practice that computerizes every aspect of running a medical facility, including patient data, electronic records, and accounting procedures, is known as a total practice management system (TPMS). A computer service bureau utilizes an outside company to coordinate data, billing services, etc. The other two options are manual methods of bookkeeping. In the single-entry system, a daily log and various records are kept and then posted to a ledger. In the double-entry system, assets are balanced against the sum of liabilities and owner's equity.

113. D: This type of accounting is financial accounting. Managerial accounting is designed to provide data that improves internal management, and a subset that focuses on what particular services cost is cost accounting. Cost analysis is the method of determining the costs of services, which are a composite of fixed and variable costs.

114. B: When using an accrual basis for income reporting, the income is recorded at the time the charges were produced. Response A describes the cash basis for income reporting, which is more commonly used.

115. C: There are three categories of fidelity bonds that can be purchased. The type that covers any employee is a blanket-position bond. A position-schedule bond pertains to a specific position but not a named employee. A personal bond covers one named employee.

116. D: When closing the facility, an administrative medical assistant should routinely do all of the things listed as well as put rooms in order for the next day. An alternative to locking up the day's receipts is to take them and a bank deposit to the bank that day.

Copyright © Mometrix Media. You have been licensed one copy of this document for personal use only. Any other reproduction or redistribution is strictly prohibited. All rights reserved. This content is provided for test preparation purposes only and does not imply an endorsement by Mometrix of any particular political, scientific, or religious point of view.

117. C: A good way of estimating the number of needed chairs in the waiting room is two seats per provider per their hourly turnover or two and a half seats per examination room. The medical assistant or receptionist must be able to see all of the people in the waiting room. Seats should not be based on the number of appointments scheduled, because that value can change significantly over time. Having as many chairs as will fit may be excessive or dangerous in terms of egress in the case of an emergency.

118. B: RAM is the type of internal memory used for temporary storage of data and programs; it can be both written to and read from. ROM is data that is permanently stored on the computer motherboard on chips. Data storage memory is also permanent memory, but it is stored in places other than the motherboard, such as internal or external hard drives, or optical drives like CDs or DVDs. RAID storage is a whole storage system.

119. D: A site address that begins with "https://" indicates a secure site. Note that a site being secure is not the same as a site being trustworthy. A site address on a .org or .gov domain may indicate trustworthiness, but does not say anything about the site's security.

120. B: An EMR is an electronic medical record from a single source, such as a medical practice, but when EMRs from various sources are combined to generate a comprehensive electronic patient database they constitute an EHS. MOSS is an available type of TPMS.

121. C: Glare from incoming light is prevented with the relative positioning described in response C. The other positions can result in some type of glare, either directly into the eyes or indirectly from reflection off the monitor. The monitor should be placed just below eye level.

122. D: A medical assistant can take a call regarding a prescription refill. However, they cannot authorize the refill themselves, so the information must be given to the provider for authorization. The other listed calls can be handled by the medical assistant.

123. A: Under the right to confidentiality, the only type of individual listed that a provider is allowed to discuss information about a patient with in all circumstances is their parent or legal guardian. A medical assistant should never discuss a patient with their employer, and discussions with insurance carriers or attorneys are allowed only if a signed release is obtained from the patient.

124. B: All of these are features of encrypted email except VPN, which is a way of increasing security using Voice over Internet Protocol (VoIP) communications.

125. C: This style is wave scheduling, a variation of which is modified wave scheduling, in which several patients are scheduled at the top of the hour plus single appointments at approximately 15-minute intervals thereafter. Double booking involves scheduling two or more patients simultaneously but performing different functions on each, such as seeing the doctor versus laboratory tests. Clustering is a style in which patients with similar types of issues are booked one after another. Stream scheduling is continuous booking of patients within discreet time frames. Other scheduling styles include open hours, in which patients are seen without appointments on a first-come, first-served basis, and customized practice-based scheduling.

126. D: Depending on whether scheduling is done on a daily appointment sheet or via computer, any combination of these things should be done. The important thing for legal and other purposes is to document cancellations and no-shows in some type of permanent record.

Copyright © Mometrix Media. You have been licensed one copy of this document for personal use only. Any other reproduction or redistribution is strictly prohibited. All rights reserved. This content is provided for test preparation purposes only and does not imply an endorsement by Mometrix of any particular political, scientific, or religious point of view.

127. C: When using an electronic medical record, this is the way of correcting errors discovered promptly. Response D describes how to make these corrections later, after the software locks out the method in response C. Responses A and B describe right and wrong ways, respectively, to make corrections on paper medical records.

128. B: An accession record is a journal or computer listing with predetermined numbers, used in a numeric filing system to assign a number (rather than a name) to a file in order to protect patient confidentiality. The alphabetic card file is used as a cross-reference and contains patient name and other information. There are two other types of filing systems, alphabetic and subject, which is useful in research settings.

129. C: Modified block letter styles put some components, including those listed, in approximately the center. The standard modified block style is described. The indented modified block differs in that paragraphs are indented five spaces. In a full block letter, every component begins flush with the left margin. A simplified letter is similar, except that the salutation and complimentary closure are left out.

130. C: All of the statements listed apply to the postal class of bulk mail, except that it must be delivered to the bulk mail entry unit at the post office and cannot be picked up.

131. A: Facilities have varying requirements, but generally a STAT report is something containing needed information, such as a laboratory report which should be transcribed and returned in less than 12 hours. The 24-hour turnaround time is generally for current reports, an example of which is a history and physical examination (H&P) report. The 72-hour turnaround is generally for old or aged reports, such as discharge summaries.

132. D: Response C applies to CDC recommendations for use of Standard Precautions, but the OSHA Bloodborne Pathogens Standard goes further to include the items in response D.

133. D: If a patient has or may have a highly transmissible disease, both Standard Precautions and the applicable type of Transmission-Based Precautions should be used. Transmission-Based Precautions depend on whether the infectious disease is spread via the airborne route, physical contact, or respiratory droplets. The hallmark of Standard Precautions is use of personal protective equipment, which includes gloves, gowns, and mouth, nose, and eye protection, but they also include proper hand hygiene and care with other potentially infectious materials like laundry.

134. B: The preferred disposal method is to put the sharp directly into a sharps container after use. Sharps and other biohazard containers have an orange or red-orange biohazard sticker. The scoop technique is a way to recap the needle for transport only if the sharps container is not nearby. Sharps and other forms of infectious waste are later burned or sterilized before disposal, usually by a company specializing in this disposal.

135. C: In the event that an employee is accidentally exposed to blood or other potentially infectious materials, they should be tested for HBV, HCV, and HIF (assuming they consent to the test) and offered prophylaxis if a test is positive. The employer must offer the employee a confidential medical evaluation, but the employee has the right to refuse this as well. The incident must be immediately reported to a superior and documented. Additional requirements include testing of the source blood if the patient consents, counseling of the employee, and submission of an OSHA 301 form.

136. C: The preferred method of hand-washing is the procedure in responses A or B. The procedure in response D is acceptable, but the use of antibacterial wipes is not.

Copyright © Mometrix Media. You have been licensed one copy of this document for personal use only. Any other reproduction or redistribution is strictly prohibited. All rights reserved. This content is provided for test preparation purposes only and does not imply an endorsement by Mometrix of any particular political, scientific, or religious point of view.

137. B: The use of chemical germicidal agents on surfaces by wiping or soaking is known as disinfection; it destroys most pathogens, but not spores. Sanitization is the use of techniques such as enzymatic detergents and ultrasonic cleaners to reduce microbial load on instruments and equipment. Sterilization is the use of techniques such as steam sterilization to kill all microbes, including spores. Antisepsis is the use of topical chemicals on the skin to kill or inhibit microbes.

138. A: The sequence recommended by the CDC for PPE removal is gown and gloves (together), then goggles, then mask, and finally washing the hands. This process is optimal for ensuring the prevention of exposure to pathogens. If taking off gown and gloves separately, gloves should be removed before the gown. After each type of PPE is removed, it should be disposed of in a biohazard container.

139. B: In order to maintain sterility, both hands should be held in front of the body, at a distance from the body, and above waist level.

140. D: Surgical hand cleansing extends further to the elbows while medical hand cleansing is focused on the hands. Surgical hand washing takes longer and hands are held up during rinsing. Hands are held down during medical hand cleansing, and lotion can be applied after. Additional differences include that alcohol-based products can be substituted for medical washing but are only used after other steps in surgical washing, and that gloves are always applied after surgical hand cleansing.

141. C: Heat-sensitive items, such as fiber-optic endoscopes, as well as certain items that will not fit in an autoclave for steam sterilization should be sterilized using chemical or so-called "cold" sterilization. In this process, the object is immersed in a chemical solution that can kill certain microorganisms and then rinsed with sterile water. The other methods are either at too high a temperature or impractical.

142. B: Response B describes the parameters that must be achieved for steam sterilization of wrapped instrument packages or trays. Response C applies if sterilizing unwrapped items (20 minutes for unwrapped objects covered with cloth). After the autoclave cycle is done, the door can be opened slightly when the temperature goes down to 212 °F, but the pressure at that point should be zero.

143. D: Use of biological indicators that are later cultured are recommended for quality control for autoclaves. These indicators contain heat-resistant bacterial spores, such as those from the thermophile Bacillus stearothermophilus, not a generic type of bacteria. Sterilization tapes, which contain a thermolabile dye that gets darker upon sterilization, do indicate that the proper parameters have been achieved but not whether spores have been killed. Autoclave tape should be placed on packages to be autoclaved; they develop stripes which indicate that a high temperature has been achieved.

144. C: Cryosurgery destroys tissues, namely things like superficial lesions, by freezing them. Usually, liquid nitrogen is used because it gets very cold, making it quite destructive. Nitrous oxide can also be utilized for most applications, except things like removal of cancerous lesions that require complete destruction. Silver nitrate and sodium hydroxide are commonly used for cautery of broken blood vessels in nosebleeds and destruction of toenail growth plates after removal of toenails, respectively.

145. B: The smallest suture material available is gauge 6-0, and it is commonly used in ambulatory settings. Gauge 0 is larger, and gauge 4 is the largest. Swaged is a term referring to suture materials that come pre-attached to a needle.

Copyright © Mometrix Media. You have been licensed one copy of this document for personal use only. Any other reproduction or redistribution is strictly prohibited. All rights reserved.
This content is provided for test preparation purposes only and does not imply an endorsement by Mometrix of any particular political, scientific, or religious point of view.

146. C: The feature described is a ratchet. Serrations are generally at the other end of the instrument and are a series of narrow slits that secure gripping without tearing the tissue; they are found on instruments like hemostats or loops. On the other hand, teeth are sharp and puncture the tissue.

147. A: Mayo dissecting scissors have beveled edges instead of some combination of blunt and/or sharp edges, characteristic of standard operating scissors. The other types of cutting instruments described are scalpels, suture or stitch removal scissors, and iris scissors.

148. B: All hemostatic forceps or hemostats, which are utilized to grasp and clamp blood vessels, have ratchets and serrations. Most, but not all, are straight, and some have teeth in addition to serrations. Response C describes several types of forceps, used for ear and nose procedures, and response D characterizes the Allis tissue forceps.

149. D: Response D is a description of sounds, which are a type of probe. Otherwise scopes have all of the characteristics listed in responses A, B, and C. Examples of scopes are otoscopes (used in the ear), proctoscopes, anoscopes, and sigmoidoscopes (used to look at the rectum, anus, and sigmoid part of the large intestine). Other types of instruments used for dilating or probing include specula, retractors, and dilators.

150. C: Of the choices, the only thing that should not be done is to mix instruments composed of different types of metals. The processing time varies depending on the instrument, but is usually at least five minutes.

151. B: The topical antibacterial cream used for burns and other abrasion wounds is silver sulfadiazine. The other choices are skin antiseptics: povidone-iodine, which can be used as a surgical scrub; chlorhexidine; and hydrogen peroxide.

152. C: Figure-eight turns, which alternate crossing on either side of the joint, should be used. Spiral turns are circular turns that overlap when going up a body part. Reverse spiral turns are turns that reverse or twist each turn on a limb that gets increasing larger. Circular turns are turns that wrap around the body part several times. All bandages are non-sterile. They may be used over a sterile dressing to anchor it, or as support.

153. A: The property of epinephrine that makes it a frequent addition to injectable anesthetics is that is a vasoconstrictor. When restricted blood flow to the area of surgery is desired, epinephrine is a good additive.

154. B: Response B describes the type of open wound known as an avulsion. A laceration is unintentional tearing of body tissue by a sharp object. A puncture is a small hole or wound caused by a pointed object. An incision is an intentional cut made during surgery with a scalpel.

155. D: This is the correct use of gloves for changing a surgical dressing, as well as for removal and wound irrigation prior to putting on a new dressing.

156. B: Fevers in which there are significant fluctuations in body temperature are either intermittent, as described here, or remittent, in which the temperature never returns to baseline. A continuous fever is one in which the body temperature stays above baseline pretty consistently. Febrile is the general term for any presence of fever, a body temperature elevated above the normal range, which for an adult is an average of 98.6 degrees Fahrenheit.

Copyright © Mometrix Media. You have been licensed one copy of this document for personal use only. Any other reproduction or redistribution is strictly prohibited. All rights reserved. This content is provided for test preparation purposes only and does not imply an endorsement by Mometrix of any particular political, scientific, or religious point of view.

157. D: Response D is the primary way in which a TA thermometer probe is used, although the probe can be used behind the earlobe if there is a great deal of perspiration on the forehead. Probe insertion into the ear is used with tympanic thermometers, which measure the aural temperature. Probe attachment to an electronic thermometer and insertion orally or rectally is commonly used today but employs a different type of thermometer.

158. B: This is the correct method for changing a temperature from Celsius to Fahrenheit. The correct formula for the opposite is expressed in response D.

159. C: During emergency situations, the pulse site used is normally the carotid pulse, which is located on either side of the front of the neck, between the larynx and sternocleidomastoid muscle. In other situations, the radial pulse above the base of the thumb on the wrist and the brachial pulse in the antecubital space on the inner side of the elbow, are commonly used sites. The apical pulse is located at the apex of the heart, can only be found using a stethoscope, and is typically used only in cardiac patients or infants. Other pulse sites include the temporal, femoral, popliteal, and dorsalis pedis artery sites.

160. A: A pulse rate of 70 beats per minute is considered a normal pulse rate for an adult (range 60-80 beats per minute). However, in infants and children this would be considered too low, because average normal pulse rates steadily decline from birth through infancy and childhood. The other choices are abnormalities. Bradycardia is a pulse rate of less than 60 beats per minute. Tachycardia is a pulse rate of more than 100 beats per minute. Arrhythmia is any abnormal electrical activity in the heart, resulting in alteration of the interval between pulsations.

161. B: Orthopnea, or labored breathing, is difficulty breathing unless standing or sitting erect; it occurs in conditions like angina pectoris, heart failure, and various pulmonary conditions. The other situations do involve a period of complete absence of breathing known as apnea. Sleep apnea is characterized by periods of more than 10 seconds in which breathing stops during sleep, depleting the brain of oxygen and potentially causing a variety of cardiac and neurologic defects. Cheyne-Stokes respiration is a respiration cycle in which there is approximately 10-60 seconds of apnea, then deep and rapid breathing, and then a decreased rate.

162. C: This is a description of rales, which is indicative of secretions in the lung passageways. Stridor and wheezing are similar in that they are high-pitched sounds caused by some type of airway obstruction; stridor sounds more like crowing, while wheezing sounds more like whistling. Stertorous respiration is labored breathing, similar to snoring, usually due to some upper respiratory obstruction.

163. D: Blood pressure is a function of how strong the heart muscle is and the elasticity of the arteries, as well as blood volume and blood viscosity. The size of the lumen of the arteries is directly related to their peripheral resistance, which also impacts blood pressure. Ejection fraction represents the volume of blood that is released from the heart with every contraction, but does not directly affect blood pressure.

164. B: The only statement that distinguishes an electronic sphygmomanometer is that it does not necessitate simultaneous use of a stethoscope because there is a digital readout. There are three types of manometers, all of which use a pressure cuff: electronic, aneroid, and the traditional mercury type, which is being phased out. Response C is true of the aneroid type, which uses a dial attached to the rubber bladder pressure cuff.

165. A: There are five phases generally observed during deflation of the pressure cuff when taking blood pressure readings. The systolic pressure is the highest pressure, representing the force

Copyright © Mometrix Media. You have been licensed one copy of this document for personal use only. Any other reproduction or redistribution is strictly prohibited. All rights reserved. This content is provided for test preparation purposes only and does not imply an endorsement by Mometrix of any particular political, scientific, or religious point of view.

exerted on arterial walls during cardiac contraction, and it is heard as the first Korotkoff sound. In subsequent phases, more blood passes through the blood vessels. Generally, the sounds heard include swishing, then rhythmic tapping, and lastly muffled tapping sounds. Sometimes there is an auscultatory gap sometime after phase I, in which no sounds are heard; but they later reappear. The diastolic pressure, which represents the force during cardiac relaxation, is taken when all sounds cease in phase V. In children, diastolic pressure may be recorded in the previous phase IV, as some tapping may be heard down to pressure zero.

166. B: A blood pressure measurement in itself is written as "systolic pressure/diastolic pressure" (for example: 110/75), but it is preferable to also note the arm used and the patient position (for example: right arm, supine).

167. B: An adult with this blood pressure (BP) reading is considered to have prehypertension, which can lead to hypertension if not controlled. Normal blood pressure for an adult is a systolic pressure less than 120 and a diastolic pressure less than 80. Any BP above 140/90 is considered hypertension. Secondary hypertension is high blood pressure due to some underlying cause, such as atherosclerosis. If atherosclerosis is treated, the BP can return to normal or close to normal.

168. D: Once the scale has been balanced, the medical assistant needs to add the number from the upper bar to that of the lower bar. This gives the patient's weight in pounds. If you need the patient's weight in kilograms, divide the number of pounds by 2.2 to convert pounds to kilograms.

169. C: This examination is auscultation. Palpation is the use of touch to feel for things like body parts, masses, and skin texture. Percussion is tapping with the fingers or a percussion hammer to listen for characteristic dull or hollow sounds. Mensuration is taking measurements such as height, weight, circumference of a body part, etc. Other examination methods are observation of things like symmetry, posture, etc., and manipulation to check for range of motion.

170. B: Patients with cardiovascular or respiratory problems should be positioned in either the semi-Fowler's or high-Fowler's positions, which are at 45- and 90-degree angles sitting up, respectively, to help them breathe. The dorsal recumbent or lithotomy position has patients lie on their back with their knees flexed and their feet either on the table or in attached stirrups. This position is used for genital and pelvic examinations, urinary catheterization, and other examinations. The Trendelenburg position has patients lie supine on their back with their feet elevated. This position is used to increase blood flow to the brain in emergencies and during abdominal or pelvic surgery. The Sims' position has patients lie laterally on their left side. This position is used for situations like vaginal and rectal exams, sigmoidoscopy, etc.

171. C: The provider can check for dental hygiene, swollen tonsils and uvula, and gag reflex using a tongue depressor and light source during the mouth and throat examination. Dental hygiene issues of note include caries and pus discharge at the gums, indicating infection. Swollen tonsils and uvula may also indicate infection. The gag reflex, a reflection of cranial nerves IX and X, should occur when the soft palate is touched; absence of the gag reflex could indicate neurologic issues. Cranial nerve XI is tested by asking the patient to shrug their shoulders.

172. B: All of these are a cause for concern, except the presence of bowel sounds if they are within expected levels.

173. C: Depending on the system used, either response A or B could be applied. Gravidity refers to the total number of pregnancies, regardless of outcome. Parity is the number of pregnancies carried to the point of viability, generally considered to be 24 weeks after conception or the attainment of one pound of body weight. Parity is not dependent on whether or not there was a live birth or the

Copyright © Mometrix Media. You have been licensed one copy of this document for personal use only. Any other reproduction or redistribution is strictly prohibited. All rights reserved. This content is provided for test preparation purposes only and does not imply an endorsement by Mometrix of any particular political, scientific, or religious point of view.

number of children born. The FPAL system for parity reflects the number of full-term deliveries (F), pre-term or premature deliveries (P), abortions prior to 20 weeks, and current number of living children (L).

174. A: A urinalysis tests for all of the listed things except VDRL, which is a blood test for syphilis. Urinalysis is done to screen for diabetes, hypertension, infection, renal disease, and pregnancy. A number of other blood tests, smears, or cultures for infectious diseases, immunity, etc., are done as part of a prenatal visit. Glucose is measured in the blood as well, to check for gestational diabetes.

175. B: This is a description of placenta previa. Eclampsia is hypertension, edema, and proteinuria induced by pregnancy, which can endanger the fetus. Placenta abruptio is sudden premature pulling away of the placenta from the uterus, which can cause fetal hypoxia and possibly death as well as maternal shock and possibly death. Incompatibility is a situation in which the mother is Rh-negative and the fetus Rh-positive and the mother develops anti-Rh antibodies to the fetus's red blood cells, which can then be depleted and cause fetal death.

176. C: The only thing listed that must be done by the provider, not the medical assistant, is swabbing of the cervix with an antiseptic and injection of a local anesthetic. The medical assistant should be prepared to assist the patient into the lithotomy position and drape them, to hand the speculum to the provider, and to document the procedure in the patient's chart.

177. A: The only false statement is that the actual breast examination should be done standing up, because it should be performed while supine in order to spread out the breast tissue. Other portions of the examination can be done standing up, such as checking in the mirror and feeling the underarm area for swollen lymph nodes.

178. C: The Bethesda System of classifying Pap tests has three categories. Category 1 is a Pap test negative for intraepithelial, precancerous, or cancerous cells or other abnormalities. Category 2 is presence of epithelial cell abnormalities; it is subdivided into four groups, of which the ones represented here are subgroup 1a (atypical squamous cells of uncertain significance) and subgroup 1c (squamous cell carcinoma). Category 3 is the presence of other malignancies such as melanoma. CIN 3 would be correct under the other classification system, which grades the amount of cervical intraepithelial neoplasia into three types of increasing dysplasia (CIN 1, CIN 2, and CIN 3).

179. B: These procedures are used to ascertain the cause of female vaginitis or male urethritis. The medical assistant often assists by mixing the discharge sample in saline and putting it on the microscope slide (wet prep/wet mount), and later adding potassium hydroxide (KOH) and preparing another slide. These are used by the provider to identify yeast, bacteria, and trichomonas, and later for fungi with KOH addition. The other choices are diagnosed using the Amplified DNA Probe Test, laparoscopy or ultrasound, and cervical punch or cervical cone biopsies.

180. B: Subcutaneous epinephrine as described is always administered until the Emergency Medical Services (EMS) arrive or symptoms subside. Diphenhydramine may also be necessary if the child is experiencing anaphylaxis, and CPR may be needed in such a case to maintain the airways.

181. C: The deltoid muscle is the preferred intramuscular site for all ages, except infants younger than 12 months, who should be vaccinated in the anterolateral aspect of the thigh or, if necessary, the gluteal muscle. The triceps muscle, which is lower along the arm, is the preferred site for subcutaneous injections. Intramuscular injections are done at a 90-degree angle to the skin, while subcutaneous ones are done at a 45-degree angle.

Copyright © Mometrix Media. You have been licensed one copy of this document for personal use only. Any other reproduction or redistribution is strictly prohibited. All rights reserved.
This content is provided for test preparation purposes only and does not imply an endorsement by Mometrix of any particular political, scientific, or religious point of view.

182. B: Growth charts up to age 36 months generally are separated according to sex and have a series of curves for both length and weight versus age in months. Typically, these measurements are recorded in one corner along with the date, age, and head (not chest) circumference. The head-circumference-for-age curves are usually on a chart that also shows percentiles for weight-for-length.

183. C: The preferred site to take a pulse rate in pediatric patients five years or younger is the apical pulse.

184. A: Prostatic ultrasound, biopsy, and prostate-specific antigen (PSA) are all used in conjunction to provide a diagnosis of prostate cancer.

185. A: All of these apply to doing a urinary catheterization on a female patient except for choice A. While the provider should use sterile gloves, only the dominant hand retains sterility throughout, because once the provider starts wiping the genitalia, the other hand becomes contaminated.

186. B: The developer in a fecal occult blood test contains guaiac, which, when combined with blood, will turn a blue color seen at the periphery within 30-60 seconds. The positive, but not the negative control, should also show this blue halo to constitute a valid test.

187. D: All of the choices are pulmonary function tests (also known as spirometry) used to assess respiration, but the PEFR is particularly useful for determining the extent of asthma or another disorder because it is depressed during an attack.

188. A: The only statement that is not universally applicable to an ESR is response A. This statement is true for all male patients and women under 50, but the normal range for women over 50 is 0-30 mm/hour. The ESR is a relatively simple test in which blood is put in a tube in an upright rack and allowed to settle, separating the plasma on top from the settled blood and red blood cells (RBCs) on the bottom; many disease states cause RBC and fibrinogen alterations that result in greater settling. There are two methods, the Wintrobe and Westergren.

189. C: The only correct way to lift a patient who cannot walk or lift themselves is by gripping their gait belt from underneath and then lifting. Injuries to the provider or the patient can result from using any of the other listed methods.

190. B: In all of these types of gaits, except the three-point gait, there is some point at which the patient is bearing weight on both legs.

191. C: This type of ROM exercise is abduction. The opposite, in which motion is toward the midline, is called adduction. Flexion is the bending of a body part, and rotation is the turning of a body part around its central axis. Other types of ROM include extension, pronation, eversion, etc. Every joint has a certain amount of ROM or amount of movement possible, and is measured in degrees using a device called a goniometer.

192. D: All of the procedures listed are part of CPR as currently recommended.

193. B: There are five schedules of drugs under the Controlled Substance Act. Schedule I applies to drugs of abuse that are not available medicinally, such as heroin. Schedule II drugs have abuse potential, but they have accepted medical uses; for example, cocaine. These drugs might be used medically, but they require the DEA form along with a non-renewable prescription. Schedules III through V drugs have decreasing potential for abuse and can be ordered via prescription.

Copyright © Mometrix Media. You have been licensed one copy of this document for personal use only. Any other reproduction or redistribution is strictly prohibited. All rights reserved. This content is provided for test preparation purposes only and does not imply an endorsement by Mometrix of any particular political, scientific, or religious point of view.

194. A: Nitroglycerin, a vasodilator, is used to treat an attack of angina pectoris or chest pain due to chronic heart disease. Atropine is used to increase heart rate. Digoxin is used in congestive heart failure or arrhythmias. Isoproterenol is used to treat heart blocks. Other types of drugs should also be available, such as albuterol (bronchodilator), epinephrine (vasoconstrictor for anaphylactic shock), prochlorperazine (an antiemetic), etc.

195. B: The correct method is response B, not the other way around, as expressed in response C. Do not convert to mg because this type of drug is a liquid and units will probably not be related to mg, a measurement of mass or weight. Multiplication by 16 is related to dose calculation in that after calculating the number of mL to administer, this can be converted to a measurement called minims; there are approximately 16 minims in a mL.

196. A: Of the choices for ECG leads given, response A describes the bipolar or standard limb leads, response B describes the augmented leads, and response D describes the chest or precordial leads.

197. C: All of the listed irregularities are types of arrhythmias. This pattern is seen in ventricular tachycardia, which is a very fast heart rate originating in the ventricles. Both ventricular tachycardia and ventricular fibrillation, which looks like an irregular up-and-down pattern on ECG, can indicate myocardial infarction and life-threatening situations. Atrial fibrillation can be associated with conditions like mitral valve prolapse, and is indicated on ECG by irregularly spaced patterns without distinguishable P waves. Paroxysmal atrial tachycardia is a sudden pattern of more rapid beating that lasts briefly; it can be seen in cardiac patients but often occurs in healthy people.

198. C: All chemical labels have composite National Fire Protection Association ratings on them in the form of four diamonds of different colors, with numbers from 0-4 on three of these diamonds indicating an increasing seriousness of the hazard. The blue diamond rates the health hazard, and "3" in that diamond means the chemical is a corrosive or toxic health hazard. Flammability is rated in the red diamond; a "3" would mean that it is a flammable liquid. Reactivity or instability is rated in the yellow diamond; a "3" would mean that it is potentially explosive near a spark or if heated. The fourth diamond is white; any symbol there would give information on a special hazard (such as W for water reactive) or appropriate protective equipment.

199. B: Response B is the approved basic metabolic panel of laboratory tests, while C is the approved comprehensive metabolic panel. Response A is the electrolyte panel, while response D is the hepatic function panel. There is often overlap between panels.

200. A: In order to collect a serum sample, the provider must use a tube that promotes clot formation, such as a red top, which contains no additives, or a red-gray mottled top, which contains a clot activator and serum separating tube. All of the other listed choices contain additives that prevent clot formation at some step in the cascade to give either plasma or whole blood.

Copyright © Mometrix Media. You have been licensed one copy of this document for personal use only. Any other reproduction or redistribution is strictly prohibited. All rights reserved.
This content is provided for test preparation purposes only and does not imply an endorsement by Mometrix of any particular political, scientific, or religious point of view.

Medical Assistant Practice Test #2

1. What does the term *edema* mean?

    a. Rash
    b. Within
    c. Vomiting
    d. Swelling

2. What is the appropriate way to take a radial pulse?

    a. Place your index finger and middle finger on the wrist, under the pinky finger
    b. Place your index finger and middle finger on the wrist, under the thumb
    c. Place your thumb on the side of the neck, next to the trachea
    d. Place your index finger on the inner portion of the cubital fossa (anterior aspect of the elbow)

3. A patient is anxious and begins hyperventilating. His hands and lips start to feel numb and tingly, and he feels lightheaded. What is the physiological cause of his symptoms?

    a. Excess carbon dioxide in the blood
    b. Excess oxygen in the blood
    c. Lack of carbon dioxide in the blood
    d. Lack of oxygen in the blood

4. Which of the following is NOT one of the five stages of grief as described by the Kübler-Ross model?

    a. Delusions
    b. Anger
    c. Denial
    d. Bargaining

5. Which of the following is tracked on a standard growth chart for patients ages 2 to 20?

    a. Age, weight, BMI
    b. Age, head circumference, height
    c. Age, height, and weight
    d. Age, head circumference, weight, height

6. A patient is upset and angry after an appointment. She is distraught and unable to pay attention when you tell her what dates are available for her follow-up appointment. This results in some confusion, and the patient accuses you of not listening. What form of defense mechanism is this patient likely demonstrating?

    a. Displacement
    b. Projection
    c. Reaction formation
    d. Denial

Copyright © Mometrix Media. You have been licensed one copy of this document for personal use only. Any other reproduction or redistribution is strictly prohibited. All rights reserved.
This content is provided for test preparation purposes only and does not imply an endorsement by Mometrix of any particular political, scientific, or religious point of view.

7. You are asked to give a three-year-old child a dose of acetaminophen (Tylenol). The child weighs 15 kg. The medication order says to give the child a dose of 15 mg/kg. The oral solution concentration is 160 mg/5 mL. What dose of the oral solution should you give the child?

a. 9 mL
b. 5 mL
c. 2 mL
d. 7 mL

8. You have finished all of your assigned tasks and are thinking of leaving a few minutes early for your lunch break when the doctor approaches you and tells you that there are patients waiting to be seen, but the exam rooms have not yet been cleaned after the last patients. You know that this is the responsibility of another medical assistant in the office, but she is on the phone dealing with an important personal problem. What should you do?

a. Explain to the doctor that cleaning the patient exam rooms isn't your assignment today, and tell the doctor where to find the appropriate medical assistant
b. Reassure the doctor that you will take care of the problem, and then quickly clean the rooms yourself
c. Wait until the other medical assistant is off the phone, and then tell her that the rooms need to be cleaned quickly
d. Ask someone else in the office to clean the patient exam rooms

9. How should you position yourself in an exam room with a patient who seems angry and potentially aggressive?

a. Position yourself between the patient and the door
b. Position yourself with a desk between you and the patient
c. Position yourself seated next to the patient
d. Position yourself as far as possible away from the patient

10. Which of the following statements about electrocardiogram (ECG) chest lead placement is TRUE?

a. V1 and V2 give information about the left side of the heart.
b. V3 and V4 give information about the interventricular septum.
c. V5 and V6 give information about the right side of the heart.
d. All of these are true.

11. You witness a patient suddenly collapse in the office. You run to the patient and realize she is unconscious, does not have a pulse, and is not breathing. While someone else calls 911, you and your coworkers begin cardiopulmonary resuscitation (CPR). At what point should you use an automated external defibrillator (AED)?

a. After one round or two minutes of CPR have been performed
b. As soon as emergency medical help arrives
c. If the patient still has no pulse after five minutes of CPR
d. As soon as possible

Copyright © Mometrix Media. You have been licensed one copy of this document for personal use only. Any other reproduction or redistribution is strictly prohibited. All rights reserved. This content is provided for test preparation purposes only and does not imply an endorsement by Mometrix of any particular political, scientific, or religious point of view.

12. What is the definition of active listening?

    a. Taking careful notes while listening to the patient in order to record important data

    b. Listening for certain key terms that will help you to quickly identify the main points that the patient is making

    c. Listening to the patient and then responding by using paraphrasing to demonstrate understanding

    d. Making use of the time during which the patient is talking to formulate your next question

13. Which of the following would be appropriate to leave in a phone message for a patient?

    a. "I am calling to let you know that your test results are positive."

    b. "I am calling for Mr. Smith from the office of Dr. Brown."

    c. "I am calling to let you know that your prescription for amoxicillin has been called into your pharmacy."

    d. "I am calling for Mr. Smith about his recent visit to Dr. Brown about his cough."

14. Which of the following is NOT a requirement to be certified as a medical assistant?

    a. Completion of an accredited medical assisting program

    b. Passing the certification examination

    c. Recertification of credentials every 60 months

    d. Work at least 10 hours per week to maintain certification

15. Which of the following would NOT be included in a living will?

    a. Whether a patient would like cardiopulmonary resuscitation (CPR) if cardiac arrest occurs

    b. If a patient would like to be kept alive with life-prolonging equipment

    c. If a patient does not want to have tube feeding

    d. How a person's assets should be distributed

16. Which of the following is considered to be one of the best overall ways to prevent the spread of infection?

    a. Always wearing gloves

    b. Thorough hand washing

    c. Wearing a respiratory mask

    d. Wearing a protective gown

17. A patient requests that you send her health records to a new physician that she is seeing. Which of the following measures should you take to follow medical privacy guidelines?

    a. Call the other physician's office to make sure they are actually seeing the patient.

    b. Ask the physician you are working with to sign a form giving permission for you to send the records to the new physician.

    c. Have the patient sign a form agreeing to the release of the medical records to the new physician.

    d. Counsel the patient that it would be safer to not have her records sent to the new physician.

Copyright © Mometrix Media. You have been licensed one copy of this document for personal use only. Any other reproduction or redistribution is strictly prohibited. All rights reserved.
This content is provided for test preparation purposes only and does not imply an endorsement by Mometrix of any particular political, scientific, or religious point of view.

18. You are working as a medical assistant for a large group of physicians. The office is located in an ethnically diverse area, and a significant portion of the patient population does not speak English. You are asked to take the vital signs and initial history of a patient who only speaks a language that you do not know. Which of the following is the best action to take?

    a.   Use the patient's nine-year-old son, who does speak English, as a translator.
    b.   Use hand gestures in order to communicate with the patient.
    c.   Use a translator phone service in order to communicate with the patient.
    d.   Use an online translator to write the patient a note explaining that they need to come back with someone who speaks English.

19. Which of the following is NOT a correct way to handle biohazardous waste?

    a.   Dispose of sharps such as glass or needles in a sharps container.
    b.   Place biohazardous materials in white plastic trash bags.
    c.   Sanitize biohazard waste containers if they become soiled.
    d.   Make sure that biohazard waste containers are all labeled with the international biohazard symbol.

20. What should you do if you become aware that a colleague is working while intoxicated?

    a.   Approach the colleague and warn them not to do it again.
    b.   Report the situation to your supervisor.
    c.   Make sure the colleague enters an appropriate treatment program.
    d.   Tell your other coworkers so you can work as a group to ensure that the colleague is able to perform his or her job sufficiently.

21. When food is traveling through the gastrointestinal system, what part of the small intestine does it enter immediately after leaving the stomach?

    a.   Jejunum
    b.   Duodenum
    c.   Ileum
    d.   Rectum

22. A six-month-old baby in the waiting room suddenly begins to choke on a small toy. The baby's mother yells for help. You run into the room to assist and see that the baby is still conscious, but she is unable to cough or make crying noises. What steps should you take to try to relieve the obstruction?

    a.   Lay the infant on the ground and give quick, consecutive thrusts on the middle of the breastbone with two fingers. After every 30 compressions, try to visualize the object that is blocking the airway.
    b.   Open the baby's mouth and sweep your finger into the back of her throat to try to dislodge the obstructing object.
    c.   Lay the infant face-down along your arm, cradling her jaw in your fingers. Using the palm of your other hand, give the baby five quick, firm blows on the back between the shoulder blades. Then, turn the infant face-up and give five quick thrusts on the middle of the breastbone with two fingers.
    d.   Hold the infant on your lap, facing away from you. Use your fist to forcefully press inward and upward just under the breastbone.

Copyright © Mometrix Media. You have been licensed one copy of this document for personal use only. Any other reproduction or redistribution is strictly prohibited. All rights reserved.
This content is provided for test preparation purposes only and does not imply an endorsement by Mometrix of any particular political, scientific, or religious point of view.

23. A patient comes into the clinic complaining of weight loss, anxiety, sweating, and diarrhea. She is diagnosed with hyperthyroidism. The thyroid gland is part of what body system?

    a. Nervous system
    b. Musculoskeletal system
    c. Digestive system
    d. Endocrine system

24. If you are asked to give the patient a referral to a cardiac specialist, what should you do?

    a. Give the patient the name and contact information of a cardiac specialist who will see him for his problem.
    b. Tell the patient to look up which cardiologists are on his insurance plan and to make an appointment with one of them as soon as possible.
    c. Send the patient's chart to a cardiologist to see if the doctor would be interested in seeing the patient.
    d. Have the patient go to the closest hospital immediately and ask to be seen by a cardiologist.

25. A patient has just been started on warfarin, and you are asked to give her further instructions on dietary guidelines that she needs to be aware of while on this medication. Which of the following is an important dietary guideline to instruct the patient about?

    a. Maintain a consistent diet
    b. Avoid eating green, leafy vegetables
    c. Avoid drinking grapefruit juice
    d. Eat double the recommended daily dose of fiber

26. Which of the following is obesity LEAST likely to play a role in?

    a. Osteoporosis
    b. Gallstones
    c. Osteoarthritis
    d. Type II diabetes

27. Which of the following locations will yield the most accurate results when taking an infant's temperature?

    a. Mouth
    b. Armpit
    c. Rectum
    d. Ear

28. What does third-party medical billing refer to?

    a. When a physician sends a bill to an insurance company
    b. When an insurance company contracts with another company to process payments
    c. When a patient has two separate forms of health insurance
    d. When a patient's insurance company handles a claim

29. If a patient is lying on their back, they are in a _____ position.

    a. Prone
    b. Prostrate
    c. Dorsal
    d. Supine

Copyright © Mometrix Media. You have been licensed one copy of this document for personal use only. Any other reproduction or redistribution is strictly prohibited. All rights reserved.
This content is provided for test preparation purposes only and does not imply an endorsement by Mometrix of any particular political, scientific, or religious point of view.

30. You are assisting a physician as he sutures a patient wound, and you inadvertently receive a needle stick. The needle had already been used on the patient, and it is therefore potentially contaminated. What action should be taken immediately?

   a. Irrigate the puncture wound.
   b. Get a tetanus shot.
   c. Call risk management.
   d. Begin HIV prophylaxis.

31. Which of the following is a federal guideline for protecting health information?

   a. HIPAA
   b. FMLA
   c. CSA
   d. HHS

32. What is the proper way to position a blood pressure cuff?

   a. Wrap the cuff loosely around the upper part of the forearm, about an inch below the elbow.
   b. Wrap the cuff snugly around the upper arm, as close to the shoulder as possible.
   c. Wrap the cuff around the elbow, just tight enough to keep it in place.
   d. Wrap the cuff snugly around the upper arm, about half an inch above the elbow.

33. Which of the following is an important and possibly life-threatening side effect of clopidogrel (Plavix)?

   a. Seizures
   b. Heart attack
   c. Bleeding
   d. Hypertension

34. Which of the following describes the correct sizing of crutches for a patient?

   a. The top of the crutches should be six inches below the armpits when the patient is standing up straight, and the handgrips should be at the level of the hips.
   b. The top of the crutches should be two inches below the armpits when the patient is standing up straight, and the handgrips should be at the level of the waist.
   c. The top of the crutches should be one inch below the armpits when the patient is standing up straight, and the handgrips should be even with the top of the hips.
   d. The top of the crutches should be four inches below the armpits when the patient is standing up straight. The handgrips can be positioned wherever the patient would like them.

35. What information should be recorded on all patient visit notes?

   a. Time and date
   b. Patient signature
   c. Patient Social Security number
   d. Physician's provider number

36. What does the prefix *dys-* mean?

   a. Discharge
   b. Around
   c. Difficult
   d. After

Copyright © Mometrix Media. You have been licensed one copy of this document for personal use only. Any other reproduction or redistribution is strictly prohibited. All rights reserved.
This content is provided for test preparation purposes only and does not imply an endorsement by Mometrix of any particular political, scientific, or religious point of view.

37. You are asked to collect a throat swab from a patient suspected of having strep throat. How should you carry out this procedure?

    a. Have the patient open his mouth just enough to fit the swab in, then move the swab back and forth until you hit the back of the throat.

    b. Depress the tongue, visualize the back of the throat, then swab the back of the throat and tonsils from side to side.

    c. Clearly visualize the back of the throat, and only take a throat swab if there are white patches visible on the tonsils.

    d. Depress the tongue, have the patient open his mouth wide, and then swab the throat, cheeks, and tongue.

38. Which of the following is NOT required to be on the label of a medical specimen?

    a. Date of collection

    b. Time of collection

    c. The patient's full name

    d. Full name and signature of the person collecting the specimen

39. Which of the following is true regarding CDC recommendations for individuals with egg allergies receiving the annual flu vaccine?

    a. Individuals who have experienced angioedema or anaphylaxis as a response to egg should not receive the flu vaccine.

    b. Individuals with a diagnosed egg allergy should not receive the flu vaccine.

    c. Individuals who have experienced hives as a reaction to eggs should receive the flu vaccine as would individuals without an egg allergy.

    d. Individuals with a diagnosed egg allergy can receive the flu vaccine regardless of their allergy severity.

40. If a patient is sitting with his arms crossed and the sides of his mouth slightly turned down while you are giving him instructions about a prescription, what would be an appropriate question to ask him?

    a. What is the problem?

    b. You don't like what I am saying?

    c. Do you want to do this appointment another time?

    d. Is there something that is bothering you?

41. What instructions should NOT be given to a female patient when a clean-catch urine sample is needed?

    a. Use a sterile wipe to clean between the labial folds, wiping from front to back.

    b. Include the initial stream of urine in the sample.

    c. Wash hands with soap and water before collection.

    d. Urinate a small amount into the toilet bowl, then collect the sample using the urine cup.

42. Which of the following would be considered an open-ended question?

    a. What brings you to the office today?

    b. Are you feeling better?

    c. Is your leg pain still bothering you?

    d. Have you been experiencing nausea?

Copyright © Mometrix Media. You have been licensed one copy of this document for personal use only. Any other reproduction or redistribution is strictly prohibited. All rights reserved. This content is provided for test preparation purposes only and does not imply an endorsement by Mometrix of any particular political, scientific, or religious point of view.

43. You are asked to take an elderly patient to get an x-ray of her chest. What should your role be in ensuring the patient's safety during the test?

  a. Make sure the patient is secured on the imaging table to reduce the risk of a fall.
  b. Hold the patient's arm during the x-ray to make sure she remains still.
  c. Check the settings on the x-ray equipment to make sure the radiation dose is correct.
  d. Make sure that the patient receives a dose of medicine for anxiety before the test.

44. What drug class does simvastatin (Zocor) belong to?

  a. Pain-relieving medications
  b. Cholesterol-lowering medications
  c. Hormone-replacement medications
  d. Antihypertensive medication

45. Which of the following is an appropriate site for an intramuscular injection?

  a. Triceps muscle
  b. Ventrogluteal muscle
  c. Quadriceps femoris muscle
  d. Soleus muscle

46. Which of the following classes of controlled substances has no currently accepted medical use in the United States?

  a. Schedule I controlled substances
  b. Schedule II controlled substances
  c. Schedule IV controlled substances
  d. Schedule V controlled substances

47. Which of the following actions does NOT help prevent the contamination of blood samples?

  a. Wiping the shaft of the needle used to draw the blood sample with an alcohol swab
  b. Disinfecting the patient's skin in the area the blood is to be drawn
  c. Washing your hands before drawing the blood sample
  d. Wearing gloves

48. Which of the following is NOT an appropriate step in the process when giving a nebulizer treatment to a patient?

  a. Verify the identity of the patient prior to dispensing any medication
  b. Check the physician's order to ensure that the correct type and dose of medication are being used
  c. Have the patient hold the face mask four to six inches away from his or her mouth
  d. Instruct the patient to take deep breaths of the medicated vapor until the medication has been fully dispensed.

Copyright © Mometrix Media. You have been licensed one copy of this document for personal use only. Any other reproduction or redistribution is strictly prohibited. All rights reserved. This content is provided for test preparation purposes only and does not imply an endorsement by Mometrix of any particular political, scientific, or religious point of view.

49. A patient runs into the office while you are in the reception area alone. He is bleeding severely from a wound to the leg. After calling for help, what should you do immediately to help the patient?

    a. Apply direct and continuous pressure to the wound with a clean cloth or bandage.

    b. Apply a tourniquet three to four inches above the wound and pull it tight until the bleeding stops.

    c. Wash the wound well with sterile water and then apply a secure bandage.

    d. Squeeze the main artery in the groin area to prevent more blood from being delivered to the lower leg.

50. What are standard precautions?

    a. Guidelines about protecting yourself from a potentially aggressive patient

    b. Guidelines about how to set up an office for patient and employee safety

    c. Guidelines about how to prevent patients from suing

    d. Guidelines about protecting yourself from potential infection

51. According to Maslow, the highest level on the hierarchy of needs that people strive to achieve is:

    a. Safety

    b. Love and belonging

    c. Esteem

    d. Self-actualization

52. Psychologist Erik Erikson developed the theory that throughout a person's life, they pass through 8 different psychosocial stages. The stage at which a young child begins to express his independence is:

    a. Stage 1 – trust vs. mistrust

    b. Stage 2 – autonomy vs. shame and doubt

    c. Stage 3 – initiative vs. guilt

    d. Stage 4 – industry vs. inferiority

53. Regarding healthcare decision-making for the Hispanic patient, the medical assistant knows that:

    a. The mother, or oldest female in the family, is likely to be the primary decision maker.

    b. The father, or oldest male in the family, is likely to be the primary decision maker.

    c. Medical decisions are likely to be made as a joint decision by all family members.

    d. Medical decisions are likely to be decided primarily by the patient, regardless of age, with the support of the family.

54. Which of the following is an example of an inappropriate exploratory question?

    a. Why were you unsure about being seen by the doctor for this condition?

    b. How are you feeling today?

    c. What changes have you noticed in your breathing?

    d. Did you realize that you were taking your medication incorrectly?

Copyright © Mometrix Media. You have been licensed one copy of this document for personal use only. Any other reproduction or redistribution is strictly prohibited. All rights reserved.
This content is provided for test preparation purposes only and does not imply an endorsement by Mometrix of any particular political, scientific, or religious point of view.

55. Which of the following is an example of a closed, or direct, question?

    a. What is your date of birth?
    b. What is the worst pain you have ever had?
    c. Why are you feeling depressed?
    d. Why is patient care your favorite part of your job?

56. When communicating with a non-English speaking patient and her family, it is best to:

    a. Have another family member serve as an interpreter, if possible.
    b. Improvise using pictures and video to teach the patient about their medical care.
    c. Hold most of the conversation through an online translating program.
    d. Arrange to have an interpreter familiar with medical terminology present.

57. When teaching a patient who has a hearing impairment, it is important to:

    a. Face him directly so your face and lips are clearly visible.
    b. Give him educational materials in print to take home and read on his own.
    c. Have the patient be the only person receiving educational material so he can feel more involved in their treatment plan.
    d. Discuss the treatment plan with the spouse or family so that they can communicate with the patient in the way that best suits his needs.

58. An effective way for the medical assistant to show that they are actively listening and understand what the speaker has said is through:

    a. Constructive criticism
    b. Asking direct questions
    c. Reflection and restatement
    d. The teach back system

59. An example of an internal distraction to communication is:

    a. Loud music in the room
    b. Pain
    c. People talking next to you
    d. The phone ringing

60. An example of an external distraction to communication is:

    a. Pain
    b. Hunger
    c. Grief
    d. Loud music in the room

61. The main difference between empathy and sympathy is:

    a. Empathy is showing no emotion and sympathy is showing emotion.
    b. Empathy is showing emotion and sympathy is showing no emotion.
    c. Empathy is becoming angry over a situation and sympathy is being happy.
    d. Empathy is placing oneself in someone else's position and sympathy is showing compassion for someone else.

Copyright © Mometrix Media. You have been licensed one copy of this document for personal use only. Any other reproduction or redistribution is strictly prohibited. All rights reserved.
This content is provided for test preparation purposes only and does not imply an endorsement by Mometrix of any particular political, scientific, or religious point of view.

62. A medical assistant works at a busy family practice office and is assigned to the prescription phone line one day. They take a call from a patient who is furious that their blood pressure medication has not yet been called in because they have been out of medication for two days. The patient is interrupting the medical assistant when trying to talk to them, yelling, and demanding the medication be called in right now. The best response is to:

   a. Calmly listen to their complaints and apologize for the delay while expressing that you can understand their frustration.
   b. Calmly explain to the patient that he or she cannot yell or insult the staff and terminate the call.
   c. Tell the patient that they are being unreasonable and remind them that the office policy is to have at least 48 hours to fill medication refills.
   d. Put the patient on hold and ask the office manager to speak with them.

63. The main difference between a power of attorney and a healthcare proxy is:

   a. A power of attorney makes all decisions for the patient when they are unable to, and a healthcare proxy serves as a backup if that person is not available.
   b. A power of attorney gives a facility the power to make decisions for the patient, and a healthcare proxy gives the physician the power to make those decisions.
   c. A power of attorney gives a family member the power to take over finances, and a healthcare proxy assigns someone to ensure they are making good decisions.
   d. A power of attorney makes financial decisions for the patient when they are unable to and a healthcare proxy is a document that assigns someone to make medical decisions for the patient.

64. A medical assistant is due for his annual performance review at work. The supervisor has told him that several staff members have come to her and complained that they do not feel he is keeping up with the work, and they often have to finish responsibilities for him. The best response is for the medical assistant to:

   a. Tell the supervisor that they are making it up because they don't seem to like you very much.
   b. Tell the supervisor that she is not very fair and seems to play favorites with other employees.
   c. Ask your supervisor for specific examples and ensure her that you will try harder to do your share of the work.
   d. Respond calmly, but then confront your co-workers after the meeting to ask why they have tried to get you in trouble.

65. The law that ensures that a patient's decisions regarding life-saving healthcare be communicated and protected is:

   a. HIPAA
   b. The Patient Self-Determination Act
   c. A Do Not Resuscitate order
   d. The Americans with Disabilities Act

Copyright © Mometrix Media. You have been licensed one copy of this document for personal use only. Any other reproduction or redistribution is strictly prohibited. All rights reserved. This content is provided for test preparation purposes only and does not imply an endorsement by Mometrix of any particular political, scientific, or religious point of view.

66. Being an organ donor or wishing to donate one's remains for medical research at the time of death, is governed by:

    a. HIPAA
    b. The Patient Self-Determination Act
    c. The Uniform Anatomical Gift Act
    d. The Joint Commission

67. Which of the following outlines the steps for effective communication?

    a. Feedback, receiver, channel, message, sender
    b. Sender, message, feedback, channel, receiver
    c. Message, feedback, channel, sender, receiver
    d. Sender, message, channel, receiver, feedback

68. The organization that works to ensure employee safety while performing job duties is:

    a. Occupational Safety and Health Administration (OSHA)
    b. The Joint Commission
    c. The Americans with Disabilities Act
    d. The Food and Drug Administration (FDA)

69. The government agency that ensures a generic drug is biologically equivalent to the brand name version of the same medication is:

    a. The Joint Commission
    b. The Clinical Laboratory Improvement Act (CLIA)
    c. The Americans with Disabilities Act
    d. The Food and Drug Administration (FDA)

70. A patient calls the office with concerns that they could be developing a rash from a new medication. When writing down the message to give to the physician, all of the following information should be included EXCEPT:

    a. The patient's name and date of birth
    b. The phone number where the patient can be reached
    c. The patient's social security number
    d. The medication they are taking and the specific symptoms they are having

71. A medical assistant is working in the lab within a busy medical practice. He is unsure of the procedure to follow when one of the physicians in the office requests a specific lab test be processed at this facility. The level of complexity for the lab, along with specific tests that can be performed at this location, is regulated by:

    a. The Joint Commission
    b. The Clinical Laboratory Improvement Act (CLIA)
    c. OSHA
    d. The FDA

72. In what year did the Americans with Disabilities Act go into effect?

    a. 1989
    b. 1990
    c. 1991
    d. 1992

Copyright © Mometrix Media. You have been licensed one copy of this document for personal use only. Any other reproduction or redistribution is strictly prohibited. All rights reserved. This content is provided for test preparation purposes only and does not imply an endorsement by Mometrix of any particular political, scientific, or religious point of view.

73. A medical assistant answers the phone at the pediatric office where she works. There is a frantic mother on the phone who says her child is having a severe asthma attack and seems to have some blue discoloration around his mouth. What steps should be taken next?

    a. Take all of the vital information necessary and tell the mother someone will call her back.

    b. Tell the mother to hang up and call 911.

    c. Alert a co-worker to call 911 and remain on the phone with the mother until paramedics arrive.

    d. Place the mother on hold and look for one of the pediatricians to take the call.

74. One of the goals of the HITECH Act is to:

    a. Enforce HIPAA regulations

    b. Encourage employee reporting of unlawful acts by their employer

    c. Decrease medication errors

    d. Increase coordination of care

75. The law that was put into place in order for drugs to be categorized based on their potential for abuse is the:

    a. Americans with Disabilities Act

    b. Controlled Substances Act

    c. Uniform Anatomical Gift Act

    d. Patient Self-Determination Act

76. All of the following duties fall under the medical assistant scope of practice EXCEPT:

    a. Interpreting lab results to a patient

    b. Performing CPR in an emergency situation

    c. Performing wound care under the direction of a provider

    d. Taking vital signs

77. The physician that a medical assistant works for has recommended to a patient that she undergo testing to determine whether she carries the BRCA gene, which places her at higher risk for developing breast or ovarian cancer. She is concerned that her health insurance carrier will cancel her policy or raise her rates if they find out the test results. The medical assistant's best response is:

    a. That is a possibility, and she should think about if she wishes to do these tests.

    b. It is illegal for an insurance company to discriminate against someone because of genetic testing.

    c. That test is not very accurate anyway, so she can hold off on having it done if she wishes.

    d. The office is required to disclose the results of the test to her health insurance carrier.

78. In the United States, the public health institute responsible for protecting public health and safety through the control and prevention of disease is:

    a. The Joint Commission

    b. OSHA

    c. The Centers for Disease Control

    d. The World Health Organization

Copyright © Mometrix Media. You have been licensed one copy of this document for personal use only. Any other reproduction or redistribution is strictly prohibited. All rights reserved.
This content is provided for test preparation purposes only and does not imply an endorsement by Mometrix of any particular political, scientific, or religious point of view.

79. The legal statute that prevents patients with outstanding medical bills from being treated unfairly or in a deceptive way in the process of debt collection is:

a. The Fair Debt Collection Practices Act
b. The Federal Trade Commission
c. The World Health Organization
d. The Truth in Lending Act

80. A patient is meeting with the Billing Supervisor at the local hospital to establish a payment plan for debt incurred from a recent Emergency Room visit. The full disclosure of any interest charges and the terms of the repayment plan are mandatory because of:

a. The Fair Debt Collection Practices Act
b. The World Health Organization
c. The Federal Trade Commission
d. The Truth in Lending Act

81. Which of the following diseases is required to be reported to the local Health Department?

a. Influenza type A
b. Gonorrhea
c. Influenza type B
d. Group B Strep in a pregnant woman

82. Of the following, the type of fracture that is very suspicious for child abuse is:

a. An ankle (lateral malleolus) fracture in a 7-year-old
b. A spiral fracture of the humerus in a 10-month-old
c. A spiral fracture of the tibia in a 3-year-old
d. A buckle fracture of the radius in a 5-year-old

83. A 16-year-old girl comes into the Urgent Care requesting STD testing. She does not want her parents to know she is being seen, and she wants to know if this is possible. The most appropriate answer is:

a. She cannot be seen without permission from her parents since she is a minor.
b. Permission for her to be seen can be obtained from another family member if she would be more comfortable with that.
c. Legally, she can be seen for STD testing without obtaining permission from her parents.
d. She is too young to have STD testing performed.

84. The document that explains what a patient should expect during their hospital stay is:

a. The Patient Bill of Rights
b. The Truth in Lending Act
c. The Fair Debt Collection Practices Act
d. The Patient Care Partnership

Copyright © Mometrix Media. You have been licensed one copy of this document for personal use only. Any other reproduction or redistribution is strictly prohibited. All rights reserved.
This content is provided for test preparation purposes only and does not imply an endorsement by Mometrix of any particular political, scientific, or religious point of view.

85. A medical assistant works in a busy family practice office. The physician has ordered an injection of Penicillin for a patient. The medical assistant accidentally gives the patient an injection of Rocephin. Who is the person ultimately responsible for this medication error?

    a. The ordering physician
    b. The medical assistant who gave the wrong medication
    c. The manager of the practice
    d. The patient for not verifying it was the correction medication

86. A patient who has been diagnosed with Lewy body dementia has reached a point at which his wife can no longer care for him at home. She is working on having financial assets placed in her name, but to do so, her attorney has told her that she will need to file the legal documents that say her husband does not have:

    a. The capacity to make financial decisions on his own
    b. The legal right to make financial decisions on his own
    c. The competency to make financial decisions on his own
    d. Children who can manage his finances for him

87. The following information should be included in an informed consent document EXCEPT:

    a. The procedure to be performed
    b. The potential risks or complications with the procedure
    c. Other procedures that could be performed instead
    d. The signatures of the provider, the patient, and a witness

88. The court order requiring someone appear in court and bring any evidence or related documents pertinent to the case with them is:

    a. Quid pro quo
    b. Documentes laborum
    c. Res ipsa loquitor
    d. A subpoena duces tecum

89. The Latin expression that literally translates to mean "let the master answer" is:

    a. Subpoena duces tecum
    b. Respondeat superior
    c. Res ipsa loquitor
    d. Respondeat inferior

90. In a medical practice case, negligence can be inferred by the effect the action had on the patient, rather than having to prove that the physician acted in a negligent manner, under:

    a. Subpoena duces tecum
    b. Res ipsa loquitor
    c. Respondeat superior
    d. Quid pro quo

91. The difference between arbitration and mediation is:

    a. An arbitration involves testimony and evidence, but is less formal than a regular trial, while mediation is a negotiation using a third party who is neutral.
    b. An arbitration is a statement handed by the court while a mediation is written by attorneys.
    c. An arbitration is a negotiation while a mediation involves formal mental health counseling.
    d. An arbitration involves children as witnesses while a mediation involves legal adults only.

Copyright © Mometrix Media. You have been licensed one copy of this document for personal use only. Any other reproduction or redistribution is strictly prohibited. All rights reserved. This content is provided for test preparation purposes only and does not imply an endorsement by Mometrix of any particular political, scientific, or religious point of view.

92. You are eating dinner at a local restaurant. A person at the next table suddenly stands, holds his hands up by his throat, and is in obvious distress. His wife says that he is choking and he is not able to breathe. Because you are trained in the Heimlich maneuver, you perform this on him. After a couple of attempts, you dislodge a piece of meat and he is able to breathe again. After a few minutes, he starts to complain of right rib pain and accuses you of breaking one of his ribs. Which legal statute will protect you against any legal action if he has a rib injury?

    a. Good Samaritan laws
    b. HIPAA
    c. The Patient Care Partnership
    d. The Nursing Practice Act

93. The difference between a misdemeanor and a felony is:

    a. A misdemeanor carries a prison sentence up to 5 years, while a felony carries a longer prison sentence.
    b. A misdemeanor is punishable with a fine, while a felony is punishable with time in prison.
    c. A misdemeanor carries a prison sentence up to 1 year, while a felony carries a longer prison sentence.
    d. A misdemeanor is punishable with community service, while a felony is punishable with time in prison.

94. The physician has asked his medical assistant to create a letter for a particular difficult patient he wishes to discharge from the practice due to multiple missed appointments and excessive rudeness to the staff. All of the following is true regarding a discharge letter EXCEPT:

    a. The letter should be sent certified, return receipt requested.
    b. The letter should state that no further appointments will be scheduled for the patient.
    c. The letter should state that acute medical care will be provided for the next 30 days.
    d. The letter should contain the reason for the discharge from the practice.

95. A patient at the practice was discharged for multiple no-show appointments, non-compliance, and abusive behavior toward the staff. The medical assistant sees on social media that he has been writing terrible things about the office, the staff, and the provider he was seeing, along with posting photos of the provider that he has digitally altered. The legal term for this is:

    a. Slander
    b. Quid pro quo
    c. Respondeat superior
    d. Libel

96. The acronym commonly used to operate a fire extinguisher is:

    a. RACE
    b. FIRE
    c. PASS
    d. PANIC

Copyright © Mometrix Media. You have been licensed one copy of this document for personal use only. Any other reproduction or redistribution is strictly prohibited. All rights reserved.
This content is provided for test preparation purposes only and does not imply an endorsement by Mometrix of any particular political, scientific, or religious point of view.

97. The medical term *osteo-* means:

a. Skin
b. Bone
c. Tissue
d. Muscle

98. The term *arthroscopy* means:

a. To look in a joint
b. Joint replacement
c. Arthritis
d. Infection in a joint

99. The medical specialty of neurology studies:

a. Bone and joint disorders
b. Connective tissue and autoimmune disorders
c. Surgery on the spine and brain
d. Disorders of the nerves or nervous system

100. A program in the work place that helps employees prevent work-related musculoskeletal disorders is:

a. Ergonomics
b. A health savings account
c. A wellness program
d. Health insurance

101. The medical assistant functions as a patient advocate by:

a. Reporting any medication errors that occur involving the patient
b. Following the Clinical Pathway for the patient's diagnosis
c. Not sharing any personal information the patient has shared
d. Protecting the health, safety, and rights of the patient

102. The criteria set forth for utilizing the electronic health record in order to provide coordinated care and improve patient quality and safety is:

a. Meaningful use
b. Health measures
c. Quality management
d. Clinical analytics

103. A medical assistant has an acquaintance who was seen for a UTI. Two days after her appointment, she sends the medical assistant a message via a social media platform requesting the results of her urine culture. The most appropriate response is for the medical assistant to:

a. Reply with the urine culture and susceptibility results but make sure it is sent as a private message that no others can view.
b. Post a public message on her account that, based on the culture results, she was prescribed the appropriate antibiotic, and she should be feeling well soon.
c. Send her a text message on her phone with the urine culture results.
d. Reply to the message that she is not able to share any personal medical information through social media and she would need to contact the office for those results.

Copyright © Mometrix Media. You have been licensed one copy of this document for personal use only. Any other reproduction or redistribution is strictly prohibited. All rights reserved. This content is provided for test preparation purposes only and does not imply an endorsement by Mometrix of any particular political, scientific, or religious point of view.

104. A patient has sent an e-mail to a medical assistant through the patient portal system associated with the electronic health record the office uses. She is describing her current symptoms and asks if it sounds like she could possibly have a urinary tract infection (UTI). The medical assistant's best response is to tell the patient that:

a. Medical conditions cannot be diagnosed through e-mail, and she will need to come in to be evaluated.

b. E-mail through a patient portal system is not secure and should not be used for sending health information.

c. Her symptoms do sound like she could have a UTI, and she should ask the provider to call in an antibiotic for her.

d. She should drink more fluids and e-mail back in a few days if her symptoms do not resolve.

105. A patient in the practice where a medical assistant works was recently hospitalized with pneumonia. The physician would like to know what antibiotic they were prescribed and if there were any medication changes when they were discharged. The document that gives the information he needs, along with the patient's course during hospitalization, is called the:

a. Admission history and physical

b. Fact sheet

c. Consent to treatment

d. Discharge summary

106. The difference between a source-oriented and problem-oriented medical record is:

a. The source-oriented record contains only the patient's subjective information, and a problem-oriented record contains only the physician's information.

b. The source-oriented record contains progress notes based on chronic medical problems, while the problem-oriented record is for acute problems only.

c. The source-oriented record contains progress notes from different healthcare providers, while the problem-oriented record is divided into separate sections of information.

d. The source-oriented record is a computerized record system, while the problem-oriented record is hand-written.

107. The scheduling template that shows dates, times, and specific slots for different activities to be scheduled is called:

a. The office template

b. The appointment matrix

c. The patient portal

d. The scheduling template

108. The medical assistant's physician likes to use his first two appointments following lunch for patients with acute illnesses. These appointment slots are to be filled that day and not before then. Which of the following patients would be appropriate to schedule in one of the acute visit appointment times?

a. A 54-year-old male who is due for his routine follow-up and medication refill

b. An 18-year-old female who needs to have a Pap smear and discuss birth control options

c. A 77-year-old male who needs to schedule a hospital follow-up appointment

d. A 32-year-old female who thinks she may have the flu

Copyright © Mometrix Media. You have been licensed one copy of this document for personal use only. Any other reproduction or redistribution is strictly prohibited. All rights reserved.
This content is provided for test preparation purposes only and does not imply an endorsement by Mometrix of any particular political, scientific, or religious point of view.

109. Accounts payable are:

a. Amounts a company owes for supplies or services purchased on credit
b. Payments received from customers who have purchased goods or services on credit from the company
c. The amount collected daily from patients in co-payment amounts
d. The deductible amount specific to each health insurance plan

110. A time-sensitive filing system to organize documents that require action on a specific date is called:

a. An appointment matrix
b. A face sheet
c. A tickler file
d. A scheduling template

111. Accounts receivable would be:

a. A liability
b. A debt
c. An asset
d. A credit statement

112. When a patient is hospitalized, Medicare calculates the payment the hospital will receive based on the:

a. DRG code
b. ICD-10 code
c. CPT code
d. Itemized billing statement

113. For Medicare reimbursement purposes, the value of a physician visit is calculated in:

a. Dollars
b. RVUs (relative value units)
c. Credits
d. Hours

114. A patient checks in to be seen in the Urgent Care. She has a high deductible insurance plan that requires she pay 100% of services received until the deductible is met. She still has $3,000 out of pocket expense to be met before she has met the deductible. On her card, it says her Urgent Care co-pay is $50. She says she would like to avoid getting a big bill after her visit and prefers to pay the amount up front. What should she pay today?

a. Nothing, just wait for it to go through insurance and then pay the bill
b. The $3,000 left for her to meet her out of pocket deductible
c. The $50 Urgent Care co-pay
d. The standard amount based on the billing code used for her visit today

115. A provider removes a 1 cm skin lesion from a patient. He enters a CPT code for the procedure that covers the removal of a skin lesion 2-3 cm. This is an example of:

a. Upcoding
b. Downcoding
c. Modifying
d. A relative value unit

Copyright © Mometrix Media. You have been licensed one copy of this document for personal use only. Any other reproduction or redistribution is strictly prohibited. All rights reserved. This content is provided for test preparation purposes only and does not imply an endorsement by Mometrix of any particular political, scientific, or religious point of view.

116. The comprehensive list of diseases and their billing codes established by the World Health Organization is:

    a. The ICD-10
    b. The ICD-9.5
    c. The ICD-9
    d. The CPT

117. The coding system used to identify those services not included in the standard list of CPT codes is:

    a. ICD-10
    b. HCPCS
    c. A DRG code
    d. A tickler

118. An example of a third-party payer is:

    a. The patient
    b. The patient's employer
    c. A health insurance company
    d. A worker's compensation coverage company

119. The statement provided to the patient from Medicare that lists the services not covered by the insurance, along with the reason why and what these services will cost, is called:

    a. An Explanation of Benefits
    b. An Advance Beneficiary Notice
    c. A credit statement
    d. An itemized bill

120. Insurance benefits for the military, retirees from the military, and their dependents is provided by:

    a. CHAMPUS
    b. CHAMPVA
    c. Medicare
    d. Tricare

121. Insurance benefits offered to dependents of certain veterans is called:

    a. CHAMPUS
    b. Tricare
    c. CHAMPVA
    d. Medicare

122. A method of reimbursement used by Medicare to provide a fixed reimbursement amount for specific services is:

    a. HIPAA
    b. PPS
    c. The Affordable Care Act
    d. CARF certification

Copyright © Mometrix Media. You have been licensed one copy of this document for personal use only. Any other reproduction or redistribution is strictly prohibited. All rights reserved. This content is provided for test preparation purposes only and does not imply an endorsement by Mometrix of any particular political, scientific, or religious point of view.

123. The medical service that is covered under Medicare Part A is:

    a. Durable medical equipment
    b. Appointments with a primary care provider
    c. Appointments with a specialist
    d. Prescription drug coverage

124. HMOs, PPOs, and Point of Service healthcare plans are all examples of:

    a. Managed care organizations
    b. Medicare
    c. Medicaid
    d. The Affordable Care Act

125. A patient calls the office with a billing question. She spoke with her insurance company about charges for a urinalysis done in the office that should have been covered by her plan. The insurance person agrees and apologizes for the error. What should be done at this point?

    a. Tell the patient she should pay the outstanding balance and seek reimbursement from her insurance carrier.
    b. Tell the patient that the office will wait until the insurance carrier pays for the test.
    c. Resubmit the charges for the urinalysis for the insurance carrier to reimburse.
    d. "Write off" the expense of the test because it will be very difficult to get the insurance carrier to pay for this.

126. A patient has been prescribed a new arthritis medication that requires prior authorization from the insurance carrier. All of the following information will need to be given to the insurance company EXCEPT:

    a. The names of other similar medications the patient has tried for this particular medical problem.
    b. A comprehensive list of all of the medications a patient is taking.
    c. The patient's symptoms that require the problem be treated with this particular medication.
    d. What other conservative (non-medication) treatments has the patient tried for this particular problem.

127. A patient is inquiring how they will know what part of their visit today will be covered by insurance. You explain to them that their insurance company will send them a (n):

    a. Beneficiary notice
    b. RVU statement
    c. Itemized bill
    d. Explanation of benefits (EOB)

128. The anatomical plane that divides the body into left and right sides is the:

    a. Coronal plane
    b. Lateral plane
    c. Sagittal plane
    d. Transverse plane

Copyright © Mometrix Media. You have been licensed one copy of this document for personal use only. Any other reproduction or redistribution is strictly prohibited. All rights reserved. This content is provided for test preparation purposes only and does not imply an endorsement by Mometrix of any particular political, scientific, or religious point of view.

129. The hand is _____ to the elbow.

   a. Distal
   b. Proximal
   c. Anterior
   d. Posterior

130. The thumb is _____ to the index finger.

   a. Distal
   b. Proximal
   c. Lateral
   d. Medial

131. The dorsal body cavity contains the:

   a. Brain and spinal cord
   b. Heart and lungs
   c. Digestive organs and kidneys
   d. Bladder and reproductive organs

132. One of the first signs of a urinary tract infection in an 86-year-old female patient is:

   a. Dysuria
   b. Confusion
   c. Urinary frequency
   d. Polydipsia

133. The neurological disease that causes destruction of the myelin sheaths surrounding the nerves is:

   a. Muscular dystrophy
   b. Multiple sclerosis
   c. Cerebral palsy
   d. Myasthenia gravis

134. The correct order in which blood flows into the heart and then to the lungs is:

   a. Inferior vena cava, superior vena cava, right ventricle, mitral valve, right atrium, pulmonary artery, lungs
   b. Superior vena cava, right atrium, right ventricle, tricuspid valve, pulmonary artery, lungs
   c. Superior and inferior vena cava, right atrium, tricuspid valve, right ventricle, pulmonic valve, pulmonary artery, lungs
   d. Aorta, right atrium, mitral valve, right ventricle, pulmonary artery, lungs

135. Where are most of the blood cells made?

   a. Bone marrow
   b. Lymph nodes
   c. Spleen
   d. Heart

Copyright © Mometrix Media. You have been licensed one copy of this document for personal use only. Any other reproduction or redistribution is strictly prohibited. All rights reserved. This content is provided for test preparation purposes only and does not imply an endorsement by Mometrix of any particular political, scientific, or religious point of view.

136. A patient is in for her regularly scheduled appointment. She has a history of COPD and has a chronic, mucus-producing cough. The medical assistant knows that the type of COPD she probably has is:

a. Emphysema
b. Asthma
c. Chronic bronchitis
d. Reactive airway disease

137. A 5-year-old child has the flu. Her mom is concerned that her 10-year-old will get the flu also, and she would like a prescription for herself and her older child for Tamiflu to take prophylactically. How should you respond to this?

a. This is reasonable and you should ask the pediatrician to write those prescriptions.
b. Routine prophylactic treatment of the flu is not recommended.
c. Under no circumstances are people treated prophylactically for the flu.
d. They would need an antibiotic to prevent getting the flu.

138. A patient recently returned from a vacation in South America. On their way home, they developed very watery diarrhea. The provider is requesting they submit a stool specimen to be tested for a parasitic infection. The patient takes the collection materials home and returns later that day with the specimen. The testing laboratory will pick up the specimen that evening. Until then, the specimen should:

a. Be left at room temperature
b. Be frozen
c. Be transferred to a microscope slide and refrigerated
d. Be refrigerated

139. Which of the following diseases can be transmitted through the airborne route?

a. Influenza
b. Chicken pox
c. Common cold
d. Pneumonia

140. Alcohol-based hand sanitizers are effective at killing all of the following EXCEPT:

a. Influenza
b. Strep throat
c. Norovirus
d. Hepatitis B

141. How does an autoclave sterilize instruments?

a. Bleach
b. Boiling water
c. Hand sanitizer
d. High-pressure steam

142. What should be worn while you are with a patient with contact precautions?

a. A gown and gloves
b. A gown, gloves, and mask
c. A gown, gloves, mask, and shoe covers
d. A self-contained oxygen suit

Copyright © Mometrix Media. You have been licensed one copy of this document for personal use only. Any other reproduction or redistribution is strictly prohibited. All rights reserved. This content is provided for test preparation purposes only and does not imply an endorsement by Mometrix of any particular political, scientific, or religious point of view.

143. A co-worker is adding a cleaning solution to a container full of used instruments when it splashes into her eyes. You would find the safety information pertaining to this particular product on the:

    a. OSHA web page
    b. Safety data sheet (SDS)
    c. Medical practice web page
    d. State medical assistant association web page

144. In what section of a patient's history and physical will one find information about alcohol use?

    a. Past medical history
    b. Past surgical history
    c. Social history
    d. Family medical history

145. A newborn weighs 6 pounds, 15 ounces. What is his weight in grams?

    a. 3000 g
    b. 3052 g
    c. 3123 g
    d. 3147 g

146. Which fingernail polish is going to affect an oxygen saturation reading obtained on a pulse oximeter?

    a. White
    b. Black
    c. Pink
    d. Fingernail polish does not affect the oxygen saturation reading on a pulse oximeter

147. A medical assistant in a busy medical practice is accidentally stuck with a contaminated needle when drawing a patient's blood. What is the FIRST thing that should be done?

    a. Exchange the gloves being worn for a new pair.
    b. Ask the patient if they have any communicable diseases that they are aware of.
    c. Remove the gloves and thoroughly wash hands with an antibacterial soap.
    d. Tell a supervisor what happened.

148. A mother calls the pediatrician's office because her 4-year-old daughter has been exposed to someone with the chickenpox. She wants to know if she can get it even though she has been vaccinated against it. Your most appropriate response would be:

    a. The chickenpox vaccine is close to 100% effective at preventing the disease, but it is possible she could still get a very mild case of the illness.
    b. The chickenpox vaccine is 100% effective and she will not get the illness.
    c. The chickenpox vaccine is about 50% effective so there is a chance she could get the illness.
    d. The chickenpox vaccine does not prevent her from getting the illness, it just ensures that it will be a milder case if she were to contract it.

Copyright © Mometrix Media. You have been licensed one copy of this document for personal use only. Any other reproduction or redistribution is strictly prohibited. All rights reserved.
This content is provided for test preparation purposes only and does not imply an endorsement by Mometrix of any particular political, scientific, or religious point of view.

149. Which of the following information is considered subjective?

a. Burning in the chest when coughing
b. A red, blistering rash on the torso
c. An elevated blood pressure reading
d. A loud, barking cough

150. In which of the following scenarios should a protective mask be worn by the medical assistant?

a. A patient with a wound infected with MRSA bacteria
b. A patient who has recently undergone cardiac bypass surgery
c. A healthy newborn in the hospital nursery
d. A pediatric patient who has been diagnosed with chickenpox

151. What is the best position for a patient having difficulty breathing?

a. Recumbent position
b. Fowler's position
c. Supine position
d. Prone position

152. What temperature should the water be when performing an ear irrigation?

a. 70 °F
b. 85 °F
c. 98.6 °F
d. 105 °F

153. For which labs tests is a nasopharyngeal swab performed?

a. Strep throat
b. Pregnancy
c. Mononucleosis
d. Influenza

154. What type of solution is added to the microscope slide to prepare a wet mount to examine vaginal discharge?

a. Hydrochloric acid
b. A salt solution
c. KOH (potassium hydroxide)
d. Baking soda and water solution

155. How should the reagent test strips used for performing a urinalysis be stored?

a. In the manufacturer's storage tube at room temperature
b. In an open container or cup at room temperature
c. In the manufacturer's storage tube in the refrigerator
d. In an open container near direct sunlight

Copyright © Mometrix Media. You have been licensed one copy of this document for personal use only. Any other reproduction or redistribution is strictly prohibited. All rights reserved. This content is provided for test preparation purposes only and does not imply an endorsement by Mometrix of any particular political, scientific, or religious point of view.

156. Which of the following results on a urinalysis would indicate a urine culture should be performed?

a. Normal study
b. Trace of protein
c. Nitrite positive
d. Elevated urobilinogen

157. A patient comes into the office to have a fasting glucose test performed. In order to ensure accurate results, how long should it have been since they have eaten or drank anything other than water?

a. 8 hours
b. 6 hours
c. 4 hours
d. No fasting is required

158. The position that is used for performing a pelvic exam is:

a. Fowler's or semi-Fowler's position
b. Knee-chest position
c. Trendelenburg position
d. Dorsal recumbent position

159. What is the proper way to measure the head circumference in a pediatric patient?

a. Use an elastic tape measure and wrap it just above the eyebrows and around the back of the head.
b. Use a paper tape measure and wrap it above the eyebrows and around the widest area of the head.
c. Use a paper tape measure and wrap it under the point of the chin and around the crown of the head.
d. Use an elastic tape measure and stretch it to wrap just above the eyebrows and around the base of the skull.

160. When the provider is performing a procedure that requires a sterile field, such as suturing, how far away should the medical assistant remain from the sterile boundaries?

a. 12 inches
b. 6 inches
c. 2 inches
d. There is no required distance the medical assistant should remain from the sterile boundary

161. When teaching a patient how to perform fingerstick tests to check their glucose level, it is important to stress that:

a. They should always apply a band-aid to the test site.
b. They should not wash their hands before performing the test.
c. That they cannot reuse the sharps in order to make them last longer.
d. They should wipe the finger being used for testing with a damp cloth.

Copyright © Mometrix Media. You have been licensed one copy of this document for personal use only. Any other reproduction or redistribution is strictly prohibited. All rights reserved.
This content is provided for test preparation purposes only and does not imply an endorsement by Mometrix of any particular political, scientific, or religious point of view.

162. When educating a patient on practicing safe sex, it is important to tell them that the best way to prevent acquiring a sexually transmitted infection is by:

   a. Using a male condom
   b. Using a female condom
   c. Using a spermicidal foam or gel
   d. Abstinence

163. You are educating a newly diagnosed diabetic patient and his family about what foods should or should not be eaten. Following the diabetic plate method, the group of foods from which the most food should come from in a day should be:

   a. Meats
   b. Non-starchy vegetables
   c. Whole grains
   d. Dairy

164. Which blood collection tubes use sodium citrate as an additive to prevent coagulation of the specimen?

   a. Light blue-top tubes
   b. Red-top tubes
   c. Gold-top tubes
   d. Lavender-top tubes

165. What instructions should a patient be given for collecting a 24-hour urine specimen?

   a. Begin collecting with the first urine specimen of the day, collect for 24 hours from that time, keep the specimen refrigerated, and take the specimen to the lab when you are finished
   b. Urinate into the toilet in the morning and then begin collecting the urine from that point on for 24 hours, leave at room temperature, and take the specimen to the lab within 24 hours
   c. Urinate into the toilet in the morning and then begin collecting the urine from that point on for 24 hours, keep refrigerated, urinate into the container the second morning, and take the specimen to the lab when you are finished
   d. Begin collecting with the first urine specimen of the day, collect for 24 hours from that time, keep the specimen at room temperature, and take the specimen to the lab when you are finished

166. All urine specimens should be:

   a. Kept at room temperature
   b. Kept at 98.6 °F
   c. Kept refrigerated
   d. Kept at room temperature or refrigerated; it does not matter

167. A patient needs to have several tubes of blood drawn. In which order should they be collected?

   a. Lavender, light blue, green, and red
   b. Light blue, red, green, and lavender
   c. Lavender, red, light blue, and green
   d. Green, red, lavender, and light blue

Copyright © Mometrix Media. You have been licensed one copy of this document for personal use only. Any other reproduction or redistribution is strictly prohibited. All rights reserved. This content is provided for test preparation purposes only and does not imply an endorsement by Mometrix of any particular political, scientific, or religious point of view.

168. Which of the following is an example of a CLIA-waived lab test?

a. Basic metabolic panel
b. Fingerstick glucose test
c. Comprehensive metabolic panel
d. Blood culture

169. A 63-year-old female develops a DVT following knee replacement surgery. She has been started on Coumadin therapy. You are educating the patient and her family on dietary restrictions with Coumadin. You explain to them:

a. She can no longer eat any green vegetables because they will increase her vitamin K level, causing the blood to thicken.
b. She needs to avoid all citrus fruit because it will cause her blood to be too thin.
c. She needs to maintain a consistent diet with some vitamin K from leafy green vegetables, but no big fluctuations in vitamin K-rich foods.
d. She should avoid red meat because of the high iron content.

170. How long can a tourniquet be left on a patient's arm for a blood draw?

a. It should be removed if the limb is becoming cool
b. 10 seconds
c. 30 seconds
d. 1 minute

171. What is the correct way to handle a blood specimen for collection of an erythrocyte sedimentation rate (ESR)?

a. Collect the blood in an ESR or red-top tube, spin in the centrifuge for 20 minutes, and keep at room temperature.
b. Collect the blood in an ESR or lavender-top tube, do not spin, and keep the specimen at room temperature or refrigerated.
c. Collect the blood in a light blue-top tube, do not spin, and keep refrigerated.
d. Collect the blood in an ESR or gold-top tube, spin in the centrifuge for 20 minutes, and refrigerate.

172. What is the correct way to handle a blood specimen for collection of a CBC?

a. Collect the blood in a red-top tube, spin in the centrifuge for 20 minutes, and refrigerate to process within 24 hours.
b. Collect the blood in a light blue-top tube, do not spin, and process immediately.
c. Collect the blood in a lavender-top tube, do not spin, and keep at room temperature to process within 24 hours or refrigerate to process within 72 hours.
d. Collect the blood in a lavender-top tube, spin in the centrifuge for 20 minutes, and keep at room temperature to process within 72 hours.

173. A patient has a lab order for a hemoglobin A1C. They have eaten breakfast that morning. What should you do?

a. Draw the specimen following protocol.
b. Tell the patient they will need to return the next day after fasting for 8 hours.
c. Call the ordering provider and ask them if the patient should be fasting for this test.
d. Draw the specimen per protocol but indicate on the tube that it is a non-fasting specimen.

Copyright © Mometrix Media. You have been licensed one copy of this document for personal use only. Any other reproduction or redistribution is strictly prohibited. All rights reserved. This content is provided for test preparation purposes only and does not imply an endorsement by Mometrix of any particular political, scientific, or religious point of view.

174. You are drawing a basic metabolic panel on a patient, and they ask you what is included in this test. Your best response is:

    a. Cholesterol and liver function tests
    b. Blood sugar and liver function tests
    c. Blood counts, kidney function, and liver function tests
    d. Blood sugar, electrolyte levels, and kidney function tests

175. A DEXA scan has been ordered for a patient. The patient asks you how this is performed. Your best response is that:

    a. An IV will be started to administer a radiocontrast agent, and the patient will be placed in a narrow tube for the test.
    b. The patient will lay down on a table for approximately 15 minutes while special x-rays are taken of the spine and hips.
    c. The patient will need to fast for at least 8 hours before a full body scan is performed.
    d. The patient will need to drink a bottle of oral contrast before x-rays are taken of the spine and feet.

176. The 5 Rights of medication administration are:

    a. The right patient, the right drug, the right dose, the right time, and the right route
    b. The right patient, the right date of birth, the right drug, the right time, and the right route
    c. The right drug, the right date, the right time, the right route, and the right response
    d. The right patient, the right route, the right action, the right time, and the right response

177. A mono test is ordered for a 17-year-old patient. This test is performed using:

    a. A urine specimen
    b. A throat swab
    c. A blood sample
    d. A nasopharyngeal swab

178. An EKG is performed in the office on a patient. The provider says that it shows the patient is in atrial flutter. You know that the appearance of the EKG will be:

    a. Wide, inverted U or V shapes
    b. A flat line
    c. Consistent narrow spikes with waves between that are sawtooth in appearance
    d. A consistent pattern of a squiggly line with narrow spikes and depressions evenly spaced apart

179. A child is in the office to have a sports physical. They achieve a 20/40 with both eyes on the vision test using a Snellen eye chart and the parent asks what the results mean. Your best response is:

    a. The child must be 20 feet from an object to see it as clear as a person with perfect vision at 40 feet.
    b. The child must be 40 feet from an object to see it as clear as a person with perfect vision at 20 feet.
    c. The child's vision is perfect.
    d. The child can see at 20 feet with his right eye what his left eye sees at 40 feet.

Copyright © Mometrix Media. You have been licensed one copy of this document for personal use only. Any other reproduction or redistribution is strictly prohibited. All rights reserved.
This content is provided for test preparation purposes only and does not imply an endorsement by Mometrix of any particular political, scientific, or religious point of view.

180. You are performing allergy testing on a patient. After the first round of allergens are injected, how long should you wait to give the second round if there is no reaction?

   a. You do not need to wait, just give each round one right after the other and then monitor for a reaction
   b. 15 minutes
   c. 30 minutes
   d. 1 hour

181. A mother calls the pediatrician's office because she wants her 4-year-old daughter checked for tuberculosis. Two days before, the child had spent the day with a family member who since had been diagnosed with TB, and the mother is concerned that her daughter will get it. Your best response is to:

   a. Tell her that she will need to come to the office for a TB skin test.
   b. Tell her that the pediatrician will call in some prophylactic antibiotics for her daughter.
   c. Reassure her that there is no cause for alarm unless her daughter begins to show symptoms with a fever/chills and bad cough.
   d. Tell her to take her daughter directly to the ER for an evaluation.

182. Which of the following is true regarding an asymptomatic patient with a positive PPD test?

   a. The patient has latent tuberculosis.
   b. The patient is contagious.
   c. Pharmacotherapy is not needed.
   d. The patient should be in respiratory isolation.

183. How should the flu vaccine be stored?

   a. In the refrigerator
   b. At room temperature
   c. Kept warm at 98.6 °F
   d. Refrigerated or room temperature, but not above 85 °F

184. What is the difference between Td and Tdap?

   a. There is no difference.
   b. Both immunize against tetanus and diphtheria, but Tdap also immunizes against pertussis.
   c. Both immunize against tetanus and diphtheria, but Tdap also immunizes against polio.
   d. Both immunize against tetanus and diphtheria, but Tdap also immunizes against measles.

185. The provider you are working with orders 100 mg of ibuprofen for a 4-year-old child. The bottle of liquid ibuprofen in the office is 200 mg/5 mL. How much should you give the patient?

   a. 1 mL
   b. 2.5 mL
   c. 5 mL
   d. 7.5 mL

Copyright © Mometrix Media. You have been licensed one copy of this document for personal use only. Any other reproduction or redistribution is strictly prohibited. All rights reserved. This content is provided for test preparation purposes only and does not imply an endorsement by Mometrix of any particular political, scientific, or religious point of view.

186. Which route is used to give a TB skin test?

    a. Intradermal
    b. Transdermal
    c. Subcutaneous
    d. Intramuscular

187. What is the purpose for using the Z-track method when giving an intramuscular injection?

    a. It is less painful for the patient.
    b. It decreases the risk of the medical assistant suffering a needle stick.
    c. It ensures you will not accidentally inject the medication into a blood vessel.
    d. It ensures the medication will be properly absorbed by preventing it from leaking out of the injection site.

188. All of the following are true regarding the mumps EXCEPT:

    a. A person cannot acquire the mumps if they have received the MMR vaccine as a child.
    b. Symptoms of the disease include a fever, swelling and tenderness along the jawline, and loss of appetite.
    c. The mumps is caused by a virus and is not treated with antibiotics.
    d. If a person has not received the MMR vaccine in the past, they should receive one injection now and another in 1 month.

189. Why is it common practice to mix Rocephin with 1% lidocaine for intramuscular injections on adults?

    a. 1% lidocaine causes vasodilation which allows for the medication to act faster.
    b. 1% lidocaine increases the rate of absorption into the muscle for the intramuscular injection of Rocephin.
    c. 1% lidocaine helps ease some of the pain involved with the intramuscular Rocephin injection.
    d. 1% lidocaine helps ease some of the common side effects of Rocephin, which include headache and joint pain.

190. You are taking vital signs on a patient who is in the office for an appointment to follow up on his diabetes. He mentions that his blood sugar has been running very high lately and he has not felt well. While you are taking his blood pressure, you notice his breath has a sweet, almost fruity smell. This can be a sign of:

    a. Diabetic ketoacidosis
    b. Common bad breath
    c. Strep throat
    d. A dental abscess

Copyright © Mometrix Media. You have been licensed one copy of this document for personal use only. Any other reproduction or redistribution is strictly prohibited. All rights reserved.
This content is provided for test preparation purposes only and does not imply an endorsement by Mometrix of any particular political, scientific, or religious point of view.

191. You are educating the parents of a patient newly diagnosed with epilepsy on what to do when their child has a grand mal seizure. All of the following are appropriate interventions EXCEPT to:

  a. Shield their body from danger by removing any obstacles, such as furniture, or place pillows around them.
  b. Monitor for any signs that the child is having difficulty breathing.
  c. Try to place a popsicle stick, tongue depressor, or other flat object into their mouth so they will not bite their tongue.
  d. Measure how long the seizure lasts and call 911 immediately if it lasts longer than 5 minutes.

192. A 3-year-old child has developed hand-foot-and-mouth disease after several other children at his daycare were diagnosed with it. Which of the following is true about this illness?

  a. It is a virus that will resolve on its own after several days and comfort measures for the symptoms are all that is necessary for treatment.
  b. This illness is not contagious and he can return to daycare tomorrow.
  c. The child will need to be seen urgently by their physician so that an antibiotic can be started.
  d. The rash with this illness must be present on the hands, feet, and in the mouth to have this diagnosis.

193. A mother brings her son in for a 5-year-old well-child visit and inquires whether he can receive the flu vaccine this year even though he has had hives from eating eggs in the past. The most appropriate response is:

  a. He cannot ever receive a flu vaccine if he has had hives from eating eggs.
  b. He can receive one of the newer formulations of the flu vaccine that is safe for those with egg allergies.
  c. It is safe for him to receive the same flu vaccine that someone without an egg allergy would receive.
  d. He can receive the flu vaccine, but it must be within a clinic setting where there is a provider who can treat an allergic reaction if he should develop one.

194. If a person thinks they may have a concussion, which symptom should be cause for them to go to the ER?

  a. Headache on and off for a week following the injury
  b. Some nausea immediately after the injury
  c. A bruise at the site where they hit their head
  d. Acute vomiting

195. The best home treatment for croup in a 2-year-old is:

  a. Antibiotics prescribed by his physician
  b. Aspirin if there is a fever
  c. Cool mist humidifier or steam therapy
  d. Over-the-counter cough syrups and decongestants

Copyright © Mometrix Media. You have been licensed one copy of this document for personal use only. Any other reproduction or redistribution is strictly prohibited. All rights reserved.
This content is provided for test preparation purposes only and does not imply an endorsement by Mometrix of any particular political, scientific, or religious point of view.

196. A 5-year-old child is diagnosed with the flu. He is asthmatic and has had frequent exacerbations of the asthma over the past year. What is the most important potential complication the parents should be monitoring?

- a. Febrile seizures
- b. Respiratory distress
- c. Intractable vomiting and/or diarrhea
- d. Severe rash

197. What information should be recorded on a multi-dose vial once it is opened?

- a. Date opened, expiration date, and initials of the person who opened it
- b. Date and time it was opened, provider that ordered the injection, and initials of the person who opened it
- c. Date it was opened and the date it will expire
- d. No information needs to be recorded on a multi-dose vial

198. A mother calls her pediatrician's office after her 5-year-old was in the day before and received the necessary immunizations before starting kindergarten. She is concerned because the child has developed a low-grade fever and redness and warmth at one of the injection sites. The most appropriate response to her is:

- a. She should bring him into the office immediately for evaluation.
- b. She should take him straight to the ER without delay.
- c. She should bring him in the next day to see the pediatrician.
- d. She should give him some ibuprofen and apply a warm compress to the area that is red.

199. What is tympanometry?

- a. A test to measure hearing acuity
- b. A test to measure visual acuity
- c. A test to assess balance and gait
- d. A test to assess mobility of the eardrum

200. What is measured with a peak flow rate?

- a. The maximum amount of air that can be exhaled
- b. The maximum amount of air that can be inhaled
- c. The amount of carbon dioxide retained in the lungs after exhaling
- d. The amount of carbon dioxide taken into the lungs during inspiration

Copyright © Mometrix Media. You have been licensed one copy of this document for personal use only. Any other reproduction or redistribution is strictly prohibited. All rights reserved. This content is provided for test preparation purposes only and does not imply an endorsement by Mometrix of any particular political, scientific, or religious point of view.

Answer Key and Explanations for Test #2

1. D: The term *edema* means swelling. The swelling is caused by an accumulation of fluid within the tissues of the body. *Exanthema* refers to a rash. The prefix *endo-* means within. *Emesis* refers to vomiting.

2. B: The radial pulse is palpated at the wrist, under the thumb. When taking a pulse, you should use the pads of your index finger and middle finger. Your thumb has a pulse beat of its own, which may interfere with feeling the patient's pulse. The carotid pulse is palpated on the side of the neck, next to the trachea. The brachial pulse is palpated on the inner portion of the cubital fossa (anterior aspect of the elbow). The ulnar artery pulse is located at the wrist, under the pinky, but it is not as commonly used as the radial pulse.

3. C: Hyperventilation refers to a patient breathing more quickly than normal. This rapid rate of ventilation results in carbon dioxide being exhaled at a higher rate than normal. This can result in respiratory alkalosis, meaning that the pH of the blood is abnormally elevated, due to rapid breathing. The symptoms that may accompany hyperventilation are related to the metabolic alkalosis that develops. The patient should be reassured in a calm manner to reduce anxiety. Have the patient sit down and instruct him to take slow, deep breaths.

4. A: The five stages of grief, as listed in the popular Kübler-Ross model, include denial, anger, bargaining, depression, and acceptance. These stages of grief may be experienced by a person facing death or by his or her survivors. They may be experienced in any order. Not everyone experiences all five stages, and some people experience other emotions not listed here. Delusions are beliefs that are held very strongly despite the fact that they are clearly false. They reflect an abnormal thought process and may be present in certain mental disorders.

5. C: Growth charts are used to track a child's growth over time. On a standard growth chart, the patient's height and weight are measured and charted according to the patient's age. Body mass index (BMI) charts may also be used, with BMI being calculated from the measured height and weight. Under usual circumstances, head circumference is not tracked in toddlers and older children. The important part of the chart is the overall pattern of growth and rate of change.

6. B: Projection is when a patient attributes their own undesired thoughts, feelings, or actions to another person. For instance, this upset patient is not listening or paying attention when you try to help her set up an appointment. She becomes more upset and then accuses you of not listening, when she is actually the one who is not listening. Displacement is when thoughts or feelings about one person are taken out on another person or object. Reaction formation is when a person converts unwanted feelings or thoughts into their opposites. Denial is when a person will not accept reality.

7. D: The child weighs 15 kg and needs to receive 15 mg of acetaminophen for every kg of body weight. The total dose should equal 225 mg (15 kg × 15 mg/kg = 225 mg). Because you know there are 160 mg/5 mL, you can calculate that there are 32 mg in every mL. In order to find out the dose in mL, divide 225 mg by 32 mg/mL, which equals 7 mL.

8. B: Teamwork is an important part of any medical career. Willingness to work as a team will help keep things running smoothly when unexpected issues arise. As part of a medical team, you will be expected to work with others to take care of patients in a safe and competent manner. In a

Copyright © Mometrix Media. You have been licensed one copy of this document for personal use only. Any other reproduction or redistribution is strictly prohibited. All rights reserved. This content is provided for test preparation purposes only and does not imply an endorsement by Mometrix of any particular political, scientific, or religious point of view.

professional work environment, you should be willing to help your coworkers when the need arises.

9. A: If you are faced with a potentially aggressive patient, it is recommended that you make sure that you are positioned between the patient and the door so you can rapidly leave the room, if necessary.

10. B: It is important to place the leads correctly and precisely so that the electrocardiogram (ECG) can be correctly interpreted. V1 and V2 give information about the right side of the heart. V3 and V4 give information about the interventricular septum. V5 and V6 give information about the left side of the heart.

11. D: Because you witnessed the collapse of the patient, the automated external defibrillator (AED) should be used as soon as possible. The AED will evaluate the patient's heart rhythm while cardiopulmonary resuscitation (CPR) is being performed, so CPR can be continued while the AED pads are being applied if there is more than one responder present. The AED will give step-by-step instructions and indicate whether the patient needs to be shocked or whether CPR alone should be continued. If a patient is found unconscious and the collapse was not witnessed, two minutes or one round of CPR should be performed before using the AED.

12. C: Active listening has been found to be a useful and empathetic way to communicate with patients. It involves listening carefully to what the patient is telling you and then restating what the patient has said back to him or her. This not only ensures that you correctly understand what the patient is saying, but it also demonstrates to the patient that they are being heard.

13. B: When leaving a phone message for a patient, you can identify who the message is for and identify yourself and the office. You can then ask the patient to return the call. You should not leave any medical information, including test results or prescription drug names, in a phone message.

14. D: In order to be certified as a medical assistant, the applicant must complete an accredited medical assisting program, pass the certification examination, and recertify his or her credentials every 60 months. In addition, the applicant must maintain current, provider-level CPR certification. The number of hours worked per week is not a specified requirement.

15. D: A living will is a written document that specifies what a patient would like to be done if he becomes unable to make healthcare decisions for himself. In a living will, the patient can express his wishes about what life-prolonging treatments he wants or does not want under various circumstances. It is a document focused on healthcare decisions, not on the patient's material assets.

16. B: Healthcare workers should thoroughly wash their hands before and after each patient contact. The Centers for Disease Control and Prevention (CDC) considers hand washing as one of the best ways to prevent the spread of infection. Hands should be washed with warm water and soap and should be vigorously rubbed together for at least 20 seconds. You should be sure to clean the back of your hands, under your nails, between your fingers, and your wrists. Hand sanitizers are another option, but they do not work as well as hand washing.

17. C: Patient records cannot be sent to other providers without the patient's consent. In order to be protected legally, you should have the patient sign an authorization form for the release of her medical records to the other physician. Ideally, this form would include a description of the information that will be released, the name and contact information of the recipient, a statement that the patient understands what will be disclosed, and the signature of the patient. It is not

Copyright © Mometrix Media. You have been licensed one copy of this document for personal use only. Any other reproduction or redistribution is strictly prohibited. All rights reserved. This content is provided for test preparation purposes only and does not imply an endorsement by Mometrix of any particular political, scientific, or religious point of view.

Mometrix

necessary for you to call the new physician or to have the physician you are working for sign a permission form. It can be very helpful and important for all of a patient's physicians to have access to the patient's previous medical records, so counseling the patient to not send the records would be inappropriate.

18. C: Ideally, you would use a translator phone service in order to communicate with the patient. Using the translator phone, you can explain to the patient what you need to do to take his or her vital signs and then ask the necessary questions for the initial patient history. In a large practice that has a diverse patient population or in a hospital setting, this type of service is often available. If the patient's young child is asked to translate, a number of problems may arise. There would be issues with patient privacy, potential problems with translation accuracy, and possible embarrassment for the parent and child. Hand gestures may be necessary, but would not be as useful as a translator phone. Asking the patient to come back with a translator should be avoided if possible.

19. B: Biohazard bags are generally red and should be labeled with the word "Biohazard" along with the international biohazard symbol. All sharps should be disposed of in appropriate sharps containers that are rigid and puncture resistant. If a biohazard container becomes soiled, guidelines should be followed to sanitize the container.

20. B: Ethically and legally, it is your duty to protect your patients. If a colleague is coming to work while intoxicated, this could place patients at risk. You should report the situation to your supervisor so appropriate action can be taken. An intoxicated employee should not be working with patients.

21. B: The small intestine is divided into three major parts. The duodenum is the first section, just distal to the stomach; the jejunum is the middle section; and the ileum is the third section that connects to the large intestine.

22. C: Answer C describes the correct way to provide choking first aid to a conscious child under the age of one. You continue to repeat the five back blows and five chest thrusts until the object is dislodged or until the baby becomes unconscious. Answer A describes infant CPR, which is what should be done if the choking baby becomes unconscious. You should not perform blind finger sweeps, as described in B because this may push the object further into the throat. If you can visualize the object, you can try to reach in and pull it out. Answer D describes how you would do the Heimlich maneuver in an older child or adult.

23. D: The endocrine system consists of a group of glands that secretes hormones into the blood. These hormones play important roles in regulating various functions of the body. With hyperthyroidism, there is excess thyroid hormone being secreted by the thyroid gland, and this can cause a number of symptoms, including weight loss, anxiety, sweating, and diarrhea.

24. A: If asked to give a patient a referral, you should give the patient the name and contact information of the type of doctor they need to see. Ideally, you will check and make sure that the referral physician takes the patient's insurance and is taking new patients, or you can tell the patient to check before his visit. Sometimes you may even make an appointment for the patient with the referral doctor. Having the patient find a doctor to see on his own is not giving him a referral. Sending the patient's chart to the specialist to see if he or she would be interested in taking the case would breach the patient's privacy and is not how referrals are made.

25. A: The most important dietary guideline to tell patients about when starting warfarin is that it is important to be consistent with their diets. Foods high in vitamin K, such as green leafy vegetables,

295

Copyright © Mometrix Media. You have been licensed one copy of this document for personal use only. Any other reproduction or redistribution is strictly prohibited. All rights reserved. This content is provided for test preparation purposes only and does not imply an endorsement by Mometrix of any particular political, scientific, or religious point of view.

can alter the effects of warfarin therapy, but as long as the patient is consistent in the intake of these foods, the medication can be adjusted accordingly.

26. A: Obesity is associated with numerous health problems. These include gallstones, osteoarthritis, type II diabetes, heart disease, hypertension, and various types of cancer. It was previously thought that obese patients were LESS likely to have osteoporosis than non-obese patients, but new research is questioning this theory. Obesity has been directly linked to the other listed health problems, but research is still ongoing about the association between obesity and osteoporosis.

27. C: A rectal temperature reading is considered the most accurate for infants. Other methods can be used to take an infant's temperature, but it is important to get the most accurate reading as possible in infants because their health is generally more delicate than that of older children. The closer the thermometer is to the inside of the body, the warmer and more accurate the temperature will be.

28. B: Third-party medical billing companies are used by insurance companies to process claims or payments. The physician may submit a claim to an insurance company, and the insurance company then passes the claim on to another company that specializes in processing that type of claim.

29. D: The definition of supine is lying on the back with the face upward. Prone is the position of lying on the stomach with the head turned to one side. Dorsal refers to the back of the body. Prostrate is defined as being stretched out, face-down.

30. A: If you receive a needle stick, you should immediately irrigate the wound with a large amount of sterile saline or another clean fluid. A tetanus shot may be necessary depending on your vaccination status, but it can be given after you irrigate the wound. After irrigating the wound, your supervisor should be informed, and you should be evaluated to determine what other tests and vaccinations are necessary. It is possible that you may need prophylaxis for human immunodeficiency virus (HIV), but this can also be done after you have washed the wound.

31. A: The Health Insurance Portability and Accountability Act (HIPAA) is a federal act that addresses the privacy of personal health information. It provides details about how personal health information must be protected.

32. D: A blood pressure cuff should ideally be placed on the upper arm, about half an inch above the elbow. The blood pressure cuff should be wrapped snugly around the arm in order to achieve proper compression of the brachial artery. You should be able to fit one finger underneath the cuff. If the cuff is too tight or too loose, the blood pressure reading may be inaccurate. Many cuffs have a brachial artery marker, which indicates how the cuff should be positioned on the arm (with the brachial artery marker just above the inner crease of the elbow).

33. C: Severe bleeding is a serious potential side effect of Plavix. Plavix is a blood thinner that is used therapeutically to prevent blood clots in high-risk patients. All patients on this medication and all healthcare providers should be aware that bleeding is one of the major risk factors associated with Plavix.

34. C: The top of the crutches should be 1 to 1.5 inches below the armpits when the patient is standing up straight. The handgrips should be even with the top of the patient's hips. It is important to size crutches correctly for a patient to avoid putting stress on other parts of the body. Improper sizing may result in discomfort and potential injury.

Copyright © Mometrix Media. You have been licensed one copy of this document for personal use only. Any other reproduction or redistribution is strictly prohibited. All rights reserved.
This content is provided for test preparation purposes only and does not imply an endorsement by Mometrix of any particular political, scientific, or religious point of view.

35. A: The correct time and date should be recorded on all patient documents. In addition, often the patient's name, birth date, and medical record number are included on documents. There are several types of documents that do require the patient's signature, Social Security number, and other personal information, but this information is not required on *all* patient visit documentation. The physician's provider number is used for health insurance purposes, and it is not required to be written on all patient visit notes.

36. C: The prefix *dys-* means abnormal or difficult. Examples include dysphagia, which means difficulty swallowing, and dysplasia, which means the abnormal growth of tissues or cells. The suffix *-rrhea* means discharge. The prefix *peri-* means around. The prefix *post-* means after.

37. B: Have the patient open his mouth wide and tilt back his head. Use a tongue depressor to depress the patient's tongue so you can see the back of the throat. Swab the back of the throat and over the tonsils from side to side. Make sure you swab any visible white patches or inflamed areas in the throat and tonsils. Avoid swabbing the tongue and cheeks because you want to focus on the bacteria collected from the throat and tonsillar area. Even if white patches are not seen on the tonsils, the patient still may have a bacterial infection and a throat swab should be taken.

38. D: When labeling medical specimens (e.g., blood, urine, or sputum) it is important to include the date and time of collection and the patient's full name and date of birth or medical record number. The lab order requisition form should accompany the lab specimen. Although the full name and signature of the person collecting the specimen are not required, the collector should include his or her initials on the label.

39. C: The flu vaccine is indeed grown in eggs, but the CDC now recommends the flu vaccine to all individuals, including those with egg allergies. Those who experience hives in reaction to egg are able to have the flu vaccine without any special monitoring. Individuals who have experienced anaphylaxis or angioedema in response to eggs are also approved to receive the annual flu vaccine, but must do so in an inpatient or outpatient setting where the administration of the vaccine can be supervised and the patient promptly treated should a reaction occur.

40. D: Many times, patients may communicate in nonverbal ways, such as using body language. It is important to pay attention to these cues because this may help you to better understand and respond to your patient. In this case, a patient who is frowning with his arms folded may indicate that he disapproves of something, does not accept what you are saying, or has another issue. When a patient displays nonverbal cues, you can use these to considerately question the patient about his feelings. Asking, "What is the problem?" would be an abrupt and possibly rude way to approach the patient. Asking, "You don't like what I am saying?" or "Do you want to do this appointment another time?" may be overinterpreting the patient's feelings.

41. B: When a clean-catch urine sample is needed from a female patient, she should be instructed to wash her hands, then sit on the toilet, spread open the labial folds with two fingers, use a sterile wipe to clean the inner folds of the labia (wiping from front to back), and use a second wipe to clean the area over the urethra. The patient should then urinate a small amount into the toilet bowl, temporarily stop the flow of urine, and then collect a urine sample using the urine cup. She should refrain from touching the inside of the sterile cup or lid.

42. A: Open-ended questions are those that encourage the patient to give full answers in their own words. Close-ended questions often result in one-word answers, and therefore they may not result in as much information being provided. It is important to use open-ended questions when performing medical interviews so the patient can give meaningful and detailed answers.

Copyright © Mometrix Media. You have been licensed one copy of this document for personal use only. Any other reproduction or redistribution is strictly prohibited. All rights reserved. This content is provided for test preparation purposes only and does not imply an endorsement by Mometrix of any particular political, scientific, or religious point of view.

43. A: When accompanying a patient to other parts of the clinic or hospital for testing, it is important to ensure that the patient remains safe and comfortable. It is your responsibility to safely transport your patient and make sure that she is securely on the imaging table to prevent falls. In general, you will be in another room when the x-ray is taken to reduce your own exposure to the radiation. You should not hold onto the patient during the x-ray. It is the radiology technician's responsibility to ensure that the equipment settings are correct. In most cases, patients do not need anxiety medication before an x-ray is performed.

44. B: Simvastatin (Zocor) is a statin. Statins are 3-hydroxy-3-methyl coenzyme A (HMG-CoA) reductase inhibitors, which work to lower cholesterol.

45. B: The three sites most appropriate for intramuscular injections are the deltoid muscle, the vastus lateralis muscle, and the ventrogluteal muscle. The deltoid muscle is located in the upper arm. The vastus lateralis muscle is located in the thigh and is commonly used for infants and toddlers because the muscle is thick and well developed. The ventrogluteal muscle is located in the hip and is the safest injection site for adults and children because it provides the greatest thickness of gluteal muscles, is free from penetrating nerves and blood vessels, and has a thin layer of fat. The dorsogluteal site is no longer recommended, due to the potential for injury to the sciatic nerve. When selecting which site to use, you should consider the age of the patient, the medication that is being injected, and the general condition of the patient.

46. A: Schedule I controlled substances are drugs that have a very high potential for abuse and have no currently accepted medical use in the United States. Schedule II drugs also have a very high potential for abuse, but they have accepted medical uses. Schedule IV and V controlled substances have a lower potential for abuse compared to Schedule I through III substances.

47. A: The needles used for blood collection come in sterile packaging. After uncapping the needle, it is best to avoid touching its shaft (the part of the needle that will puncture the patient's skin). Wiping the needle with an alcohol swab is unnecessary because the needle is already sterile. Disinfecting the patient's skin, washing your hands, and wearing gloves will all help prevent contamination of blood samples.

48. C: During a nebulizer treatment, the patient should have the face mask placed securely over his or her mouth and nose in order to ensure that the majority of the medication is inhaled. If the face mask is held several inches away, the medication may disperse into the air rather than being inhaled by the patient. It is important to always verify a patient's identification before giving any treatments. It is also essential to check that the correct type and dose of medication are being given, exactly as ordered by the physician. The patient should be instructed to take deep breaths so the nebulized medication is carried into the lungs.

49. A: When a patient presents with severe bleeding from a wound, continuous pressure should be applied directly to the wound for at least 20 minutes. If the blood seeps through the bandage, more material should be added on top without taking off the first bandage. If applying direct pressure to the wound does not stop the bleeding, the main artery supplying the area can be occluded (at the "pressure point") by squeezing the artery against the bone. If a patient is bleeding severely, you should not take time to clean the wound, but first focus on stopping the bleeding. Applying a tourniquet should not be the immediate reaction to severe bleeding because this can have significant adverse effects.

50. D: Standard precautions are a set of medical practice guidelines that are meant to protect healthcare workers from infection. Healthcare workers are instructed to use standard precautions

Copyright © Mometrix Media. You have been licensed one copy of this document for personal use only. Any other reproduction or redistribution is strictly prohibited. All rights reserved. This content is provided for test preparation purposes only and does not imply an endorsement by Mometrix of any particular political, scientific, or religious point of view.

to prevent contact with blood and all other potentially infectious substances. In any situation where there may be exposure to bodily fluids (e.g., blood, cerebral spinal fluid, vaginal secretions), employees should wear personal protective equipment (e.g., gloves, masks, gowns, and eye protection) and wash their hands. These guidelines apply to the care of all patients, regardless of status.

51. D: Psychologist Abraham Maslow developed a 5-level hierarchy of human needs. The most basic are physiological needs and safety, followed by being loved and belonging to a social group. These are followed by feelings of accomplishment and self-esteem. The highest level in Maslow's hierarchy is achieving self-actualization, when a person reaches their full potential and has mastered the lower levels.

52. B: The 1-1/2 to 3-year-old child is starting to make their own decisions by walking away from a parent or choosing which toy to play with or food he would like to eat. Erikson has called this Stage 2 of development, a period during which the child experiences autonomy vs. shame and doubt when they begin to exercise their independence.

53. B: Within the Hispanic culture, men are the primary decision makers and the leaders of the family. Men are usually the providers for the family and will often make the medical decisions for all family members. While this is a general cultural quality for the medical assistant to be aware of, it may not be practiced by all Hispanic families.

54. A: An exploratory question is an open-ended question that offers the patient the opportunity to give a full, complete answer. Answer options A, B, and C all exemplify exploratory questions in their nature, but using the word "why" (as is used in answer option A) when asking exploratory questions is considered nontherapeutic language as it may be perceived as judgmental. This may result in the individual actually closing up in their response. Answer option D also exemplifies nontherapeutic therapeutic communication, but it is not exploratory in nature. Rather, it is a close-ended question meant to elicit a yes or no answer in response.

55. A: A closed, or direct, question is direct and seeks information. An example is asking a person for their date of birth. This type of question does not open the door for a long explanation, but rather, is used when seeking specific information from the patient. It is the type of question that is used when the patient does not need to explain a problem or their emotions. The answers are usually short and succinct.

56. D: Whenever possible, have an interpreter present in these types of situations, ideally one who has undergone some training in medical terminology. Using a family member is not ideal because it is not known if they are able to translate medical terms correctly. Online software may not be accurate and there is no way to verify that the terms and concepts are being interpreted appropriately. Pictures and videos will enhance communication provided through an interpreter.

57. A: Having a patient with a hearing impairment offers the opportunity to utilize different forms of teaching. Some of these patients may have some degree of hearing acuity left, but most have learned to adapt and read lips. It is important to be aware of any distracting background noises and to face the patient directly so that the face and mouth are clearly visible. Care should be taken not to turn away when talking or cover the mouth with a hand or clipboard, as these actions will also make it difficult for the patient to understand.

58. C: When listening to someone explain something, it is important to internally reflect on what they are saying to actively listen and understand what is being said. Restating what has been said is

Copyright © Mometrix Media. You have been licensed one copy of this document for personal use only. Any other reproduction or redistribution is strictly prohibited. All rights reserved. This content is provided for test preparation purposes only and does not imply an endorsement by Mometrix of any particular political, scientific, or religious point of view.

a way to verify understanding of the information that was given. This is especially important with complex material or when learning a new skill.

59. B: An internal distraction to communication can be anything that is happening within a person that takes their attention away from the conversation that is being held. This can include pain, hunger, being too cold or too hot, or having other stressors on their mind. Loud music, a TV, or other voices in the area are all considered external distractors.

60. D: An external distraction to communication is anything that is happening in the environment around a person that interferes with their ability to communicate or receive information without being distracted. This can include loud music, a TV playing, or loud voices in the room. Pain, hunger, or internal emotions are all internal distractions to communication.

61. D: Empathy and sympathy are frequently confused. Empathy is placing oneself in someone else's shoes to understand what they must be going through when in a stressful or sad situation. Sympathy, on the other hand, is feeling compassion, sorrow, or pity for that person, despite the inability to relate to what they must truly be feeling.

62. A: When dealing with an irate patient, it is important to maintain a calm demeanor even when that is not felt internally. Often, the patient simply needs to express their frustration to someone who will listen. Calmly listen to the patient, restate their frustrations and let them know you can understand why they are so angry, and then assure them you will help to fix the problem if it is an issue that can be handled over the phone.

63. D: A power of attorney is someone that is assigned by the patient to have the legal authority to make financial decisions on their behalf when they are unable to. The healthcare proxy is a legal document that assigns all healthcare decision-making to a person when the patient is unable to. These can be the same person or two different people. It is ideal to have two people in these roles who can communicate and work well together as their decision-making can affect the care that a patient receives.

64. C: Receiving constructive criticism is a necessary part of improving in all aspects of our lives. Receiving feedback at work, whether it is positive or negative, can help to identify areas of strength and weakness that can be used to make a person a better employee. In this case, identifying specific areas of the job in which there seems to be room for improvement can help to improve patient satisfaction, improve office relationships, and decrease stress on the job when the medical assistant feels more efficient at completing his or her work.

65. B: The Patient Self-Determination Act was put into place in 1990 to ensure a patient's decisions regarding the care they receive is communicated to members of the healthcare team. The wishes of a patient are outlined in advance directive documents, and these wishes must be communicated to all members of the healthcare team. For example, if a patient wishes to have specific life-saving interventions in the event of an emergency, these wishes must be carried out under federal law. This also includes any requests to avoid extensive life-saving measures if the patient wishes.

66. C: The Uniform Anatomical Gift Act was established in 1968 and has undergone two revisions since then. It was put into place in order to outline the specific procedures that need to be followed in the event of transportation of an organ for transplantation. It also includes the procedures that must be followed for someone to donate their remains to medical science for research purposes. It allows for any adult to choose to donate all or a portion of their body for transplantation or research purposes.

Copyright © Mometrix Media. You have been licensed one copy of this document for personal use only. Any other reproduction or redistribution is strictly prohibited. All rights reserved. This content is provided for test preparation purposes only and does not imply an endorsement by Mometrix of any particular political, scientific, or religious point of view.

67. D: The order in which effective communication occurs is sender, message, channel, receiver, and feedback. The sender communicates the message, orally or in writing. The channel through which the message is carried can be verbally face-to-face or over the phone. It can be written in an interoffice memo, e-mail, or text message. The receiver then interprets the message internally. Feedback is then given by the receiver to restate the message and show that it was communicated correctly. Feedback may also be an explanation or question, if clarification is needed.

68. A: Occupational Safety and Health Administration (OSHA) was signed into law by President Richard Nixon in 1970. It was established to ensure that employees are provided with the training necessary to perform their job duties safely while offering a safe work environment in which to do so. The agency is also responsible for protection to employees who enact the whistleblower action to report unsafe conditions at the place of their employment.

69. D: The Food and Drug Administration (FDA) was established in 1906 to regulate the research, development, production, and distribution of medications. It has extended its role to include monitoring drug effectiveness, generic and brand name medications, prescription and over-the-counter medications, cosmetics, veterinarian medications, and the health effects of tobacco use. The FDA has field offices throughout the country and has employees placed in several foreign countries.

70. C: All of the information listed is vital except for the patient's social security number. The name and date of birth are to ensure the correct patient chart is accessed. The phone number where the patient can be reached that day is essential so instructions can be called back to the patient. The medication, whether it is prescription or over-the-counter, along with the specific symptoms they have been having should also be included in order for the provider to make a decision as to what should be done for the patient.

71. B: The Clinical Laboratory Improvement Act (CLIA) falls under the regulation of the FDA and the Center for Medicare and Medicaid Services. It regulates all medical laboratory facilities in the collection of, handling of, and processing of human blood and tissue. It also establishes the complexity of specific laboratory tests and determines if a test can be performed at different facilities based on its level of complexity and the abilities of a specific lab. All CLIA-certified laboratory facilities must undergo regular inspections to ensure they are meeting the standards set forth for their facility.

72. B: The Americans with Disabilities Act became a law in 1990. It prohibits discrimination against anyone who has a disability in all areas of public life. The purpose of the law is to ensure all people with disabilities have the same rights and opportunities as everyone else. Amendments to the Act were signed into law in 2009 to further clarify the definition of disability.

73. C: In an emergency situation, it is very important to remain calm. In this situation, keep the mother on the phone and have a co-worker nearby call 911 to have emergency personnel sent immediately to their house. Try to encourage the mother to remain as calm as possible in order to try to calm the child in distress. Let her know that emergency help is on the way and remain on the phone with her until they arrive.

74. D: The HITECH Act (Health Information Technology for Economic and Clinical Health) was created in 2009 to expand the use of computer record keeping to help meet meaningful use goals. It is designed to help meet the 5 goals of healthcare in the United States for meaningful use. These goals are to improve quality, safety, and efficiency of healthcare; ensure patient privacy; facilitate patient involvement in their care; improve the health status of the population; and increase coordination of care.

Copyright © Mometrix Media. You have been licensed one copy of this document for personal use only. Any other reproduction or redistribution is strictly prohibited. All rights reserved.
This content is provided for test preparation purposes only and does not imply an endorsement by Mometrix of any particular political, scientific, or religious point of view.

75. B: The Controlled Substances Act was placed into law in 1970 in order to categorize medications based on their potential for abuse. It also established guidelines for the manufacture, possession, use, and distribution of certain medications. This created 5 schedules, or categories, under which drugs can be placed based on their medical use and abuse potential.

76. A: The medical assistant's scope of practice varies from state to state, but there are some generalities that can be made across the board. A medical assistant cannot independently interpret lab or other test results. This information must first be received from the provider. They also cannot give out any medical advice or treatment advice over the phone without being instructed to do so by a provider. The medical assistant can take vital signs, perform specific tasks as outlined by the provider, and perform minor procedures (suture removal, venipuncture). Work duties differ from practice to practice, and it is important to know the laws in the state in which one works.

77. B: The Genetic Information Nondiscrimination Act (GINA) was established in 2008. It forbids health insurance carriers and employers to discriminate against people based on genetic testing. It does not protect against discrimination based on genetic information from life insurance carriers, disability insurance, or long-term care insurance.

78. C: The Centers for Disease Control, or CDC, was established in 1946 and is headquartered in Atlanta, Georgia. Not only does it focus on disease control and prevention, but it also coordinates educational efforts to promote health in U.S. citizens. The CDC collaborates with many international health organizations to assist with disease control and prevention throughout the world. The Director of the CDC is appointed by the President of the United States.

79. A: While the Federal Trade Commission is the agency that protects the nation's consumers, it also enforces the Fair Debt Collection Practices Act to prevent deceptive or unfair debt collection processes and prevents abusive methods being used to collect debt. This is enforced for any debts being collected for personal expenses such as credit cards, medical bills, auto loans, and mortgages. It does not include any debts incurred from running a business.

80. D: The Truth in Lending Act was established in 1968 as a federal law in the United States. It was established to mandate complete disclosure in any lending practices. This requires businesses that offer credit or a structured payment settlement for a debt to disclose the full terms of the agreement, including interest charges, penalties, fees, and the full amount of the structured payments.

81. B: Gonorrhea is a communicable disease that is required to be reported to the local Health Department. Health Departments gather information regarding influenza outbreaks and reports these to the CDC, but a positive flu test does not require a report to be filed with the Health Department. Group B Strep is a common infection that pregnant women are tested for before delivery. Some of the other communicable diseases that require reporting are chlamydia, trichomoniasis, HIV, hepatitis, Legionnaire's disease, and mumps.

82. B: Spiral fractures occur when one end of an extremity is fixed in place and the rest of the extremity continues to move. For example, a "toddler's fracture" of the tibia occurs when a young child falls a short distance onto an outstretched leg. In the child who is not yet walking, a spiral fracture occurs when a limb is held in place and then twisted or jerked hard.

83. C: Based on federal regulations, a minor can be seen for STD counseling, pregnancy testing, and requests for birth control without obtaining permission from their parents or guardian. This also applies to parental requests for medical records pertaining to this visit, which cannot be released without permission from the patient.

Copyright © Mometrix Media. You have been licensed one copy of this document for personal use only. Any other reproduction or redistribution is strictly prohibited. All rights reserved.
This content is provided for test preparation purposes only and does not imply an endorsement by Mometrix of any particular political, scientific, or religious point of view.

84. D: The Patient Care Partnership replaced the American Hospital Association's Patient Bill of Rights. It outlines what the patient should expect during their hospital stay regarding their rights and responsibilities. It states that the patient will receive a high quality of care, involvement in their care, protection of their privacy, assistance with filing insurance claims, and preparation for discharge.

85. A: As "the captain of the ship," the ordering physician is the one ultimately responsible for a patient receiving an incorrect medication. The medical assistant committed a medical error, but the physician is responsible for all of those who work under him or her in following through on their orders. The medical assistant would be named in any legal proceedings that could result from this error, but the physician is responsible for overseeing all medical procedures that take place in the office.

86. C: Competency is the legal term used to mean a person does not have the mental ability to make decisions for themselves, such as managing finances. It is often confused with capacity, which is determined by a physician, often a psychiatrist, after a series of mental status tests are performed. The legal system is responsible for deeming someone incompetent to make his or her own decisions.

87. C: The informed consent document is a legal document that must be completed before a medical procedure. This document includes the procedure to be performed, the potential risks of the procedure, the risks of not having the procedure performed, the date and time the document was reviewed with the patient, and the signatures of the provider performing the procedure, the patient, and a witness.

88. D: A subpoena duces tecum (Latin: under penalty to bring with you) is used most often when a person is summoned to participate in a deposition. The order requires that the person bring any pertinent documents with them that contain information necessary during the information-gathering portion of a legal case. If the documents are not produced, the person must show good reason why they are not available.

89. B: Respondeat superior literally means "let the master answer." It refers to the legal action that the person in charge is responsible for the actions of those under him or her. It is commonly referred to as "the captain of the ship" rule. If someone in a medical office makes a mistake that results in, or has the potential to result in, injury to the patient, the supervising physician is the person who is ultimately responsible for the mistake.

90. B: Under res ipsa loquitor (Latin: the thing speaks for itself), there is not a burden of proof to show the physician acted in a negligent manner. Rather, the results of his or her actions can be enough to show negligence or malpractice. Examples include leaving a foreign object in a patient after surgery, operating on the wrong patient, performing the wrong procedure on a patient, or operating on the wrong part of the patient.

91. A: An arbitration involves the same elements as a regular court trial, such as testimony and the presentation of evidence, but is usually on a less formal basis. Mediation is used to settle a dispute using a neutral third party. With mediation, one side is not ruled right and one wrong, rather, it is a negotiation process in order to reach an agreement. In arbitration, the proceedings are overseen by an arbitrator who makes a ruling on the case that is legally binding.

92. A: Good Samaritan laws are in place to prevent legal consequences for someone who acts in good faith to help save another person. This includes rib injuries while performing the Heimlich maneuver or CPR. The thought is that the act was performed with good intentions to save the life of

Copyright © Mometrix Media. You have been licensed one copy of this document for personal use only. Any other reproduction or redistribution is strictly prohibited. All rights reserved. This content is provided for test preparation purposes only and does not imply an endorsement by Mometrix of any particular political, scientific, or religious point of view.

another person. Any injury or negative outcome that results from this occurred in the act of good intentions, so the person should not be held liable.

93. C: In the United States, a misdemeanor is punishable with up to 1 year in jail or prison. A felony is a crime that is punishable with prison time longer than 1 year. Examples of a misdemeanor include petty theft, prostitution, public intoxication, and possession of marijuana. Examples of felonies include homicide, kidnapping, involuntary manslaughter, and burglary.

94. B: When discharging a patient from the practice, the written notification of this decision should be sent certified with a return receipt for proof of delivery. In order to avoid charges of patient abandonment, the provider will need to offer care on an urgent or emergent basis only for 30 days following receipt of the letter. Ideally, this would have been discussed with the patient in the office already, but the decision to discharge should also be communicated in writing.

95. D: Libel is defamation of character in written form, such as public posts on social media. This is easier to prove in court than slander, because there is written proof of the transgression. Slander is when character is defamed via the spoken word. Libel is illegal in the United States and subject to punishment.

96. C: The acronym PASS is commonly used to provide basic instructions for operating a fire extinguisher. PASS stands for Pull the pin on the extinguisher, Aim the nozzle at the base of the fire, Squeeze the trigger on the extinguisher, and Sweep from side to side when spraying.

97. B: The medical term *osteo-* means bone. It is most often used to describe a specific illness or condition, such as osteoarthritis, osteomyelitis, or osteosarcoma.

98. A: *Arthroscopy* contains the roots *arthro-*, meaning joint, and *–scopy*, meaning viewing or observing. This is a procedure in which small incisions are made through which a small camera can be inserted so the surgeon can visualize the space within a joint on a monitor. It is frequently used for shoulder and knee procedures.

99. D: Neurology is the specialty that studies disorders of the nerves and nervous system. Though the spine and brain are part of the nervous system, any surgery on this system would be performed by a neurosurgeon, not a neurologist.

100. A: Ergonomics is the study of design with the goal of increasing productivity at work while decreasing excessive stress on the musculoskeletal system. Examples of tools that are used include ergonomic chairs that have multiple adjustments for comfort and lumbar support or a padded roll in front of a keyboard or mouse to prevent hand fatigue and carpal tunnel syndrome.

101. D: The medical assistant functions as a patient advocate through many different actions, but the overall goal is to keep the patient safe and ensure they are receiving the highest quality of care possible. This can involve providing necessary education about a disease state or coordinating efforts with many providers for the patient to receive all of the necessary care they need.

102. A: Meaningful use was established to provide an incentive through Medicare and Medicaid by utilizing the electronic health record to its fullest potential. It sets forth specific objectives and goals to improve the quality of patient care, patient safety, and result in better patient outcomes. It has been released in three separate stages. The American Recovery and Reinvestment Act of 2009 authorized Medicare and Medicaid to offer these incentives to those healthcare professionals who meet the criteria for meaningful use.

Copyright © Mometrix Media. You have been licensed one copy of this document for personal use only. Any other reproduction or redistribution is strictly prohibited. All rights reserved. This content is provided for test preparation purposes only and does not imply an endorsement by Mometrix of any particular political, scientific, or religious point of view.

103. D: With social media being used by most people, it is frequently misinterpreted as a means of communication for all aspects of our lives. It is important to note, however, that only secure methods should be used for discussing healthcare issues with a patient in order to prevent the violation of privacy laws. In this case, the patient should be informed that her lab results cannot be discussed through social media, and she will need to contact the office.

104. A: The best response is that medical conditions cannot be diagnosed through e-mail, and she will need to be seen in person. E-mail messages sent through a patient portal system are usually secure, but a diagnosis cannot be made this way. The medical assistant does not have the authority within his or her scope of practice to give independent medical advice to the patient.

105. D: The discharge summary outlines the full course of the patient's hospital stay from admission through discharge. It includes the history of their present illness along with a summary of any tests and labs that were performed during the stay. It will also include a list of the medications with which the patient was discharged home. Most hospitals have strict requirements for the time frame in which the discharge summary must be completed following discharge of the patient.

106. C: The source-oriented record organizes patient information into the source of the documents it contains. For example, it contains progress notes from each member of the health care team outlining their evaluation and plan for the patient. The problem-oriented medical record is divided into 5 sections: initial and annual assessments, problem list, care plans, progress notes, and discharge summary.

107. B: The appointment matrix is a linear schedule that lists the date and times of appointments. The time slots on the matrix are identified as being open or full and any time slots that are blocked for either administrative time or lunchtime are visible. The matrix can also be formatted to identify which time slots should be used for annual physicals or same day acute visits.

108. D: The patient who thinks she may have the flu would be the most appropriate choice and characterized as an acute illness. Many offices will set aside a set number of appointment times for their patients who need to be seen on an acute basis. All of the other choices are routine appointments that should be scheduled in other appointment times.

109. A: Accounts payable are those payments that need to be made by a company to pay for supplies or services that were purchased on credit. In an office, there may be several accounts established for office supplies, office cleaning services, and certain medication or medical supply companies that are paid monthly. These would be the accounts payable.

110. C: A tickler file is used to organize documents that are time-sensitive and need to be addressed by a certain date. This can include items that need follow-up attention to check their status. A tickler file is set up with one file for each day of the month (1-31) along with one file for each month of the year. Using this system ensures that nothing will be missed on a specific date that it may be due.

111. C: Accounts receivable are those payments that are due to a company in return for goods and services that were given. This is on a credit basis. A payment received would be classified as an asset since it increases income to the company.

112. A: The DRG, or diagnosis related group, determines the payment a hospital will receive from Medicare for a hospitalization. In the past, hospital bills were itemized with every single supply that was used, including everything from toothbrushes to syringes. Medicare now uses DRGs, which

Copyright © Mometrix Media. You have been licensed one copy of this document for personal use only. Any other reproduction or redistribution is strictly prohibited. All rights reserved.
This content is provided for test preparation purposes only and does not imply an endorsement by Mometrix of any particular political, scientific, or religious point of view.

identify the patient's diagnosis or surgery. The payment made to the hospital is a set price based on that DRG. This is calculated based on the average cost that a hospitalization incurs for a specific diagnosis or procedure.

113. B: A relative value unit, or RVU, is the value assigned to a physician visit or specific procedure. The more complex the visit or procedure, the more RVUs it is worth. The RVU values are used to calculate the cost of a specific visit or procedure. This scale is often used, at least partially, in determining provider salaries or a bonus structure.

114. D: When an insurance company requires all of the deductible, or out of pocket expense, to be met before anything will be covered, the patient should pay the amount of their appointment based on the visit code. This code is determined by the provider based on the level of complexity of the office visit. In this case, she still has to meet $3,000 in out of pocket expense before her insurance will cover anything. The $50 Urgent Care co-pay applies once she has met her deductible. Otherwise, she will need to pay the cost of the visit depending upon office policy.

115. A: Upcoding is the practice of billing for a more complex procedure or diagnosis than was actually treated. This is considered a fraudulent practice and can lead to charges of billing fraud. Oftentimes, it is done accidentally when the time is not taken to search for the correct CPT code based on the actual service provided.

116. A: The International Statistical Classification of Diseases and Related Health Problems (ICD) is now in its 10th revision. The ICD was created by the World Health Organization. Work on the 10th version started in 1983 and was finished in 1992. The United States adopted this version for use in 2015. The ICD-10 contains over 14,000 disease states and symptoms for which there is a diagnosis code.

117. B: HCPCS, or the Healthcare Common Procedure Coding System, is used to identify those services or supplies that are not included in the standard CPT code list. This includes ambulance services, prosthetics, and other durable medical equipment.

118. C: A third party payer is an organization that pays for the medical expenses of a person. This is usually a health insurance company such as Medicare, Medicaid, or private health insurance. The patient is the first party payer who purchases the health insurance policy.

119. B: The Advance Beneficiary Notice supplied by Medicare identifies which services Medicare will not pay for. Included in this statement is what the estimated cost will be to the patient along with an explanation of why the service is not covered. This is provided to the patient prior to a procedure or specific services that are recommended so that the out of pocket cost is disclosed.

120. D: Tricare is the carrier that offers medical insurance benefits to the military, retirees, and their dependents. This program was formerly known as CHAMPUS, or the Civilian Health and Medical Program of the Uniformed Services.

121. C: CHAMPVA is the program that offers medical benefits to the spouse and dependents of certain veterans. There are specific qualification criteria. The veteran must be deemed totally disabled due to a service-connected condition, have died from a service-connected condition, have died in combat, or have been rated totally disabled due to a service-connected condition at the time of their death.

122. B: The Prospective Payment System is a method of reimbursement established by Medicare to provide a predetermined, fixed amount of payment to facilities and organization offering specific

Copyright © Mometrix Media. You have been licensed one copy of this document for personal use only. Any other reproduction or redistribution is strictly prohibited. All rights reserved.
This content is provided for test preparation purposes only and does not imply an endorsement by Mometrix of any particular political, scientific, or religious point of view.

services. The patient's classification is determined using the IRF-PAI tool to classify patients in a specific category that identifies which services they will need while undergoing skilled or rehabilitative nursing care. The fee for these services varies depending upon the type of facility offering the services, but it ensures that specific services will be reimbursed appropriately.

123. A: Medicare Part A covers the services available outside of a physician's office. This includes hospitalization, skilled nursing home care for the first 100 days after a 3-day hospital stay, hospice care, home care, and durable medical equipment. Medicare Part B covers the care provided within the physician's office.

124. A: Managed care organizations were established in the 1970s in an effort to control the costs of healthcare. With a managed care organization, the insured patient has a pool of providers to choose from when seeking healthcare. The PPOs tend to be more flexible, but HMOs are very strict with specific in-network providers that must be seen to avoid higher out of pocket expenses. Reimbursement rates for providers are controlled and based on flat rates for specific services provided.

125. C: Once a specific claim for a service or diagnostic test has been declined by the insurance carrier, it must be resubmitted for re-evaluation. In this case, it would be important to have the name of the person the patient spoke with at the insurance company so it can be used for future reference. The charges should be resubmitted to the patient's insurance by the practice, and if they are declined a second time, the person the patient spoke to at the insurance company should be contacted directly.

126. B: The insurance company is going to need a list of medications that the patient has tried for this particular problem in the past, but not a comprehensive list of all of the medications the patient is taking. Often, it needs to be proven that either other treatments have not helped or there were uncomfortable side effects that affected the patient. Depending upon the nature of the problem, the insurance carrier may require that more conservative treatments, such as therapies, be tried before approving an expensive medication.

127. D: The explanation of benefits (EOB) statement from the insurance company explains what the total charge was for the services provided at a medical appointment. It outlines how much of each charge is covered by insurance and what amount is the policyholder's responsibility. It will also give an explanation of why any charges were not covered.

128. C: There are 3 main anatomical planes, or imaginary lines that divide the body into 2 sections. The sagittal plane divides the body into left and right sides. The coronal plane divides the body into front (anterior) and back (posterior) sections. The transverse plane divides the body in half to separate top and bottom sections.

129. A: The hand is distal to the elbow. The further a point is from the center of the body, the more distal it is. Proximal anatomical landmarks are those that are closest to the core. When comparing 2 points, the one furthest away from the core is distal to the more proximal point.

130. C: When the human body is in anatomic position, the palms are facing forward. In that position, the thumb is further away from the rest of the hand, so it is more lateral. While in this position, the fingers are closer to the body so they are more medial.

131. A: The dorsal body cavity contains the brain and spinal cord. The heart and lungs are found in the thoracic cavity. The digestive organs and kidneys are found in the abdominal cavity. The

Copyright © Mometrix Media. You have been licensed one copy of this document for personal use only. Any other reproduction or redistribution is strictly prohibited. All rights reserved. This content is provided for test preparation purposes only and does not imply an endorsement by Mometrix of any particular political, scientific, or religious point of view.

bladder and reproductive organs are found in the pelvic category. These cavities can be further broken down into subcategories that contain specific organs within the larger cavity.

132. B: A urinary tract infection will usually cause dysuria, urinary frequency, and urinary urgency. These classic symptoms are usually not very pronounced, though, in the elderly population. Confusion is very common, especially in those with underlying dementia, along with other behavior changes.

133. B: Myelin is a white fatty substance that coats nerve cells and makes it easier for the cells to communicate messages to the brain. With multiple sclerosis, this myelin sheath is destroyed, which interferes with neurologic function, movement, and sensation. There are currently no treatments that stop this process, but there are some medications that can help slow down the progression and prolong the patient's ability to maintain functionality and independence.

134. C: Blood enters the right atrium through the superior and inferior vena cava. It then passes through the tricuspid valve into the right ventricle. It flows through the pulmonic valve to the pulmonary artery where it is transported to the lungs to receive oxygen.

135. A: Most of the body's blood cells are made in the bone marrow. There are certain types of white blood cells that are made within the lymph nodes and spleen, but most of the white blood cells, red blood cells, and platelets are made within the bone marrow. When a patient is suspected to have a disease affecting blood cell formation, such as certain types of cancers, a bone marrow biopsy is performed to further analyze the cells being produced.

136. C: There are 2 main types of COPD: chronic bronchitis and emphysema. Chronic bronchitis is characterized by a productive cough for several months. As its name implies, this is a long-term illness and often not something curable. Symptoms can be controlled, however, with the use of inhalers and smoking cessation.

137. B: The Centers for Disease Control does not recommend the routine use of antivirals for flu prophylaxis due to the risk of promoting viral resistance to the medication. Tamiflu is recommended for prophylactic therapy for those who are immunocompromised, those who could potentially suffer great complications if they were to contract the flu, and in a group living situation in which there is a flu outbreak. Even for these patients, prophylaxis is only recommended if it can be given within 48 hours of their first exposure to the person who had the flu.

138. D: A stool specimen for laboratory testing should be refrigerated until the testing can be completed. In rare cases, the specimen is frozen, but only if it will be at least 48 hours before it can be sent to the testing laboratory. The specimen will be invalid if it is left to sit at room temperature for more than an hour.

139. B: Of these illnesses, only the chicken pox is transmitted through the air. The other diseases listed are transmitted via droplets from the respiratory tract or mucous membranes that settle on surfaces and come in contact with individuals. Other airborne diseases include tuberculosis, measles, and severe acute respiratory syndrome (SARS).

140. C: Alcohol-based hand sanitizers will kill most bacteria, viruses, and fungi that cause infection. The norovirus, which is responsible for a gastrointestinal illness that causes vomiting and diarrhea, is often not affected by hand sanitizers. Hand washing with soap and water is the best way to kill the norovirus if you come in contact with it.

Copyright © Mometrix Media. You have been licensed one copy of this document for personal use only. Any other reproduction or redistribution is strictly prohibited. All rights reserved. This content is provided for test preparation purposes only and does not imply an endorsement by Mometrix of any particular political, scientific, or religious point of view.

141. D: An autoclave is a machine that is used to sterilize instruments. It uses high-pressure steam to kill organisms, viruses, and spores and to sterilize instruments and other medical equipment. Depending upon the model and size of the autoclave, the high-pressured steam can reach up to 120-°F for 15-20 minutes in order to adequately sterilize items.

142. A: When you are around a person on contact precautions, a gown and gloves are required. The infection is not airborne, so a mask is not necessary. Some of the infections that require contact precautions include MRSA, VRE, infectious diarrhea, and open wounds.

143. B: The Material Safety Data Sheet (MSDS) contains all of the information pertaining to safety for a specific product used within the office. These were created to promote safety and prevent injury to staff, and patients, in the office. Everything from printer ink toner to the dish soap found in the clinic break room has an MSDS. These are required to be kept in one location within the office to be reviewed in case of a spill or accidental exposure.

144. C: The social history contains information about alcohol use. The other information included in that part of the patient note is tobacco use, employment, illicit drug use, high-risk sexual behavior, and hobbies or interests.

145. D: The conversion from pounds to grams is 1 pound = 453.59 grams and 1 ounce = 28.35 grams. This child weighs 6 pounds, 15 ounces, therefore the calculation is as follows:

$$(6 \text{ pounds} \times 453.59 \text{ grams}) + (15 \text{ ounces} \times 28.35 \text{ grams}) \approx 3147 \text{ grams}$$

146. B: According to the National Institutes of Health, dark fingernail polish had the most impact on an oxygen saturation reading obtained via pulse oximetry. Black and brown fingernail polishes can cause a significantly lower oxygen saturation reading on the pulse oximeter and should be removed when it is critical to get an accurate reading.

147. C: In the event of an accidental needle stick, or other type of exposure to body fluids, the affected area should be thoroughly washed immediately. If there is a splash exposure on the face, the eyes should be thoroughly flushed at an eye washing station. Once that has been done, the person should tell their immediate supervisor. Each facility is different in how they handle exposure to blood and body fluids, but a process will be in place that should be followed when this happens.

148. A: The chickenpox vaccine is 98% effective and will usually prevent a child from getting the illness. There is still a chance that she could get chickenpox, but let the mother know that she would not get as many skin lesions and the fever would be less than if she had not been vaccinated.

149. A: Subjective information is the information given by the patient. It is information in their own words pertaining to their health. Subjective information can include the patient's explanation of how they feel, if something hurts, or a description of pain. Objective information is the information that is gathered through assessment and physical exam. Vital signs, the sound of a cough, or the description of a rash can be examples of objective data.

150. D: A protective mask should be worn whenever there is exposure to an illness that is airborne, like chickenpox, or when there is a risk of coming into contact with respiratory droplets, such as with the flu. MRSA is an infection that requires contact protections, so a mask is not necessary unless the patient has pneumonia caused by MRSA.

Copyright © Mometrix Media. You have been licensed one copy of this document for personal use only. Any other reproduction or redistribution is strictly prohibited. All rights reserved.
This content is provided for test preparation purposes only and does not imply an endorsement by Mometrix of any particular political, scientific, or religious point of view.

151. B: A Fowler's position is when a patient is sitting with the head of the bed in a semi-upright, position. The head of the bed should be in a 45-60° angle. The patient's legs can be bent or straight. This position helps to relax the abdominal muscles to make breathing easier. This position can also decrease the risk of aspiration in patients who are at risk.

152. C: Ear irrigation, or ear lavage, is performed to help remove earwax or certain foreign bodies. The water should be at body temperature, or 98.6 °F. If the water is too cold or too warm, it can be very painful to the patient or cause them to have significant dizziness.

153. D: A nasopharyngeal swab is used to test for influenza. It is also used to test for RSV, pertussis (whooping cough), and MRSA colonization. The patient should be sitting down or be upright in bed. Their chin is slightly elevated and the swab is passed into the nostril along the floor of the nose, not straight up. Once resistance is met, slightly depress the tip of the patient's nose and the swab will slide easily into the nasopharyngeal space. Rotate the swab a few times and then withdraw the swab.

154. B: To examine vaginal discharge in order to diagnose the cause of the discharge, a wet mount slide may be performed. The provider will obtain a swab of the vaginal discharge and transfer this onto a microscope slide. A salt solution is then added to the slide. When checking for a yeast infection only, KOH (potassium hydroxide) may be added because it will kill all of the bacteria present and leave only the yeast behind. The most common diseases diagnosed using a wet mount slide are bacterial vaginosis, gonorrhea, chlamydia, and trichomoniasis.

155. A: The reagent test strips used for urinalysis should not be exposed to moisture, direct sunlight, or noxious fumes. They should be left in the original storage tube provided by the manufacturer and kept at room temperature. If they are exposed to cold temperatures, direct sunlight, or noxious fumes, the results of the urinalysis will not be accurate.

156. C: The presence of nitrites on a urinalysis indicates the presence of a urinary tract infection. A urine culture should be performed on this specimen to determine the specific organism causing the infection and a susceptibility test to determine if the appropriate antibiotic is being used to treat the infection. Per provider discretion, a urine culture may also be performed for the presence of blood or leukocytes in the specimen.

157. A: A person should have fasted for at least 8 hours before having fasting blood work. This would be for a fasting glucose test or cholesterol check. If a chemistry panel is being performed to assess other electrolyte levels, fasting is not required.

158. D: The patient should be in a dorsal recumbent position for a pelvic exam. The patient is lying on their back with their knees bent and angled at an outward position. The feet are planted flat on the exam table, bed, or in stirrups. This allows for the pelvic area to be easily seen and examined.

159. B: A paper tape measure should be used to measure head circumference, or one that is made out of a non-flexible material. The tape measure should be placed approximately 1-2 inches above the eyebrows and wrapped around the back of the head at its widest point. An elastic tape measure should not be used because it can stretch and give an inaccurate reading.

160. A: Unsterile personnel should maintain a distance of at least 12 inches from the sterile field. This is to ensure there is no accidental contamination to the instruments used or the sterile field in which the procedure is being performed. In the office, a sterile field is required for suturing, removal of a skin lesion, or for some wound care procedures.

Copyright © Mometrix Media. You have been licensed one copy of this document for personal use only. Any other reproduction or redistribution is strictly prohibited. All rights reserved.
This content is provided for test preparation purposes only and does not imply an endorsement by Mometrix of any particular political, scientific, or religious point of view.

161. C: It should be stressed that the patient should not reuse the sharps used for glucose testing. There is a risk of infection at the testing site when a previously used sharp is used, plus the puncture point is dulled after it is used, which can make testing more difficult. Of note, the patient should also be instructed that needles used for insulin injections should also not be reused for these same reasons. The patient should wipe their finger being used for testing with an alcohol pad to minimize infection risks, not a damp cloth.

162. D: Abstaining from sexual activity all together is the best way to prevent acquiring a sexually transmitted infection. A male or female condom acts as a barrier method to avoid exposing a partner to bodily fluids, but these are not reliable and can break. Certain diseases, such as herpes or syphilis, may also still be transmitted despite using a condom.

163. B: According to the American Diabetes Association, the diabetic patient should fill half a plate with non-starchy vegetables, such as broccoli, squash, or salad greens. One quarter of the plate should be lean protein foods such as chicken, fish, or lean beef. The remaining quarter of the plate should be filled with carbohydrate foods such as whole grains, starchy vegetables, fruits, or dairy products. Fatty foods and those with refined sugar should be very limited or avoided all together.

164. A: Light blue-top tubes contain sodium citrate to prevent coagulation of the specimen. These tubes are used for coagulation studies, such as a PT or PTT. When performing any coagulation studies, a light blue-top tube is the only tube that should be used.

165. C: There are important steps that must be followed for a 24-hour urine specimen to be collected correctly. The patient should be instructed to urinate into the toilet when they wake up in the morning. Then, the patient should urinate into the collection container for the next 24 hours and keep the specimen in the refrigerator. The next morning, the patient should urinate into the container. The collection container should then be returned to the lab or office as instructed.

166. C: All urine specimens should be kept refrigerated. If kept at room temperature or warmer, bacterial growth can occur in the urine and this can alter the test results. If a specimen is left at room temperature or warmer for more than one hour, the specimen is considered invalid and will need to be recollected.

167. B: The order in which blood specimens are collected for specific tests is very important. Specimens that are drawn in tubes that contain anticoagulants must be drawn first. If a blood culture is ordered (yellow-top tube or special manufacturer's collection container), this should be drawn first to avoid any possible contamination from other specimen tubes.

168. B: CLIA is the organization that is responsible for the licensing of medical laboratories. Certain tests are considered at very low risk for being performed inaccurately, thereby reducing the risk of any harm to the patient. These tests are considered CLIA-waived since they can usually be performed by the patient with accurate results. These tests include fingerstick glucose tests, home pregnancy tests, home urine drug testing, and urine ketone testing strips.

169. C: A common misconception in the dietary needs of patients taking Coumadin is that they are not allowed to eat leafy, green vegetables. This is not true. If they very rarely eat any of these types of vegetables, and suddenly greatly increase their intake of them, the INR level used to measure the therapeutic level of Coumadin will be decreased. The best advice is to continue with their normal diet without any great fluctuations in the amount of leafy greens they eat to maintain a consistent INR reading. Citrus fruits and red meat do not have an effect on the INR value.

Copyright © Mometrix Media. You have been licensed one copy of this document for personal use only. Any other reproduction or redistribution is strictly prohibited. All rights reserved.
This content is provided for test preparation purposes only and does not imply an endorsement by Mometrix of any particular political, scientific, or religious point of view.

170. D: A tourniquet used during blood collection should not be left on for more than one minute. If selecting a vein takes longer than that time, the tourniquet should be removed and left off for 1-2 minutes before reapplying and collecting the specimen. The risk of leaving the tourniquet on too long is that the blood can become more concentrated distal to the tourniquet site, which may affect the results of the lab test.

171. B: To check an erythrocyte sedimentation rate (ESR), the blood should be collected in a special ESR tube or a lavender-top tube. This specimen is not spun in the centrifuge and can be kept at room temperature or refrigerated until it is processed.

172. C: A complete blood count (CBC) should be drawn in a lavender-top tube. This specimen should not be spun in the centrifuge. The specimen is stable at room temperature for 24 hours before it needs to be processed, or it can be refrigerated to be processed within 72 hours.

173. A: A hemoglobin A1c is a blood test used to look at the average blood sugar level of a patient over the past 2-3 months. Because it is an average and not a test of blood sugar at a specific point in time, it is not necessary for the patient to fast before having this test performed.

174. D: A basic metabolic panel (BMP) is a blood test that checks a blood sugar level, electrolyte levels, and kidney function. The electrolytes checked include sodium, potassium, and calcium, among others. The BMP does not include a test to check liver function. The comprehensive metabolic panel (CMP) includes everything in a BMP in addition to tests to check liver function.

175. B: A DEXA scan is an easy, noninvasive test of bone density. It is used to assess the density of the spine and hipbones to assess for osteopenia or osteoporosis. The patient lies down on a table and x-rays are taken of the spine and hips. It takes approximately 15 minutes. There are no IV or oral contrast agents given beforehand.

176. A: The 5 Rights of medication administration are a tool to help the nurse reduce medication errors when administering medications to patients. They include the right patient, right drug, right dose, right time, and right route. Doing this can decrease the risk of adverse patient reactions due to a medication error.

177. C: Testing for mononucleosis is done with a blood specimen. There is a rapid in-office test called a Mono-Spot that can be performed, or the specimen can be collected and sent to a lab for the test. A throat swab is used to test for strep throat and may also be performed as the two illnesses can have similar symptoms. Though not conclusive for testing for mono, a CBC may also be performed to assess for any elevations in white blood cells.

178. C: Atrial flutter has consistent narrow spikes with waves between that are sawtooth in appearance on an EKG. The patient may be in atrial flutter and have no symptoms at all. More likely, they will be experiencing a rapid heart rate or palpitations, dizziness or lightheadedness, and shortness of breath.

179. A: When using a Snellen eye chart, the result gives the distance at which a person needs to stand from an object compared to the distance at which a person with normal vision would need to stand. If 20/20, the vision is normal. If the second number is greater than 20, that indicates the person being tested needs to be 20 feet from an object while a person with normal vision can be further (>20 feet). If the result gives a number less than 20, such as 20/15, the person being tested has greater than normal vision and can be at 20 feet to see an object while others with normal vision need to be closer (15 feet).

Copyright © Mometrix Media. You have been licensed one copy of this document for personal use only. Any other reproduction or redistribution is strictly prohibited. All rights reserved. This content is provided for test preparation purposes only and does not imply an endorsement by Mometrix of any particular political, scientific, or religious point of view.

180. B: When allergy skin testing is performed, a small amount of different allergen solutions are injected just under the surface of the skin. Approximately 15 minutes should go by to see whether there is a reaction at any of the injection sites. If there is no reaction, another round of injections is given with a slightly larger amount of the allergens. This continues for several rounds, with approximately 15 minutes of time between each round. Once a localized reaction occurs for an allergen, the testing for that allergen is stopped.

181. A: Tuberculosis is a serious lung infection that is transmitted via the airborne route. A TB skin test, or PPD, is performed to check if a person has been exposed to the disease. The time of exposure until the time that a skin test will convert to a positive result is approximately 2-12 weeks. The CDC recommends testing immediately and retesting 8-10 weeks after the last known exposure. Once a person develops a positive skin test, their chance of developing an active TB infection is greatest within the first 2 years.

182. A: A positive PPD test indicates that the patient has been exposed to someone with tuberculosis, not that they have an active infection themselves. It is recommended that they be further evaluated with a chest x-ray and be treated with medications to prevent activation of the infection.

183. A: The flu vaccine needs to be kept refrigerated at 35-46 °F. It should be kept in the central part of the refrigerator rather than up against a wall or back of the refrigerator where temperatures can become cooler. It should not be stored in the door of the refrigerator due to greater temperature fluctuations in that location.

184. B: Both Td and Tdap immunize against tetanus and diphtheria. Tdap also immunizes against pertussis, or whooping cough. When a patient requires an updated tetanus shot, it may be more beneficial for them to receive Tdap. This is especially true for those patients who have young children or grandchildren, or who are around children frequently through their job.

185. B: If the patient needs to receive 100 mg of ibuprofen and the concentration available is 200 mg per 5 mL, you would give 2.5 mL of the liquid. To calculate this amount, first divide the 200 mg by 5 mL to find that the bottle's concentration of ibuprofen is 40 mg/mL. Because the child was prescribed 100 mg, divide 100 mg by 40 mg (the amount in 1 mL) to get the number of mL needed to provide this 100 mg dose: 2.5 mL.

186. A: The PPD skin test to check for TB exposure is given intradermally. A special TB syringe is used. The needle should be placed bevel-side up almost parallel to the surface of the skin on the inside of the forearm. The needle is then inserted just under the surface of the skin, and the PPD solution is injected. This should form a bleb, or small bump, just under the surface of the skin.

187. D: The Z-track method of giving an intramuscular injection ensures absorption of the medication because it prevents the medication from leaking out of the injection site. When an IM injection needs to be given, apply firm pressure with your thumb and then slide the tissue a couple of inches to the side. Give the injection and then slowly remove the needle as you release the tissue that was being held to the side. Never massage the site after giving a Z-track injection because it can cause the medication to be absorbed in the subcutaneous tissue rather than the muscle.

188. A: The MMR vaccine originally started in 1988 as a single dose injection to provide immunity to measles, mumps, and rubella. The requirements for this vaccine were changed in 1996 when a second dose was added to the vaccine schedule. Because of this, many adults have never received the second injection, so they do not have full immunity against these diseases. If both injections were not received, those who only received one injection can still acquire these diseases.

Copyright © Mometrix Media. You have been licensed one copy of this document for personal use only. Any other reproduction or redistribution is strictly prohibited. All rights reserved.
This content is provided for test preparation purposes only and does not imply an endorsement by Mometrix of any particular political, scientific, or religious point of view.

189. C: Rocephin (ceftriaxone) is a third-generation cephalosporin antibiotic used to treat a variety of infection. Mixing Rocephin with 1% lidocaine helps ease some of the pain involved with the injection, which requires a deep intramuscular injection, preferably using the Z-track method, for appropriate administration. Rocephin comes in powder form and must be reconstituted with either 1:1 water or 1% lidocaine in order to be prepared for injection.

190. A: Diabetic ketoacidosis is a condition in which the blood sugar becomes dangerously high. It can lead to a diabetic coma and even death if it is not treated urgently. This elevation in blood sugar and ketones causes the breath to have a sweet or fruity smell. These observations should be shared with the provider.

191. C: It is appropriate to use your finger to gently sweep in the mouth if vomit or another object is visible, but nothing should be forced into the mouth of a person having a seizure. This will increase the risk of choking on the foreign object.

192. A: Hand-foot-and-mouth disease is a relatively common illness, frequently seen as it spreads through daycare settings. It is caused by Enteroviruses, most frequently the Coxsackie virus. Since this is a viral infection, antibiotics are not effective at curing the illness. Controlling the symptoms with ibuprofen or acetaminophen for pain and fever and offering cool liquids and soft foods until the lesions resolve are helpful.

193. C: In the past, those with any allergy to eggs were advised to not receive a flu vaccine. New guidelines from the CDC have stated that if a person has only a hive-type reaction to eggs, without any respiratory or cardiac complications, and they do not require treatment with epinephrine, they can safely receive the same flu vaccine that is given to those without an egg allergy. There are 2 new formulations of the flu vaccine that do not contain egg protein, but these are only for those 18 years and older. If a person has had an allergic reaction to eggs in the past that has required treatment with epinephrine, they can receive the flu vaccine but should do so under the supervision of a trained medical professional who can treat an allergic reaction should one occur.

194. D: A concussion occurs when there is sufficient trauma to a person that the brain is traumatized from the force of the injury. It is common to have a headache on and off, sometimes lasting for a few weeks after the injury. Some dizziness and nausea may also occur after the injury. If vomiting, a change in mental status, lethargy, or visual changes occur, however, the person should be evaluated in the ER to determine whether testing needs to be performed to assess for any bleeding around the brain.

195. C: A cool mist humidifier or placing the child in a steam-filled room, such as a bathroom with a hot shower running, can help to moisten the airway and thin thick mucus secretions. Antibiotics are not usually prescribed with croup unless there is another underlying bacterial infection accompanying this. Aspirin should never be given to a child due to the risk of Reye's syndrome. Over-the-counter cough syrups and decongestants should not be given to children this age.

196. B: This particular child is at an increased risk of developing significant respiratory complications due to his history of unstable asthma. His parents should be instructed to monitor his respiratory status very closely and report to the ER immediately if he should have an increase in asthma symptoms.

197. A: When a multi-dose vial is opened, it should be labeled with the date it was opened, the date it will expire, and the initials of the person who opened it. Depending upon the facility, there may be other requirements to include on the vial. It is important to note that the expiration is not necessarily the date on the vial posted by the manufacturer. Most facilities have as protocol to only

Copyright © Mometrix Media. You have been licensed one copy of this document for personal use only. Any other reproduction or redistribution is strictly prohibited. All rights reserved. This content is provided for test preparation purposes only and does not imply an endorsement by Mometrix of any particular political, scientific, or religious point of view.

keep open vials or bottles for 30 days after they have been opened. Always refer to the facility's policy.

198. D: This is a normal reaction for an immunization injection. Applying a warm compress to the area can be soothing and help to relieve the discomfort. Ibuprofen or Tylenol can help with a low-grade fever. The mother should be told that any severe redness or blistering at the site of the injection, along with a fever >101 °F that does not respond to antipyretics should be evaluated.

199. D: Tympanometry is not a test of hearing acuity, but it is usually used in conjunction with a standard hearing test. Tympanometry is a test to determine the level of mobility of the eardrum. The ear is monitored while a sound is made. The degree of mobility from vibrations on the eardrum, and the movement of the small bones in the middle ear is measured. If the vibration is decreased, it can be a sign of conductive hearing loss.

200. A: Peak flow rate is the measurement of the maximum amount of air that can be exhaled after a patient has taken in a large breath. It is used to assess the degree of obstruction in the airway with asthma. It is dependent upon the patient's ability to use their core muscles to force out all of the air they can, so it can be affected by their ability to perform this test. It is used frequently to assess progression of asthma.

Copyright © Mometrix Media. You have been licensed one copy of this document for personal use only. Any other reproduction or redistribution is strictly prohibited. All rights reserved.
This content is provided for test preparation purposes only and does not imply an endorsement by Mometrix of any particular political, scientific, or religious point of view.

Tell Us Your Story

We at Mometrix would like to extend our heartfelt thanks to you for letting us be a part of your journey. It is an honor to serve people from all walks of life, people like you, who are committed to building the best future they can for themselves.

We know that each person's situation is unique. But we also know that, whether you are a young student or a mother of four, you care about working to make your own life and the lives of those around you better.

That's why we want to hear your story.

We want to know why you're taking this test. We want to know about the trials you've gone through to get here. And we want to know about the successes you've experienced after taking and passing your test.

In addition to your story, which can be an inspiration both to us and to others, we value your feedback. We want to know both what you loved about our book and what you think we can improve on.

The team at Mometrix would be absolutely thrilled to hear from you! So please, send us an email at tellusyourstory@mometrix.com or visit us at mometrix.com/tellusyourstory.php and let's stay in touch.

Copyright © Mometrix Media. You have been licensed one copy of this document for personal use only. Any other reproduction or redistribution is strictly prohibited. All rights reserved. This content is provided for test preparation purposes only and does not imply an endorsement by Mometrix of any particular political, scientific, or religious point of view.

Additional Bonus Material

Due to our efforts to try to keep this book to a manageable length, we've created a link that will give you access to all of your additional bonus material:

mometrix.com/bonus948/ncctncma

317

Copyright © Mometrix Media. You have been licensed one copy of this document for personal use only. Any other reproduction or redistribution is strictly prohibited. All rights reserved.
This content is provided for test preparation purposes only and does not imply an endorsement by Mometrix of any particular political, scientific, or religious point of view.